∪482990

Posttraumatic Stress Disorder: Etiology, Phenomenology, and Treatment

Posttraumatic Stress Disorder: Etiology, Phenomenology, and Treatment

Edited by

Marion E. Wolf, M.D.
Chief, Tardive Dyskinesia Program
North Chicago V.A. Medical Center
North Chicago, Illinois; and
Clinical Professor of Psychiatry
Loyola University Stritch School of Medicine
Maywood, Illinois

Aron D. Mosnaim, Ph.D.
Professor of Pharmacology and Molecular Biology
University of Health Sciences/
The Chicago Medical School
North Chicago, Illinois

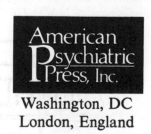
American Psychiatric Press, Inc.
Washington, DC
London, England

Note: The authors have worked to ensure that all information in this book concerning drug dosages, schedules, and routes of administration is accurate as of the time of publication and consistent with standards set by the U.S. Food and Drug Administration and the general medical community. As medical research and practice advance, however, therapeutic standards may change. For this reason and because human and mechanical errors sometimes occur, we recommend that readers follow the advice of a physician who is directly involved in their care or the care of a member of their family.

Copyright © 1990 American Psychiatric Press, Inc.
ALL RIGHTS RESERVED
Manufactured in the United States of America
First Edition

93   4   3   2

American Psychiatric Press, Inc.
1400 K St., N.W., Suite 1101, Washington, D.C. 20005

The paper used in this publication meets the minimum requirements of the American National Standard for Information Sciences—Permanence of Paper for Printed Library Materials, ANSI Z39.48—1984.   ∞

Library of Congress Cataloging-in-Publication Data

Posttraumatic stress disorder: etiology, phenomenology, and treatment
  / edited by Marion E. Wolf, Aron D. Mosnaim.
        p.   cm.
    "This book was developed from the symposium . . . held at the Annual Meeting of the American Psychiatric Association, San Francisco, May 1989"—Introd.
    Includes bibliographical references.
    ISBN 0-88048-299-0
    1. Post-traumatic stress disorder—Diagnosis—Congresses. 2. Post-traumatic stress disorder—Etiology—Congresses. 3. Post-traumatic stress disorder—Treatment—Congresses. I. Wolf, Marion E., 1945–   . II. Mosnaim, Aron D., 1940–   . III. American Psychiatric Association. Meeting (142nd : 1989 : San Francisco, Calif.)
    [DNLM: 1. Stress Disorders, Post-Traumatic—Diagnosis—Congresses. 2. Stress Disorders, Post-Traumatic—Etiology—Congresses. 3. Stress Disorders, Post-Traumatic—Therapy—Congresses.   WM 170 P858 1989]
RC552.P67P668   1990
616.85′21–dc20
DNLM/DLC
for Library of Congress   90-68
                                                                                                          CIP

British Library Cataloguing in Publication Data

A CIP record is available from the British Library.

Contents

Contributors

Paul Bartone, Ph.D.
Walter Reed Army Institute of Research, Washington, D.C.

Avraham Bleich, M.D.
Department of Mental Health, Israel Defense Forces, Tel
Hashomer, Israel

Bruce Boman, M.B.B.S., F.R.A.N.Z.C.P., Ph.D.
Department of Veterans' Affairs, Repatriation Hospital, Concord,
Sydney, Australia

Etzel Cardeña, Ph.D.
Department of Psychiatry and Behavioral Sciences, Stanford
University School of Medicine, Stanford, California

Elisheva Dan, P.A.
Department of Psychiatry, V.A. Medical Center, West Haven,
Connecticut

Wolter S. de Loos, M.D., Ph.D.
War and Violence Stress Unit, Department of Medicine, Leiden
University Hospital, Leiden, The Netherlands

Seymour Diamond, M.D.
Diamond Headache Clinic, Chicago, Illinois; University of Health
Sciences/The Chicago Medical School, Chicago, Illinois

Richard P. Ebstein, Ph.D.
Research Division, Ezrath Nashim Hospital, Jerusalem, Israel;
Department of Psychiatry, Hebrew University Medical School,
Jerusalem, Israel

Charles K. Embry, M.D.
Department of Psychiatry, V.A. Medical Center, Louisville,
Kentucky; Department of Psychiatry, University of Louisville
School of Medicine, Louisville, Kentucky

Frederic Flach, M.D.
Department of Psychiatry, Cornell University Medical College,
New York, New York; Payne Whitney Clinic of the New York
Hospital, New York, New York

Julia B. Frank, M.D.
Department of Psychiatry, University of Texas at Austin,
Austin, Texas

Matthew J. Friedman, M.D., Ph.D.
National Center for Posttraumatic Stress Disorder Studies, V.A.
Medical Center, White River Junction, Vermont; Departments of
Psychiatry and Pharmacology, Dartmouth Medical School,
Hanover, New Hampshire

Earl L. Giller, Jr., M.D., Ph.D.
Department of Psychiatry, University of Connecticut Health
Center, Farmington, Connecticut; V.A. Medical Center, West
Haven, Connecticut

Mark S. Greenberg, Ph.D.
Department of Psychiatry, Harvard Medical School, Boston,
Massachusetts; New England Deaconness Hospital, Boston,
Massachusetts

Larry Ingraham, Ph.D.
Walter Reed Army Institute of Research, Washington, D.C.

Terence M. Keane, Ph.D.
Boston Psychology Service, V.A. Medical Center, Boston,
Massachusetts; Tufts University School of Medicine, Boston,
Massachusetts

Thomas R. Kosten, M.D.
Department of Psychiatry, V.A. Medical Center, West Haven,
Connecticut; Department of Psychiatry, Yale University School of
Medicine, New Haven, Connecticut

Bernard Lerer, M.D.
Research Division, Ezrath Nashim Hospital, Jerusalem, Israel;
Department of Psychiatry, Hebrew University Medical School,
Jerusalem, Israel

Steven Lipper, M.D., Ph.D.
Department of Psychiatry, V.A. Medical Center, Durham, North
Carolina; Department of Psychiatry, Duke University Medical
Center, Durham, North Carolina

Michael Maliszewski, Ph.D.
Department of Behavioral Medicine, Diamond Headache Clinic,
Chicago, Illinois

John W. Mason, M.D.
Department of Psychiatry, V.A. Medical Center, West Haven,
Connecticut; Department of Psychiatry, Yale University School of
Medicine, New Haven, Connecticut

**Alexander C. McFarlane, M.B.B.S. Hons., Dip. Psychother.,
F.R.A.N.Z.C.P.**
Department of Psychiatry, Flinders Medical Centre, The Flinders
University of South Australia, Bedford Park, Australia

James L. Meyerhoff, M.D.
Neurochemistry and Neuroendocrinology Branch, Walter Reed
Army Institute of Research, Washington, D.C.

Aron D. Mosnaim, Ph.D.
Department of Pharmacology and Molecular Biology, University of
Health Sciences/The Chicago Medical School, North Chicago,
Illinois

Edward H. Mougey, M.S.
Neurochemistry and Neuroendocrinology Branch, Walter Reed
Army Institute of Research, Washington, D.C.

Scott P. Orr, Ph.D.
Research Service, V.A. Medical Center, Manchester, New
Hampshire; Department of Psychiatry, Harvard Medical School,
Boston, Massachusetts

Bruce D. Perry, M.D., Ph.D.
Harris Center for Developmental Studies, Chicago, Illinois;
Department of Child and Adolescent Psychiatry, University of
Chicago School of Medicine, Chicago, Illinois

Roger K. Pitman, M.D.
Research Service, V.A. Medical Center, Manchester, New
Hampshire; Department of Psychiatry, Harvard Medical School,
Boston, Massachusetts

James H. Reich, M.D., M.P.H.
Department of Psychiatry, V.A. Medical Center, Brockton,
Massachusetts; Department of Psychiatry, Harvard Medical
School, Boston, Massachusetts

Arik Shalev, M.D.
Department of Psychiatry, Hadassah University Hospital, Jerusalem, Israel

Zahava Solomon, Ph.D.
Mental Health Department, Medical Corps, Israel Defense Forces, Tel Hashomer, Israel

Steven Southwick, M.D.
Department of Psychiatry, V.A. Medical Center, West Haven, Connecticut; Department of Psychiatry, Yale University School of Medicine, New Haven, Connecticut

Landy F. Sparr, M.D.
Department of Psychiatry, V.A. Medical Center, Portland, Oregon; Department of Psychiatry, School of Medicine, Oregon Health Sciences University, Portland, Oregon

David Spiegel, M.D.
Department of Psychiatry and Behavioral Sciences, Stanford University School of Medicine, Stanford, California

Robert J. Ursano, M.D.
Department of Psychiatry, The Uniformed Services University of the Health Sciences, Bethesda, Maryland

Bessel A. van der Kolk, M.D.
Trauma Center, Massachusetts Mental Health Center, Boston, Massachusetts; Department of Psychiatry, Harvard Medical School, Boston, Massachusetts

Victor Wahby, M.D., Ph.D.
V.A. Central Office, Education Service, Washington, D.C.

Marion E. Wolf, M.D.
Department of Psychiatry, V.A. Medical Hospital, North Chicago, Illinois; Department of Psychiatry, Loyola University Stritch School of Medicine, Maywood, Illinois

Jessica Wolfe, Ph.D.
Psychology Service, Boston V.A. Medical Center, Boston, Massachusetts; Tufts University School of Medicine, Boston, Massachusetts

Kathleen Wright, Ph.D.
Walter Reed Army Institute of Research, Washington, D.C.

Rachel Yehuda, Ph.D.
Department of Psychiatry, V.A. Medical Center, West Haven, Connecticut

Dedication

T his book is dedicated to all those men, women, and children who have suffered from atrocities inflicted upon them by other human beings. It is written in remembrance of my father, Jochnan Wolf, M.D. (1911–1986), born in the Warsaw Ghetto, and the only survivor of his family from Nazi extermination, his parents, brother, other relatives, and close friends having been murdered in the concentration camp Treblinka.

Marion E. Wolf, M.D.
Highland Park, Illinois
November 8, 1989

Introduction

This book was developed from the symposium "Posttraumatic Stress Disorder: Biological Mechanisms and Clinical Aspects" held at the annual meeting of the American Psychiatric Association, San Francisco, May 1989. It also incorporates manuscripts from other research groups in an attempt to present an up-to-date, balanced view of recent developments in the field of posttraumatic stress disorder (PTSD).

The book is organized into three sections: (1) etiology, (2) phenomenology, and (3) treatment. The first section contains three chapters in which psychological factors of importance in the etiology of PTSD are addressed. In Chapter 1, Dr. McFarlane offers a comprehensive view of the role of vulnerability factors in determining the psychological consequences of traumatic stress, an issue of controversy in which political and sociological forces surrounding the problem have at times obscured the scientific investigation of this matter. Drs. Spiegel and Cardeña, in Chapter 2, focus on dissociative mechanisms in PTSD and also discuss therapeutic interventions that are useful in the treatment of dissociative symptoms. In Chapter 3, Dr. Flach deals with the resilience hypothesis of PTSD. Little is known about the adjustment of individuals who have been exposed to trauma but who do not develop PTSD. This chapter, by shifting away the focus from pathology and stressing dynamic changes, opens a window to studies in this important new direction.

The second section, on phenomenology, includes a review by Drs. Wolfe and Keane in Chapter 4 of recent validational and diagnostic efforts in PTSD that have promoted a better understanding of this disorder. In the next chapters, comorbidity of PTSD with Axis I, Axis II, and Axis III diagnoses is addressed. Dr. Reich focuses on personality disorders and PTSD in Chapter 5. There seems to be a general agreement that PTSD is associated with deleterious personality changes. However, the nature of this association has been subject to major controversy. Nevertheless, although the evidence for personality to predispose to PTSD is fragmentary, it shows a trend in a positive direction. In Chapter 6, Dr. Boman contrasts the general public's image and the clinician's view of Vietnam veterans. The medical sequelae of PTSD are addressed in Chapters 7 and 8. Dr. de Loos describes the interaction of psychological and organic factors that complicate the management of patients with this condition. Drs. Diamond and Maliszewski describe the frequent pain complaints, including headache, among PTSD subjects, stressing the need for a multidimensional approach to the management of chronic pain in individuals with PTSD. In Chapter 9, Dr. Solomon addresses the effects of repeated exposure to stress and describes a new variety of PTSD: the reactivated form. Dr. Wright and colleagues, in Chapter 10, deal with PTSD as seen in civilian life and illustrate the impact of an aircraft disaster on the individual and the community. These chapters focusing on the clinical phenomenology of PTSD are followed by three chapters that focus on the biological characterization of this condition, including the special features of opiate-mediated analgesia (Dr. Pitman et al., Chapter 11), the role of platelet adenylate cyclase activity as a possible biologic marker for PTSD (Dr. Lerer et al., Chapter 12), and recent psychoendocrinologic studies in PTSD (Dr. Giller et al., Chapter 13).

The third section, on treatment, includes chapters on pharmacotherapy and psychotherapy in the treatment of PTSD. In Chapter 14, Dr. Frank and colleagues address the use of antidepressants in the treatment of PTSD. Although the authors' findings indicate that antidepressants are of significant benefit in the treatment of this condition, other studies do not support the view that antidepressants are efficacious in relieving specifically the symptoms of chronic PTSD. In Chapter 15, Dr. Lipper discusses the use of carbamazepine in the treatment of PTSD and elaborates on the implications of the therapeutic use of this agent for the "kindling hypothesis" of PTSD. Dr. Friedman, in Chapter 16, presents a comprehensive overview of biological aspects of PTSD and concurrent psychiatric diagnoses and their implications for pharmacotherapy. In Chapter 17, Dr. Embry addresses psychotherapeutic interventions in PTSD, describing parameters for effective psychotherapy and illustrating these with various case examples. In the last chapter, Dr. Sparr addresses legal aspects of PTSD, discussing uses and misuses of this diagnostic entity.

Several chapters in this book deal specifically with Vietnam veterans, and the reader is cautioned about generalizations from combat-related PTSD to PTSD as seen in civilian patients.

The integration of the various manuscripts into a cohesive volume is intended to bridge the gap between the views of some practitioners who deny the existence of this disorder and the views of those who idealize the PTSD patient, by recognizing that we are not dealing with "perfect heroes" but with real, human, imperfect PTSD casualties.

Marion E. Wolf, M.D.
Aron D. Mosnaim, Ph.D.

Etiology of Posttraumatic Stress Disorder

Chapter 1

Vulnerability to Posttraumatic Stress Disorder

Alexander C. McFarlane, M.B.B.S. Hons.,
Dip. Psychother., F.R.A.N.Z.C.P.

The role of personality and vulnerability factors is one of the major controversies that has surrounded the psychological effects of extremely traumatic events. This issue has tended to be polarized according to the prevailing attitudes and the dominant theory of psychopathology of the time. The political and social ferment that surrounded the Vietnam War played a major role in changing the tone of the debate. The classification of the psychiatric disorders following traumatic stress changed with time and has reflected the existing views about the relative contribution of vulnerability factors and, prior to DSM-III (American Psychiatric Association 1980), separated the acute reactions to stress from the more enduring effects of combat and other types of catastrophic stress. The research examining these issues has been subject to a number of methodological biases that have influenced the interpretation and analysis of the available data. These inconsistencies are frequently ignored, and few attempts have been made to resolve or confront the conflicting opinions in the literature.

One important dynamic influencing this debate has been the clinical issues involved in the treatment of the effects of traumatic stress. The need for social justice and the prevention of the stigmatization of victims has been a major concern of some clinicians, aware of how the victims of traumatic stress can all too easily be blamed for their disorder. This clinical dilemma also raises theoretical concerns. As Spiegel (1988) has noted:

> Traditional psychiatric theory has been especially weak in dealing with posttraumatic stress disorders, because developmental dynamic theories are unequipped to account for the sudden intrusion of major life stress. In fact, to apply traditional techniques to individuals suffering from a rape or combat experience is by its very nature to belittle the importance of the trauma and attempt to interweave it into a pattern of the person's development. Many patients with post-traumatic stress disorders find this demeaning and humiliating since it relegates to the periphery the importance of their emotional reactions to the trauma itself. Further, it reinforces the common irrational belief that they are somehow responsible for the tragedy which befell them, and thereby encourages them to avoid working through the helplessness which is at the core of PTSD symptomatology. (p. 18)

Despite the importance of this perspective, it is essential that this concern with inappropriate blame does not interfere with the scientific examination of the role of vulnerability and personality in the etiology of posttraumatic stress disorder (PTSD).

CLASSIFICATION AND VULNERABILITY

The classification of psychiatric disorders that follow in the wake of extremely traumatic events has been greatly influenced by the uncertainty about the role of personality and other predisposing factors in the etiology of these disorders. The inclusion of PTSD in DSM-III arose from a consensus that the nature and intensity of the stressor was the primary etiologic factor determining the symptoms that people develop in the setting of extreme adversity. When discussing the role of vulnerability factors in the etiology of PTSD, it is necessary to examine the historical origins of this uncertainty about the nature and phenomenology of the effects of traumatic stress. Earlier systems of classification were influenced by several issues.

First, the predominance of psychoanalytic theory in determining the early classification of neurotic disorders and its emphasis on intrapsychic factors as etiologic determinants of anxiety and depression inevitably focused on the role of character pathology in posttraumatic symptoms. This theoretical perspective has colored the debate about the role of personality to a greater extent than the empirical evidence would warrant (Boman 1986). While the psychoanalytic school saw both early traumas of a developmental origin and external stressors experienced in childhood as critical determinants of adult psychopathology, ironically it minimized the possibility that extreme stresses in adulthood could in their own right be equally destabilizing to an individual's psychological functioning.

Second, earlier systems of classification separated the issues involved in the development of acute symptoms from more enduring patterns of psychopathology, in contrast to the more recent discussions about the effects of traumatic stress. For example, the previous systems of classification tended to assume that symptoms would be time limited unless some preexisting character pathology was present that would contribute to their maintenance (Green et al. 1985). In DSM-I (American Psychiatric Association 1952), "gross stress reaction" was a disorder that was thought to resolve rapidly unless perpetuated by premorbid personality pathology. Similarly, DSM-II (American Psychiatric Association 1968) categorized the effects of traumatic stress under the diagnosis "transient situational disturbance" if the symptoms were short lived, and then would use the category of "anxiety neurosis" for more enduring symptoms. This implied that the stress response was transient in nature unless the individual had some particular preexisting vulnerability. Thus the notion that very traumatic events in adult life could have prolonged adverse psychological consequences represents a recent change in the formulation of the effects of traumatic stress.

Follow-up studies of the survivors of concentration camps (Ettinger 1961) and the atomic bomb blasts (Lifton 1967) of World War II perhaps first initiated the shift in focus from the individual to the inescapable consequences of the horror of these calamities. This shift in emphasis was not necessarily in response to empirical evidence about the unimportant role of premorbid personality, but rather reflected a repugnance with the barbarity of the Nazi regime and recognition of the enormous threat that nuclear war posed to all humanity. The dehumanizing role of social systems and the danger posed by unchecked scientific and technological developments made people concentrate on external threats because the victims could not be individually held responsible for their suffering.

Finally, clarification of the role of personality factors in the etiology of PTSD has been hampered by the inadequate discussion of what constitutes a normal response to an extremely traumatic event (McFarlane 1988b, 1988c, 1988d). Most clinicians working with the victims of traumatic stress will have heard the claim that PTSD is a normal response to an abnormal stress. This mirrors how some professionals dealing with the victims of trauma are uncertain about whether PTSD is a psychopathologic state, particularly in close proximity to the stressor (Rahe 1988). This confusion is also reflected in the research literature, where sociologists such as Quarantelli (1985) have argued that traumatic events such as disasters have little or no long-term effects on the mental health of the victims, although Quarantelli sees such events as an important cause of distress and problems with living.

The psychiatric literature does little to clarify this uncertainty; available systems of classification have generally not examined the distress response and its differentiation from pathological depression and anxiety. This is partly because most behavioral and psychodynamic theories of etiology do not distinguish between clinical disorder and the minor psychopathology of everyday life. This has meant that there is relatively little theoretical or phenomenological investigation of the initial distress response in individuals according to their personality and vulnerabilities. It is obvious that there will be a blurred division between those people who experience the normal stress response and those who have an established PTSD, particularly in the weeks immediately after the event.

This is reflected in the current diagnostic criteria for PTSD, where the intrusive imagery does not have a one-to-one relationship with the disorder (McFarlane 1988c). Intrusive imagery is commonly observed in victims of disasters who do not have any numbing or other disturbance of mood arousal or attention, and may be as much an indicator of distress due to exposure to extreme adversity as a marker of PTSD. In populations who have been traumatized, these recurring recollections may have a relatively low specificity for PTSD, which contrasts with a more typical outpatient setting in which such imagery would be a highly specific marker for PTSD.

This confusion is also embodied in the current DSM-III-R (American Psychiatric Association 1987) diagnostic criteria, where PTSD is a legitimate diagnosis only if an individual has experienced an event that would be "markedly distressing to almost anyone" (p. 250). One example of such an event is assumed to be a natural disaster. In a study of a massive Australian bushfire disaster (McFarlane 1988d), data collected on 469 fire fighters revealed that there was a significant group who were not particularly distressed, as measured by the Impact of Event Scale (Horowitz et al. 1979), despite having had an intense exposure to the fires. Also, based on detailed interviews with more than 300 victims of this disaster, it is apparent that the range of immediate reactions is considerable, with some seeing the experience as a personal challenge for survival, which at one level they found stimulating. Thus an external threat of considerable magnitude is not necessarily distressing, and the individual's response is determined to a significant degree by the personal meaning of the event and a range of other premorbid characteristics, an issue that has lead to ambiguity and confusion in the interpretation of the DSM-III-R criteria.

Thus, historically, the classification of the psychiatric disorders following traumatic stress has been intimately bound up with the question of the role of personality and predisposing factors in the etiology of individual stress responses. The current system represents a focusing away from the individual to the role of the trauma. The debate about the problem continues to attract attention and a diversity of opinions. Breslau and Davis (1987a, 1987b) reviewed the available literature that challenged the current conceptualization of PTSD, indicating that many contradictions and uncertainties remain to be clarified.

BACKGROUND ISSUES

Historically, the debate about the role of the trauma and individual vulnerability has been an emotive issue for moral and legal reasons. This has, at times, made it difficult to examine the scientific validity of the various claims. Issues of cowardice and moral inferiority have sometimes become confused with the notion of vulnerability because of the problems that decompensation on the battlefield poses for the military, the setting where the answer to this question of vulnerability has particular relevance. Any discussion of the issue of vulnerability as a cause of PTSD in war veterans is therefore one of considerable sensitivity and has implications for policy about armed services recruitment.

The interest in Vietnam veterans' long-term psychiatric morbidity contrasts starkly with the initial claim during the war that there were very few psychiatric casualties (Boman 1982). The reason why the role of individual vulnerability has been played down in this group, in contrast to the veterans of other wars, has complex origins. This relates as much to the political and social conflict that surrounded that war as to the objective scientific data. The unpopularity of the Vietnam War contrasts to attitudes about the other major wars of this century. The community's guilt about the effects of this antiguerrilla war on a generation of conscripted soldiers has led to a wish to compensate these individuals for the long-term scars they bear. This has influenced the attitudes and emphasis of researchers, because to investigate the role of vulnerability factors can be interpreted as blaming the soldier rather than the war.

An atmosphere of suspicion and prejudice often surrounds the victims of accidents who seek financial compensation for psychiatric disorders. In this setting, the question of legal liability directly confronts the question about whether the accident can account for the symptoms experienced or whether the individual's vulnerability is the critical issue. This can shift the balance of legal argument against the victims in determining the size of a damages settlement.

The investigation of the role of personality has also been hampered by several other issues. The populations that have been studied have often been screened in a variety of ways. For example, combat servicemen in World War II in various allied armies went through a range of screening procedures in an attempt to decrease the number of cases of shell shock, which had at times seriously debilitated the fighting capacity of the armed forces in World War I (Boman 1986). Similarly, the men on oil rigs in the North Sea are a highly preselected group (Weisaeth 1985). This means that many of the obvious vulnerability factors such as a personal history of psychiatric illness will already have been used to screen out the potential victims of the several accidents that have been studied. Emergency service personnel tend to be similarly vetted.

This will have several effects that will tend to decrease the chance of finding that predisposing factors play an important role in the etiology of PTSD. Researchers will obviously tend to look at the role of the same personality and vulnerability factors that are used in the screening procedures, as the researcher and the personnel managers will have access to the same knowledge base. This means that these variables will have a low incidence in the traumatized population and, as a result, will have little probability of being identified as playing a significant role. As well, the subjects may have withheld information during the selection process that they anticipated may have led to their preclusion from being selected for their particular job. In the event of some major trauma, they are unlikely to volunteer this information because it could interfere with any compensation claim that may arise.

Furthermore, the very decision to choose a position that potentially puts oneself at risk also means that many personnel chosen for combat roles have a particular character type. Thus the study of servicemen and highly selected occupational groups may lead to quite atypical results that could minimize the role of vulnerability factors in PTSD. This possibility is seldom discussed in the literature but raises the importance of methodology in the investigation of this issue.

CONFLICTING ISSUES

The role of personality in determining the response to traumatic stress has been a difficult problem to study for a variety of reasons. This further complicates the interpretation of much of the available information.

Life events research has been bedeviled by the fact that many life events can be the result of the individual's illness rather than its cause, and much effort has been spent trying to define those events that are "independent" of the person's control (Brown and Harris 1978). Natural disasters and wars are events that are beyond the individual's control. Therefore, much research into the etiology of PTSD has used the intensity of the traumatic stress and the nature of the person's experience as independent variables. However, close examination of this issue suggests that the picture is somewhat more complicated.

People's mental state at the time of the trauma can have a significant impact on their behavior during the impact of the stressor. Studies of military conflict have generally found that there is a direct relationship between the number of psychiatric disorders and the intensity of the conflict (Artiss 1963; Levav et al. 1979; Reid 1948). This has been used as evidence about the direct effect of the stress of combat as a cause of PTSD. An examination of the relationship between combat exposure and psychological stress came up with a challenging finding (Palinkas and Coben 1987). It confirmed that United States Marines injured in Vietnam had a significantly increased risk of psychiatric hospitalization. However, most of the first psychiatric hospitalizations occurred before the patients were wounded in action. Furthermore, psychiatric patients who were treated and then returned to duty had a significantly greater than expected risk of subsequently being wounded. These data suggested that psychiatric casualties had a significantly greater risk of being wounded. Therefore these findings call into question the validity of using combat casualties as a measure of combat exposure.

Similarly, it is possible that the probability of being injured in a natural disaster may be partly a measure of the individuals' mental state at the time as well as the intensity of the disaster. Deaths in disasters may also be at times a consequence of the individual's mental state. For example, one study described the case of a woman with agoraphobia who died in a bushfire because she was unwilling to leave her house despite the fact that it was ablaze (McFarlane 1986). Weisaeth's (1984) study of a factory explosion demonstrated that at least 20% of people behave in ways that do not optimize their survival. McFarlane's (1989a) study of a group of volunteer fire fighters found that panicking or coming close to panic was related to the personality trait of neuroticism. These findings indicate how personality factors influence people's capacity to survive in the face of danger and that their experience and perception of the event is not an entirely independent event.

The potentially confounded relationship between combat and PTSD comes from studies which revealed that participation in atrocities increased the risk of psychological and behavioral disturbance above and beyond the cumulative exposure to combat. Breslau and Davis (1987a) found that involvement in atrocities accounted for 29% of the variance of PTSD and that other combat stressors accounted for only a further 6% of the variance. They concluded that "the participation in atrocities conferred a uniquely strong risk for PTSD" (p. 581). The reasons for being involved in atrocities are complex. Lifton (1973) suggested that to resist requires an exceptionally well-grounded sense of right and wrong. Against this background, however, it is important to consider that such behavior involves the choice of the individual at one level and cannot be seen as independent of personality (Hendin and Haas 1984). As well, Yager et al. (1984) pointed out that individual reactions to atrocities vary widely, again stressing personality differences. Therefore a strong association between measures of combat stress and PTSD in the Vietnam War does not resolve the issue about the possible etiologic role of personality factors.

The problem of accurate recall is another issue that can be a source of error in the investigation of the etiology of PTSD and can minimize the role of vulnerability factors. One study that investigated the impact of a natural disaster examined the reporting of injury 4 months after the event and then again 1 year later (McFarlane 1988b). In contrast to a chronically symptomatic group who all recalled their experience with perfect accuracy, only 43% of a group without symptoms continued to report that they were injured. The victims who were not disordered seem to have forgotten the personal trauma involved, in contrast to the PTSD group whose memories were intrusively and vividly imprinted. Hence any investigation that does not collect quantitative data about the event in close proximity to the event may exaggerate the size and nature of the association between the stressor and the disorder because of the lower rates of recall of the group that was not disordered, and, as a consequence, minimize the role of other factors. This is an important issue because of the significant amount of research into the etiology of PTSD that has looked at populations of Vietnam veterans more than a decade after they returned from combat. In other life events research, the accuracy of recall has been found to decay significantly once the event occurred more than 6 months before the time of questioning (Henderson et al. 1981; Paykel 1983).

The method of analyzing and presenting the data can significantly influence the interpretation of the relative role of the stressor. There are many studies of Vietnam veterans that have compared PTSD patients with a variety of other groups, often inpatients with other diagnoses. These studies have generally concluded that combat exposure has played a central role in the onset of chronic PTSD. These populations are often highly selected, and the validity of the control groups has been questioned (La Guardia et al. 1983). This strength of association between combat and significant symptoms is less clear-cut in carefully designed studies where nonpatient samples have been examined (Helzer et al. 1979; Yager et al. 1987). The latter studies have used correlational analyses in contrast to between-group comparisons. The assumptions and biases about the character of the relationship implicit in these different methods of analysis are seldom articulated.

The data from studying a variety of traumatic stresses suggest that even the most devastating trauma seldom leads to more than 50% of the population developing PTSD (Green 1982; Lystad 1988; Sethi et al. 1987). As the intensity of exposure increases, the number of victims who develop PTSD increases progressively (e.g., Shore et al. 1986). Such findings are used as an example of a "distinct linear dose-response relationship" (Snow et al. 1988, p. 175) between the impact of the trauma and PTSD, and are presented as evidence for the primary role of the stressor in PTSD. However, a dose-related effect makes no comment about the strength of that relationship. Particularly if the relationship is relatively weak in terms of the amount of variance accounted for, a number of other etiologic variables will be required to explain the onset of symptoms. The fact that generally at least half the people exposed to traumatic events do not develop PTSD despite the experience of extreme danger, loss, and threat emphasizes that variables other than the event are also required to explain the onset of PTSD.

If a group of victims who have a similar exposure to the trauma are studied and if those who have PTSD are compared with those who do not have PTSD, such a method of analysis is likely to highlight the role of personality and other predisposing factors. An approach that would be of considerable interest is not to ask the question of whether vulnerability factors play a role, but rather to ask what is the relative risk that they predict and at what intensity of trauma do they cease to have predictive capacity. These are important questions because there is no stressor that invariably leads to disorder. In other words, the question exists as to whether the prevalence of PTSD in an exposed population is the same as the prevalence of vulnerability factors or whether a further group of individuals in whom such risk factors do not operate decompensate in an extremely traumatic setting.

The DSM-III-R criteria also create the possibility of some bias in any examination of the role of personality in the etiology of PTSD (Burges-Watson 1987). By focusing on the withdrawal from social relationships and avoidance, the DSM-III-R group C criteria for PTSD are more likely to be endorsed by any individual who is premorbidly an introvert and/or avoidant.

In this way, the very definition of PTSD as it currently stands means the diagnosis is likely to be made in individuals of a certain constellation of personality traits independent of whether these characteristics do, in fact, increase the probability of intrusive memories and disturbed arousal and attention. Conversely, the individual who does not respond to the intrusive memories by withdrawal and avoidance will not attract a diagnosis of PTSD even though he or she is significantly impaired.

RESEARCH EVIDENCE

The research evidence about the impact of the relative role of the trauma and personality factors is conflicting: some studies emphasize the role of the event, whereas others focus on the contributing role of vulnerability. In essence, no hypothesis is sustainable if contradictory evidence exists, and any conclusion needs to take account of both bodies of data once the evidence has been examined in the light of the various methodological issues discussed.

The Stressor

Combat. The data about the effects of combat and the role of vulnerability factors are contradictory. Although there have been a large number of studies examining this issue after the Vietnam War, all cannot be examined in the context of this review. Some investigators have failed to find any relationship between preservice or service adjustment and postservice difficulties (e.g., Card 1987; Figley 1978; Kadushin et al. 1981; Laufer et al. 1984; Penk et al. 1981). Card (1987) argued that these studies were conducted at a later time than the studies that demonstrated the role of predisposing factors and that they utilized more sophisticated research designs and sampling methods.

However, the results from some well-designed studies suggest that the role of combat alone is not large (Andrew et al. 1985). For example, Helzer et al. (1979) found that postservice depression was more frequent in those who showed defects in personality, parenting, education, and alcohol intake prior to service. Van Putten and Yager (1984) pointed out that, despite the suffering of veterans of the Vietnam War, many had similar combat experiences and remained well adjusted.

Studies from other wars similarly suggest that vulnerability factors may play a role. Kettner (1972) studied a group of Swedish soldiers serving in the United Nations Forces in the Congo and found that soldiers who did succumb to combat exhaustion were defined by several vulnerability factors, such as a family psychiatric history. A similar study of the Yom Kippur War demonstrated that, while the intensity of battle was an important predictor of the number of psychiatric casualties, personality factors influenced who decompensated and the rate of recovery (Levav et al. 1979). In a follow-up study of World War II veterans, Brill and Beebe (1955) found participation in combat not to be predictive of the veterans' later mental health, but preservice personality disturbance was highly associated with illness at follow-up. Perhaps the most carefully conducted study looking at these issues has been conducted by Solomon et al. (1987, 1988). Their findings show that a number of different factors—age, education and economic status, previous war-related psychological problems, battle experiences, and the extent of the combat stress reaction—made independent contributions to the prediction of PTSD. Postwar social functioning was mainly related to the demographic variables. These authors concluded that the more vulnerable soldiers suffered more severe PTSD a year after the Lebanon War. They argued for the generalizability of their findings because, in contrast to many studies of the Vietnam War (e.g., Foy et al. 1984; Penk et al. 1981), they drew their subjects from a fairly representative group of soldiers. These studies that have shown that predisposition plays a role in the onset of PTSD indicate also that preexisting psychiatric illness is neither necessary nor sufficient for the diagnosis of psychiatric morbidity after massive trauma (Ursano and Holloway 1985).

Disasters. In 1982, Green reviewed the literature examining the psychological consequences of disasters and concluded that the methodological problems were sufficiently extensive to prevent any accurate generalizations. Much of the research published since that time has been affected by the same problems of sampling, and some of the better studies have not examined the role of vulnerability (e.g., Shore et al. 1986). For example, a study conducted by Green et al. (1986) found that PTSD in the victims of a supper club fire was largely accounted for by the traumatic experience of the disaster (60% of the variance), with vulnerability factors playing a minor role. However, this investigation examined only 117 of the 2,500 affected people, and the representativeness of the sample could not be defined.

Two studies have examined the issue of vulnerability in a more systematic manner. Weisaeth (1984) successfully followed up all the victims of a huge Norwegian factory paint fire in a study that commenced several days after the accident. He found that the prevalence of acute PTSD was determined by the initial intensity of the exposure. However, the prognosis at 4 years was more influenced by pre-accident psychological functioning than by the intensity of exposure to the explosion.

McFarlane investigated this issue in two ways in a longitudinal study of a representative sample of 469 fire fighters who had a particularly intense exposure to an Australian bushfire disaster. When the relative contribution of the disaster experience and vulnerability factors to the symptoms in this group were compared over time, the role of the threat experienced and the losses incurred progressively decreased over a 29-month period (McFarlane 1989a). In contrast, the longer the symptoms of posttraumatic morbidity remained, the greater the role played by several vulnerability factors, such as neuroticism, a family or personal history of psychiatric illness, and a tendency not to confront conflicts. Because the measures used in this study had also been used in several other epidemiological studies in Australian populations, it was possible to compare the contribution of these vulnerability factors to the development of symptoms in populations unaffected by disaster. The contribution of neuroticism to symptoms was less than half that found in an average urban population, suggesting that vulnerability factors play a significantly smaller role in the onset and maintenance of posttraumatic morbidity than in the other types of psychiatric impairment more commonly present in nontraumatized populations.

A selected subsample of this population were interviewed using the Diagnostic Interview Schedule (Robins et al. 1981), and the determinants of acute, delayed onset, and chronic PTSD were examined. The acute PTSD group had no major vulnerability factors and seldom had a coexistent psychiatric disorder. In contrast, the chronic PTSD group scored significantly higher on a number of the vulnerability factors, such as concurrent psychiatric disorder, a positive family history for psychiatric disorder, avoidance as a personality trait, as well as being older and having panicked more during the disaster. The combined data from this study suggest that while the disaster event plays a critical role in the onset of PTSD, its chronicity is predicted to a significant degree by a variety of premorbid factors, but that these probably exert a lesser impact than in other psychiatric disorders.

The Three Mile Island nuclear incident was also extensively investigated. Whether this event would qualify for the type of stressor required to cause PTSD is a moot point. Although there was no loss of life or destruction of property, the effects of this event had much more to do with the psychological impact of a potential rather than a real threat or any confrontation with immediate death. The absence of any significant increase in the population of psychiatric patients exposed to the nuclear accident (Bromet et al. 1982) would suggest that this was not a pathogenic stressor. However, Bromet et al.'s data suggested that the patients' perception of danger and their perception of the adequacy of their social supports (Henderson et al. 1981) indicate the importance of the meaning to the individual rather than the real threat involved.

Other Stressors. A variety of other individual traumas have been studied, such as rape (Steketee and Foa 1987) and other violent crimes (Kilpatrick et al. 1989). While many of the studies examining these groups were not specifically studying PTSD, the evidence tends to suggest that a variety of vulnerability factors appear to operate, such as prior psychiatric disorder (Atkeson et al. 1982) and drug and alcohol abuse (Ruch and Leon 1983). On the other hand, other accounts do not support the role of vulnerability (Kilpatrick et al. 1989).

In summary, looking across a range of stressors, the evidence is conflicting, with many studies suggesting that personality and other vulnerability factors predict the onset of PTSD, while others have failed to demonstrate the role of factors other than the intensity of the stressor. It is not possible at this stage to reach a definite conclusion. Any interpretation of the data needs to take into account the problems of conducting research in this area. Inevitably, it would seem probable that the answer falls somewhere between the poles of opinion. In addition, the role and effects of an acute and short-lived stressor have not been adequately compared with the more enduring traumas, such as being in repeated heavy combat or being a concentration camp victim.

Family History

Both Slater (1943) and Symonds (1943), in their investigation of World War II veterans, thought that genetic factors were important in soldiers who broke down under minor stress. They found that severe stress was necessary to bring out symptoms in those without a positive family history of psychiatric disorder.

The one published systematic study examining this issue in a patient group found that 66% of the PTSD veterans gave a family history of psychiatric disorder (Davidson et al. 1985). When the relative prevalence of anxiety and depression was examined in these patients' families, the data supported the view that PTSD is one form of pathological anxiety. The incidence of anxiety and depression was very similar to that in the relatives of patients with generalized anxiety disorder.

Interestingly, similar findings emerged in a study of a community sample of emergency service workers, where 55% were found to have a positive family history (McFarlane 1988a). Unpublished data from a latter stage of this study revealed that a higher incidence of a family history was found in the more chronic cases. These findings suggest that Davidson et al.'s (1985) conclusions were not simply a product of the fact that they were studying a patient population. Thus these family studies suggest that PTSD sufferers have a pattern of psychiatric morbidity in their families similar to that in other patient groups where a family history is thought to be a significant vulnerability factor.

Concurrent Psychiatric Disorder

The diagnostic parsimony of some clinicians means that coexisting disorders are often underdiagnosed, a practice that was encouraged by the use of hierarchical diagnosis prior to the publication of DSM-III-R. The concurrence of PTSD has now been studied in several patient populations, and more than 50% are found to be suffering from another psychiatric disorder (Davidson et al. 1985; Escobar et al. 1983; Sierles et al. 1983). This raised the important and unanswered question about whether similar etiologic pathways exist in these disorders. This degree of concurrence has also been found in McFarlane's (1989a) sample of fire fighters, suggesting that this finding in patient populations is not simply the product of concurrent disorders increasing the severity of symptoms and increasing the likelihood of becoming a patient.

These data suggest that PTSD probably shares common etiologic processes with both the anxiety disorders and depression and hence may share some of the same vulnerabilities.

CLINICAL PERSPECTIVE

Inevitably, a clinician cannot assess or treat a patient with PTSD without considering the issues of personality and individual meaning. To focus solely on the impact of the trauma fails to deal with the personal context of an event that requires consideration in the treatment process. It is the uniquely individual perceptions of the experience that determine reality for the victim. This was graphically demonstrated by a patient who had been brutally tortured and survived the experience to live in Australia as a refugee. His most traumatic and distressing memories were not of the physical or psychological abuse he suffered but rather the delusions and hallucinations he experienced when he became delirious because of the physical consequences of his torture. The most distressing intrusive memory was a hallucination that his father was also being tortured.

The exploration of the individual's perceptions inevitably requires focusing on a range of issues that may have heightened the person's vulnerability to particular aspects of the trauma. Horowitz (1986) proposed that in PTSD there is a blocking of the cognitive and affective process that involves the integration of the representations of the trauma with the individual's preexisting schemata. This is particularly likely if the individual had conflictual schemata prior to the trauma that were defended against, but were brought to awareness by the event. For example, the recognition of not being in control and the intense feeling of helplessness when trapped in a bushfire with flames 800 feet high were devastating to a man who had fought throughout his adult life to assert his independence and control.

Paradoxically, the psychotherapeutic treatment of PTSD often focuses on an attempt to decrease the patients' sense of responsibility for their trauma and on the external reality of the situation. This can be done only by understanding the individual vulnerability to internalizing the horror of the trauma. Thus while treatment aims to focus on the external event and minimize the individual's responsibility for his or her symptoms, in contrast to neurotic disorders, this does not mean that the issue of personality or vulnerability is unimportant to the etiology. In fact, patients with PTSD are frequently poorly treated because clinicians fail to recognize the way a major stressful event in adult life can organize internal perceptions and the phenomenology of PTSD. Such clinicians inappropriately blame the symptoms on some earlier trauma in the developmental period. At the same time, it is necessary to examine the way that the meaning of a trauma can be molded by some previous event with which the person had otherwise successfully coped.

PTSD frequently coexists with a number of other DSM-III-R Axis I disorders. This again raises the issue of vulnerability and the probability that the trauma alone does not account for the pattern of response in a number of patients. These other disorders require treatment if there is to be a successful therapeutic intervention for the PTSD symptoms, an issue seldom mentioned in the literature (McFarlane 1989b).

Thus the management of patients with PTSD requires a delicate balance between acknowledging the central role of the trauma in causing the intrusive thinking and avoidance and the part played by vulnerability factors in determining the meaning of the trauma and pattern of disordered mood and arousal. The consideration of premorbid vulnerability factors does not mean that the clinician either blames the patient or minimizes the importance of the trauma in molding the clinical picture.

CONCLUSIONS

The understanding of the role of personality and vulnerability factors in determining the psychological consequences of traumatic stress remains an issue of controversy. The political and sociological forces surrounding the problem have, at times, obscured the scientific investigation of the dilemma. One important factor is that researchers often become advocates for the victims they have studied and may also be called on to defend claims for compensation in court (e.g., Gleser et al. 1981). Similarly, researchers who wish to continue studying groups, such as the Vietnam veterans, must be careful not to alienate their subjects by publishing data that may disadvantage the veterans' cause. The investigation of the effect of critical incident stress debriefing has been significantly hampered because of the delicate issue of not wanting to alienate emergency service personnel, which could occur if the issue of vulnerability was raised. The participation of compensable injury victims in research programs in Australia has often been discouraged by solicitors who are concerned that the findings may not necessarily assist their clients' claims.

Therefore, researchers need to be aware of the factors that might bias the way they formulate the problem of vulnerability and personality in PTSD, the method of analysis they choose to examine their data, and the emphases and interpretations they place on positive and negative findings.

REFERENCES

American Psychiatric Association: Diagnostic and Statistical Manual of Mental Disorders. Washington, DC, American Psychiatric Association, 1952

American Psychiatric Association: Diagnostic and Statistical Manual of Mental Disorders, 2nd Edition. Washington, DC, American Psychiatric Association, 1968

American Psychiatric Association: Diagnostic and Statistical Manual of Mental Disorders, 3rd Edition. Washington, DC, American Psychiatric Association, 1980

American Psychiatric Association: Diagnostic and Statistical Manual of Mental Disorders, 3rd Edition, Revised. Washington, DC, American Psychiatric Association, 1987

Andrews G, Christensen H, Hadzi-Pavolovic D: Exhibit 1452: Royal Commission on the Use and Effects of Chemical Agents on Australian Personnel in Vietnam. Canberra, Australia, Australian Government Printing Service, 1985

Artiss KL: Human behaviour under stress: from combat to social psychiatry. Milit Med 128:1011–1014, 1963

Atkeson BM, Calhoun KS, Resick PA, et al: Victims of rape: repeated assessment of depressive symptoms. J Consult Clin Psychol 50:96–102, 1982

Boman B: The Vietnam veteran twenty years on. Milit Med 150:77–79, 1982

Boman B: Early experiental environment, maternal bonding and the susceptibility to post-traumatic stress disorder. Milit Med 151:528–531, 1986

Breslau N, Davis GC: Posttraumatic stress disorder: the etiological specificity of wartime stressors. Am J Psychiatry 144:578–583, 1987a

Breslau N, Davis GC: Posttraumatic stress disorder: the stressor criterion. J Nerv Ment Dis 175:255–264, 1987b

Brill NQ, Beebe GW: A follow-up study of war neuroses (Veterans Administration medical monograph). Washington, DC, U.S. Government Printing Office, 1955

Bromet E, Schulberg HC, Dunn L: Reactions of psychiatric patients to the Three Mile Island nuclear accident. Arch Gen Psychiatry 39:725–730, 1982

Brown GW, Harris T: The Social Origins of Depression. London, Tavistock, 1978

Burges-Watson IP: Posttraumatic stress disorder in Japanese prisoners of war (letter). Am J Psychiatry 144:1110, 1987

Card JJ: Epidemiology of PTSD in a national cohort of Vietnam veterans. J Clin Psychol 43:6–17, 1987

Davidson J, Swartz M, Storck M, et al: A diagnostic and family study of posttraumatic stress disorder. Am J Psychiatry 142:90–93, 1985

Ettinger L: Pathology of the concentration camp syndrome. Arch Gen Psychiatry 5:371–379, 1961

Escobar JI, Randolph ET, Pruente G, et al: Posttraumatic stress disorder in Hispanic Vietnam veterans. J Nerv Ment Dis 171:585–596, 1983

Figley CR (ed): Stress Disorder Among Vietnam Veterans. New York, Brunner/Mazel, 1978

Foy DW, Sipprelle RC, Rueger DB, et al: Etiology of posttraumatic stress disorder in Vietnam veterans: analysis of premilitary, military and combat exposure influences. J Consult Clin Psychol 52:79–87, 1984

Gleser GC, Green BL, Winget C: Prolonged Psychosocial Effects of a Disaster: A Study of Buffalo Creek. New York, Academic, 1981

Green BL: Assessing the levels of psychiatric impairment following disaster. J Nerv Ment Dis 170:544–552, 1982

Green BL, Linday JD, Grace MC: Post-traumatic stress disorder: toward DSM IV. J Nerv Ment Dis 173:406–411, 1985

Green BL, Grace MC, Gleser GC: Identifying survivors at risk: long term impairment following the Beverly Hills Supper Club fire. J Consult Clin Psychol 53:672–678, 1986

Helzer JE, Robins LBN, Wish E, et al: Depression in Vietnam veterans and civilian controls. Am J Psychiatry 136:526–529, 1979

Henderson S, Byrne DG, Duncan-Jones P: Neurosis and the Social Environment. Sydney, Academic, 1981

Hendin H, Haas AP: Combat adaptations of Vietnam veterans without posttraumatic stress disorder. Am J Psychiatry 141:956–960, 1984

Horowitz M: Stress Response Syndromes, 2nd Edition. Northvale, NJ, Jason Aronson, 1986

Horowitz M, Wilner N, Alvarez W: Impact of Event Scale: a measure of subjective distress. Psychosom Med 41:209–218, 1979

Kadushin C, Boulanger G, Smith JR: Long-term stress reactions: some causes, consequences and naturally occurring support systems, in Legacies of Vietnam. Edited by Egendorf A, Kadushin C, Laufer RS, et al. Washington, DC, U.S. Government Printing Office, 1981

Kettner B: Combat strain and subsequent mental health: a follow-up of Swedish soldiers serving in the United Nations forces in 1961–1962. Acta Psychiatr Scand [Supp] 230:1–112, 1972

Kilpatrick DG, Saunders BE, Amick MC, et al. Victims and crime factors associated with the development of crime-related posttraumatic stress disorder. Behavior Therapy 20:199–214, 1989

La Guardia RL, Smith G, Francois R, et al: Incidence of delayed stress disorder among Vietnam veterans: the effect of priming on response set. Am J Orthopsychiatry 53:18–26, 1983

Laufer RS, Gallops MS, Frey-Wouters E: War stress and trauma. J Health Soc Behav 25:65–85, 1984

Levav I, Greenfeld H, Baruch E: Psychiatric combat reactions during the Yom Kippur War. Am J Psychiatry 136:637–641, 1979

Lifton RJ: Death in Life: Survivors of Hiroshima. New York, Random House, 1967

Lifton RJ: Home From War. New York, Simon & Schuster, 1973

Lystad M (ed): Mental Health Response to Mass Emergencies. New York, Brunner/Mazel, 1988

McFarlane AC: Posttraumatic morbidity of a disaster: a study of cases presenting for psychiatric treatment. J Nerv Ment Dis 174:4–14, 1986

McFarlane AC: The aetiology of post-traumatic stress disorders following a natural disaster. Br J Psychiatry 152:116–121, 1988a

McFarlane AC: The longitudinal course of posttraumatic morbidity: the range of outcomes and their predictors. J Nerv Ment Dis 176:30–39, 1988b

McFarlane AC: The phenomenology of posttraumatic stress disorders following a natural disaster. J Nerv Ment Dis 176:22–29, 1988c

McFarlane AC: Relationship between psychiatric impairment and a natural disaster: the role of distress. Psychol Med 18:129–139, 1988d

McFarlane AC: The aetiology of post-traumatic morbidity: predisposing, precipitating and perpetuating factors. Br J Psychiatry 154:221–228, 1989a

McFarlane AC: Treatment of post-traumatic stress disorder. Br J Med Psychol 62:81–90, 1989b

Palinkas LA, Coben P: Psychiatric disorders among United States Marines wounded in action in Vietnam. J Nerv Ment Dis 175:291–300, 1987

Paykel ES: Methodological aspects of life events research. J Psychosom Res 27:341–352, 1983

Penk W, Robinowitz R, Roberts WA, et al: Adjustment differences among male substance abusers varying in degree of combat experience in Vietnam. J Consult Clin Psychol 49:426–437, 1981

Quarantelli EL: An assessment of conflicting views on mental health: the consequences of traumatic events, in Trauma and Its Wake. Edited by Figley CR. New York, Brunner/Mazel, 1985, pp 173–215

Rahe RH: Acute versus chronic psychological reactions to combat. Milit Med 153:365–372, 1988

Reid DD: Sickness and stress in operational flying. British Journal of Social Medicine 2:123–131, 1948

Robins LN, Helzer JE, Croughan J, et al: National Institute of Mental Health Diagnostic Interview Schedule. Arch Gen Psychiatry 38:381–389, 1981

Ruch LO, Leon JJ: Sexual assault trauma and trauma change. Women Health 8:5–21, 1983

Sethi BB, Sharma M, Singh T, et al: Psychiatric morbidity of patients attending clinics in gas affected areas in Bhopal. Indian J Med Res [Supp] 86:45–50, 1987

Shore JH, Tatum EL, Vollmer WM: Psychiatric reactions to disaster: the Mount St. Helen's experience. Am J Psychiatry 143:590–595, 1986

Sierles FS, Chen J, McFarland RE, et al: Posttraumatic stress disorder and concurrent psychiatric illness: preliminary report. Am J Psychiatry 140:1177–1179, 1983

Slater E: The neurotic constitution. Journal of Neurology and Psychiatry 6:1–6, 1943

Snow BR, Stellman JM, Stellman SD, et al: Post-traumatic stress disorder among American Legionnaires in relation to combat experience in Vietnam: associated and contributing factors. Environ Res 47:175–192, 1988

Solomon Z, Mikulincer M, Jakob BR: Exposure to recurrent combat stress: combat stress reactions among Israeli soldiers in the Lebanon war. Psychol Med 17:433–440, 1987

Solomon Z, Benbenishty R, Mikulincer M: A follow-up of the Israeli casualties of combat stress reaction (battle shock) in 1982 Lebanon war. Br J Clin Psychol 27:125–135, 1988

Spiegel D: Dissociation and hypnosis in post traumatic stress disorders. Journal of Traumatic Stress 1:17–33, 1988

Steketee G, Foa EB: Rape victims: posttraumatic stress response and their treatment. Journal of Anxiety Disorders 1:69–86, 1987

Symonds CP: The human response to flying stress. Br Med J 30:1081–1083, 1943

Ursano RJ, Holloway HC: Perspectives on posttraumatic stress disorder. Am J Psychiatry 142:1526, 1985

Weisaeth L: Stress reactions in an industrial accident. Unpublished doctoral dissertation, Oslo University, Oslo, Norway, 1984

Weisaeth L: Psychiatric studies in victimology in Norway: main findings and recent developments. Victimology 10:478–487, 1985

Van Putten T, Yager J: Posttraumatic stress disorder: emerging from the rhetoric. Arch Gen Psychiatry 41:411–413, 1984

Yager T, Laufer R, Gallops M: Some problems associated with war experience in men of the Vietnam generation. Arch Gen Psychiatry 41:327–333, 1984

Chapter 2

Dissociative Mechanisms in Posttraumatic Stress Disorder

David Spiegel, M.D.
Etzel Cardeña, Ph.D.

Trauma, such as a natural disaster, crime victimization, or combat, can be understood as a sudden extreme discontinuity in a person's experience. Physical threat and damage undermine many basic assumptions by which people live: their sense of control over their bodies and physical environment and their myth of invulnerability (Yalom 1980). Traumatic events commonly bring about extensive alterations of emotional, cognitive, and volitional processes (Horowitz 1976), so it is not surprising that the psychological reaction to trauma should incorporate fundamental discontinuities of experiences that cannot be fully integrated into the ordinary personal consciousness of the individual. In his work with war veterans, Erikson (1968) deemed the impact of repeated and/or traumatic violent events to effect a "distinct loss of ego identity. The sense of sameness and continuity and the belief in one's social role were gone" (p. 67). Thus dissociative reactions (e.g., depersonalization and derealization) are not uncommon during and immediately after trauma. In some more extreme cases, the discontinuity of experience results in a fragmentation of memory (e.g., psychogenic amnesia or fugue) or identity (e.g., multiple personality disorder), which threatens the self as a coherent whole.

DISSOCIATION DURING TRAUMA

Dissociation is a special form of consciousness in which events that would ordinarily be connected are divided from one another. Clinical examples include psychogenic fugue, in which patients may suddenly travel to another town, losing awareness of their ordinary store of memories and identity, and start a new life until suddenly, sometimes weeks or months later, they regain a coherent memory of their previous life and lose their new orientation and store of memories.

Dissociative processes are characterized by sudden discontinuities or switches in states of consciousness and psychological subsystems that seem not to relate in any direct way to one another. Another clinical example is the different personality states of a patient with multiple personality disorder. Each personality system may have varying degrees of amnesia for what goes on when other personality systems have access to consciousness. Each personality seems to act as though it were in full charge of the person, even though it is only one piece of the patient's personal history and total pattern of consciousness. Thus the defense is primarily one of separating into pieces what is normally a continuous pattern of consciousness and memory, for example, to dissociate present experience from past memory or one aspect of personality from another.

There is a consistent literature supporting the notion that a significant number of individuals experience dissociative phenomena during and/or shortly after the traumatic episode. These episodes may be short lived and do not necessarily culminate in posttraumatic stress disorder (PTSD) symptoms, although the latter have received greater theoretical and clinical attention. Various forms of depersonalization, derealization, and numbing have been reported by victims of life-threatening danger (Noyes and Kletti 1977)—for instance during the Hyatt Regency Hotel skywalk collapse (Wilkinson 1983) and in a combat situation (Solomon et al. 1988). Dissociative alterations of perception (e.g., physical numbness, time distortion, and hallucinatory phenomena) have been reported in connection with hostage situations in adults (Hillman 1981; Siegel 1984) and in children (Terr 1979), and with concentration camp experiences (Jaffe 1968). Finally, dissociative alterations in memory in the form of amnesia or as an isolated memory of the traumatic event as an unwilled but recurrent experience are frequent experiences of, for instance, victims of bushfires (McFarlane 1988a), tornadoes (Madakasira and O'Brien 1987), and the Hyatt Hotel collapse (Wilkinson 1983).

Despite its possible complications and ultimate negative effects, dissociation can be thought of as a process with some adaptive value, from the automatization of behaviors that do not require careful surveillance, to a psychological escape from intolerable circumstances (Hilgard 1970; Ludwig 1983; Spiegel 1984, 1986). Dissociative defenses, which allow individuals to compartmentalize and separate aspects of experience, seem to perform two main functions during a traumatic event. They help individuals separate themselves from the full impact of physical and emotional trauma while it is occurring. They also help isolate the catastrophic experience from the continuous account of personal identity by, for example, totally or partially separating the episode from memory. Although these functions help preserve the integrity of an ego that is being overwhelmed by an intolerable traumatic episode (Freud 1926), they exact a high price by delaying the necessary working through and putting into perspective of traumatic experiences after they have occurred (Lindemann 1944). There is evidence that avoidance of thinking about a natural disaster (e.g., Australian bushfires) may be the best predictor of an acute maladjustment reaction (McFarlane 1988b).

Dissociative defenses help the trauma victim maintain a sense of detachment during an episode of physical and emotional helplessness. However, these same defenses may later become a mechanism by which the individual quite literally loses psychological mastery of a very important episode in his or her life. The traumatic episode, and its consequent reliving, are dissociated from the general mode of conscious experience with which the individual has a greater familiarity and sense of control. The common phenomenon of intrusive imagery—for example, visual or auditory flashback

(Burstein 1985; Horowitz 1976; Mueser and Butler 1987)—exemplifies both the intense reexperiencing of the trauma and the apparent lack of control over the content of the individual's consciousness. Thus the physical helplessness experienced at the time of the trauma is replaced by psychological helplessness over intrusive, unbidden images, reliving of the trauma, and startle reactions.

A traumatic episode seems to create an intense focusing of attention on the essential aspects of the event and a parallel disregard for peripheral aspects (Christianson 1987). For instance, hyperalertness is one of three common experiential factors reported in life-threatening situations (Noyes et al. 1979). The unremitting attention to urgent stimuli facilitates an initial full absorption in the event, with a greatly diminished sense of reflective mentation. This form of continuous attention or absorption has been shown to facilitate the appearance of altered states of consciousness, involving changes in self schemata and emotional and cognitive processing, even within a benign context (Cardeña 1988; Deikman 1966).

The very effectiveness of the dissociative defense at isolating strong affect associated with trauma may produce posttraumatic numbing and hamper necessary working through of affect-laden memories (Lindemann 1944; Scheff 1979). The response to a traumatic event, therefore, commonly involves an altered state of consciousness partly brought about by the unusual demands of focused attentional deployment. Although this mental state remains isolated from more ordinary cognition, the experience during the traumatic episode can be reevoked by external (e.g., sounds) or internal (e.g., moods) events associated with the trauma, consistent with the postulates of state-dependent memory (cf. Bower 1981). The main problem, therefore, is not that responses to traumatic events are dissociated and thereby kept out of awareness, but that they are instances of state-specific knowledge (Tart 1975) that remain unintegrated and unprocessed within more ordinary contextual and reflective modes of conscious awareness. Therefore, flashbacks and other common manifestations of PTSD can be understood as manifestations of more general attentional and memory processes (McGee 1984).

In summary, it is quite common for trauma victims to report dissociative responses during traumatic experiences, which are often extremely helpful in allowing the person to process overwhelming fear, pain, and helplessness (Spiegel 1986, 1988a). This adaptive aspect of traumatic dissociation is illustrated in the following case:

A young man's car broke down on a heavily traveled freeway. As he was trying to examine the car, he was struck by an intoxicated motorcyclist attempting to escape the pursuing highway patrol. He was severely injured, both legs were broken, and one later required amputation. He lay injured on the freeway in the midst of oncoming traffic. His friends were begging him to get off the road, and at first he protested that he could not move, but at the suggestion of a friend he started to think about one of his favorite places, a fishing lodge where he and his father went. He found himself concentrating almost entirely on the experience of fishing, got up, and walked off the freeway on his badly injured legs. He experienced no pain at all until several hours later when his leg was being manipulated for X-ray at a hospital emergency room.

This unfortunate young man had clearly separated, or dissociated, himself from the traumatic experience while it was occurring, keeping his shock, pain, and fear out of conscious awareness, even though he at no time lost consciousness. Similarly, many rape victims report that they experience the rape as if they were floating above their own bodies, feeling sorry for the person undergoing the sexual assault (Rose 1986). It has been well demonstrated that hypnotizable individuals can employ dissociative mechanisms to provide partial or complete relief of pain (Hilgard and Hilgard 1975; Spiegel and Bloom 1983). It would be surprising indeed if people did not spontaneously use this capacity to reduce their perception of pain or extreme anxiety during acute trauma. Many subjects report a strange kind of unreality to a traumatic experience, a form of discontinuity in their consciousness that mirrors the sudden discontinuity in their physical reality.

Hypnosis and Dissociation

Hypnosis can be understood as controlled and structured dissociation (Nemiah 1980; Spiegel and Spiegel 1978). There are three prominent components to the hypnotic experience. The first is absorption, or total involvement in one perception, idea, or memory at the expense of others (Tellegen 1981). The second is dissociation, a compartmentalization of experience, which is a complementary attribute to the absorption. The more intensely one focuses on one aspect of consciousness, the more other aspects are likely to be relegated to the periphery of awareness. Events that would ordinarily be conscious are now relegated to the periphery of awareness, if at all. Thus a hypnotized individual may respond to a series of instructions without any conscious recollection of having heard the instructions (Hilgard 1986; Spiegel and Spiegel 1978). The third main component of hypnotic experience, suggestibility, is a heightened responsiveness to social cues (Orne 1959). Because a person in a hypnotic state is fully absorbed in only one or two aspects of awareness, such a subject is less likely to judge or evaluate the meaning of the experience critically. Thus if given an instruction in a hypnotic state, the individual is less likely to question the motivation of the person giving the instruction or to think through the consequences of acting on it. It is not that hypnotized individuals are in any way deprived of their will, but they are less likely to act on it or be aware of it. Indeed, they may come to experience an instruction from someone else as if it were their own idea (Evans 1979). This process lends a sense of involuntariness to hypnotic experiences. Even though people choose to act in hypnotic and dissociative states, they may experience their actions as somehow mysteriously imposed from outside; while they might ultimately attribute the idea to themselves, they experience their action as relatively automatic. This sense of involuntariness associated with hypnotic phenomena fits naturally with the sense of involuntariness imposed on a victim of trauma.

Indeed, the three major DSM-III-R categories of symptomatology of PTSD (American Psychiatric Association 1987) are quite analogous to the extreme major components of hypnotic dissociation. First, the sudden reliving of a traumatic event, not as a memory but as if it were recurring in the present tense, is very much like hypnotic absorption, in which the memories are so vivid they are not experienced as memories but rather as a reexperiencing of the trauma with the associated intense affect. Second, the loss of pleasure in usually pleasurable activities, or numbing of responsiveness, carries with it the flavor of dissociation. The dissociated traumatic memories tend to remove from PTSD patients the full range of affective response. What is left seems to them not quite whole and does not express a full engagement into pleasurable activities and experiences. Thus the defensive compartmentalization of traumatic memories has as its price a loss of the full range of affective responses. Finally, PTSD symptoms include startle responses and other exaggerated sensitivities to stimuli reminiscent of the traumatic experience. These can be viewed as analogous to suggestibility, which can be thought of as a heightened and uncritical response to social cues. For instance, the woman who is raped in an elevator finds the environment of an elevator enough to provoke a full-scale reenactment of the assault; associated cues, then, become strongly "suggestive" of the traumatic episode.

A number of converging lines of research strongly point to a link between traumatic symptomatology and hypnosis. Hypnotizability is a normal form of dissociative response, but a strong correlation between hypnotizability and pathologic dissociation (e.g., multiple personality disorder) has recently been observed. Individuals with these disorders also commonly report having been exposed to a traumatic experience at an early age. These findings support a relationship between hypnotic capacity and traumatic experience. Two studies have now shown that Vietnam veterans with PTSD are more hypnotizable than normal subjects. Stutman and Bliss (1985) compared the hypnotizability of those veterans responding to a newspaper ad who were high in PTSD symptoms with those who were low and found that the symptomatic group was more hypnotizable. Our group (Spiegel et al.

1988) compared the hypnotizability of 65 Vietnam veterans with PTSD to that of a normal comparison population and to patients with schizophrenia, affective disorders, and generalized anxiety disorder. The PTSD group had higher hypnotizability scores than all of the other groups. Indeed, their scores were twice the mean scores obtained for schizophrenic patients on the Hypnotic Induction Profile (Spiegel and Spiegel 1978).

Patients with pathological dissociation such as multiple personality disorder also report a very high prevalence of repeated childhood trauma, particularly physical and/or sexual abuse. Reports of the prevalence of childhood trauma among patients with multiple personality disorder range from 85% to 95% (Boor 1982; Coons et al. 1988; Putnam et al. 1986). That these reports have a basis in external reality has been supported by Coons and Milstein's (1986) study in which they were able to confirm through records, witnesses, and so on, a history of childhood physical and/or sexual abuse in 17 (85%) of 20 patients with multiple personality disorder. This group of patients, like those with PTSD, have also been found to be very highly hypnotizable (Spiegel et al. 1989).

Clinically, these patients will often report that they first dissociated when the physical abuse began. A so-called protector personality emerged to take over from the patient, who was allowed to escape psychologically from the punishment. One such personality emerged during a first episode of sexual abuse by the patient's father. The personality said, "You don't want to be with him. You come and be with me." It is interesting that often such protector personalities turn on the primary personality after the physical abuse stops (Watkins and Watkins 1988). They cease to be defenders and become identified with the aggressor, thereby perpetuating the unconscious belief that the punishment inflicted on the child was deserved rather than unwarranted. Their very ability to absorb repeated abuse from parents comes to imply to such patients that they somehow deserved it, or even encouraged and participated in it. The rage expressed by the protector personalities turned enemies might also be increased by the anger felt toward the perpetrators of the original abuse, an anger that could not find free expression during childhood because of the fear of emotional and/or physical retaliation. The guilt, then, can also be interpreted as inward-deflected rage. Very often these patients report having provoked assault as a way of protecting younger siblings from similar abuse; or it may be that such reports are their way of controlling in fantasy what they were helpless in fact to protect themselves from. Clearly, again, dissociative capacity emerges as a means of coping with trauma and as a posttraumatic symptom. Indeed, multiple personality may be conceptualized as a chronic, severe PTSD (Spiegel 1984).

Herman et al. (1989) studied traumatic histories in borderline patients. They found a high prevalence of such trauma but, in particular, noted that dissociative symptoms were strongly predicted by a traumatic history, even more so than a borderline diagnosis per se. These recent findings are congruent with Hilgard's (1970) early observations that normal hypnotizable students had a history with more frequent reports of punishment than low hypnotizable students. Indeed, she noted that it was possible that hypnotic or dissociative capacity might be useful in "escaping from an otherwise unpleasant reality."

TREATMENT CONSIDERATIONS

The treatment of PTSD patients using hypnosis must take into consideration the type of trauma, the type of PTSD symptomatology, dispositional characteristics, current environmental stresses, and secondary gains (Denny et al. 1987; Spiegel 1988b). PTSD patients suffer radical discontinuities in their conscious memories of trauma in such a manner that these memories are kept separate from other memories or components of the patient's identity. The way one feels about oneself when one is being abused is and should be radically different from the way one feels in more protected and safe circumstances. Such patients need help in integrating these disparate views of self.

A crude analogy to computers can be drawn (Spiegel 1989). A dissociative disorder is a bit like files in different directories of a DOS-type computer system. Under most circumstances, when one is looking for a file in another directory, the computer feigns ignorance, stating that no such file is available. One must then go back to the root directory and into the other directories to retrieve it. In the same sense, a patient reexperiencing trauma does so as if it were the only memory about self available. The degradation and helplessness seem total, despite a majority of life experiences that suggest otherwise. Psychotherapy is in a sense like writing a "PATH" command in a DOS-type computer, telling it that it can find access to the other files even if they are in a different directory.

Thus various dissociated states can be accessed in a controlled way, for example, using hypnosis, and linked in hypnosis with information from other nontraumatic states or information, leading to a different conclusion about the self from the traumatic experience. One useful technique is a split-screen technique. For example, a rape victim is taught to picture the assailant on one side of the screen while in hypnosis and to relive aspects of the assault. At the same time, on the other side of the screen, she is instructed to picture what she was doing to protect herself, to humanize herself to the assailant, to fight him off, to get help. Thus she comes away with a more complex view of the scene. A related technique is described by Grigsby (1987), who used imagery to provoke in his patient more intense flashbacks "under control" until the patient was able to have cathartic release and to entertain different outcomes to the event imaged.

The usefulness of hypnosis in helping patient and therapist access and integrate previously dissociated information relevant to a traumatic experience is illustrated in the following case:

> A Vietnam veteran suffered spontaneous intrusive episodes of uncontrolled crying regarding the death of a friend who had gone with him to Vietnam. He had handed the friend his orders, they parted, and he learned from family at home 6 weeks later that his friend had been killed 3 days after they separated. He was overwhelmed with sadness and guilt about the friend's death.
> Using hypnosis, he tearfully relived receiving the bad news about his friend. He was then asked to relive a happier time with him. He recalled a walk down the beach, noting that his friend told him he did not expect to return alive from Vietnam, and that he seemed very much at peace.
> He emerged from the hypnosis and said: "I have not been able to think of those memories for 15 years." He was taught to use self-hypnosis to work through both aspects of the loss.

Hypnosis was used to help this patient access dissociated memories for the purpose of helping him tolerate painful affect while restructuring his memory of the event. The newly associated material helped him experience the loss of his friend as an affirmation of his relationship with him at the same time, thereby making the loss more tolerable.

Uses of hypnosis in the treatment of trauma have four main components.

Access Dissociated Material. Hypnosis provides a controlled means of retrieving and storing memories kept out of conscious awareness. It can thus temporarily bypass defenses, yet leave them relatively intact if the affect associated with memories is overwhelming. Patients may or may not remember memories uncovered during hypnotic regression. This provides some reassurance that they need not be overwhelmed by them.

Provide Cognitive Restructuring of the Memories. It is not enough to retrieve dissociated memories and facilitate expression of affect. It is important that patients emerge from the experience with a broader perspective, integrating the trauma into their personal history in a way that makes it real but less all-encompassing. This helps them to see it as a real part of their past rather than experiencing it as though it were present. The latter may be necessary at first to help them place the events into historical context.

Impart Control in the Process of Therapy. It is crucial that patients work through material with a sense of control, since helplessness is the primary feeling defended against. Thus it is helpful to have the patient pace the therapy and learn to use self-hypnosis to work through memories with a sense of mastery rather than revictimization.

Establish a Supportive Relationship With the Therapist. It is not uncommon for a traumatic transference to emerge in which the patient projects feelings about the traumatic event or about those individuals (if any) responsible for it onto the therapist. The therapist's desire to work through traumatic memories can seem to the patient like a desire to reinflict suffering. Furthermore, such patients often feel ashamed and unworthy of caring because of the image of the self created during the trauma. Once they reveal these feelings, they expect rejection from the therapist. Demonstrating concern concretely and working through transference issues is an important way in which the process of therapy counters aftereffects of the trauma (Brende and Benedict 1980; Haley 1978).

CONCLUSIONS

Dissociative symptoms are a prominent component of the response to trauma as it is occurring and its immediate aftermath as well as of PTSD. Symptoms such as depersonalization and derealization, psychogenic amnesia, and numbing of responsiveness serve to defend against overwhelming feelings of helplessness and fear. However, they may prevent or delay working through of the traumatic experience, leading to further symptomatology. These dissociative symptoms are amenable to therapeutic intervention, including techniques employing hypnosis, a structured and controlled dissociation. Treatment involves accessing and restructuring dissociated memories, helping patients manage painful affect, and using the therapeutic relationship to provide support and reassurance. Dissociative symptoms represent both a problem and an opportunity in the treatment of trauma-related disorders.

REFERENCES

American Psychiatric Association: Diagnostic and Statistical Manual of Mental Disorders, 3rd Edition, Revised. Washington, DC, American Psychiatric Association, 1987

Boor M: The multiple personality epidemic. J Nerv Ment Dis 170:302–304, 1982

Bower GH: Mood and memory. Am Psychol 36:129–148, 1981

Brende JO, Benedict BD: The Vietnam combat delayed response syndrome: hypnotherapy of dissociative symptoms. Am J Clin Hypn 23:34–40, 1980

Burstein A: Posttraumatic flashbacks, dream disturbances, and mental imagery. J Clin Psychiatry 46:374–378, 1985

Cardeña E: The phenomenology of quiescent and physically active deep hypnosis. Paper presented at the 39th annual meeting of the Society for Clinical and Experimental Hypnosis, Asheville, NC, 1988

Christianson SA: Emotional and autonomic responses to visual traumatic stimuli. Scandanavian Journal of Psychology 28:83–87, 1987

Coons PM, Milstein V: Psychosexual disturbances in multiple personality: characteristics, etiology and treatment. J Clin Psychiatry 47:106–110, 1986

Coons PM, Bowman ES, Milstein V: Multiple personality disorder: a clinical investigation of 50 cases. J Nerv Ment Dis 176:519–527, 1988

Deikman A: De-automatization and the mystic experience. Psychiatry 29:329–343, 1966

Denny N, Robinowitz R, Penk W: Conducting applied research on Vietnam combat-related post traumatic stress disorder. J Clin Psychol 43:56–66, 1987

Erikson EH: Identity: Youth and Crisis. New York, WW Norton, 1968

Evans FJ: Contextual forgetting: posthypnotic source amnesia. J Abnorm Psychol 88:556–563, 1979

Freud S: Inhibitions, symptoms and anxiety (1926), in The Standard Edition of the Complete Psychological Works of Sigmund Freud, Vol 20. Translated and edited by Strachey J. London, Hogarth Press, 1959, pp 77–175

Grigsby JP: The use of imagery in the treatment of posttraumatic stress disorder. J Nerv Ment Dis 175:55–59, 1987

Haley SA: Treatment implications of post-combat stress response syndrome for mental health professionals, in Stress Disorders Among Vietnam Veterans. Edited by Figley CV. New York, Brunner/Mazel, 1978

Herman JL, Perry JC, van der Kolk BA: Childhood trauma in borderline personality disorder. Am J Psychiatry 146:490–495, 1989

Hilgard ER: Divided Consciousness (expanded edition). New York, John Wiley, 1986

Hilgard ER, Hilgard JR: Hypnosis in the relief of pain. Los Altos, CA, William Kaufmann, 1975

Hilgard JR: Personality and Hypnosis: A Study of Imaginative Involvement. Chicago, IL, University of Chicago Press, 1970

Hillman RG: The psychopathology of being held hostage. Am J Psychiatry 138:1193–1197, 1981

Horowitz MJ: Stress Response Syndromes. New York, Jason Aronson, 1976

Jaffe R: Dissociative phenomena in former concentration camp inmates. Int J Psychoanal 49:310–312, 1968

Lindemann E: Symptomatology and management of acute grief. Am J Psychiatry 101:141–146, 1944

Ludwig AM: The psychobiological functions of dissociation. Am J Clin Hypn 26:93–99, 1983

Madakasira S, O'Brien K: Acute post traumatic stress disorder in victims of a natural disaster. J Nerv Ment Dis 175:286–290, 1987

McFarlane AC: The longitudinal course of posttraumatic morbidity: the range of outcomes and their predictors. J Nerv Ment Dis 176:30–39, 1988

McFarlane AC: The aetiology of post-traumatic stress disorders following a natural disaster. Br J Psychiatry 152:116–121, 1988a

McGee R: Flashbacks and memory phenomena. J Nerv Ment Dis 172:273–278, 1984

Mueser KT, Butler RW: Auditory hallucinations in combat-related chronic post traumatic stress disorder. Am J Psychiatry 144:299–302, 1987

Nemiah JC: Dissociative disorders (hysterical neurosis, dissociative type), in Comprehensive Textbook of Psychiatry, Vol 3. Edited by Kaplan HI, Sadock BJ. Baltimore, Williams & Wilkins, 1980

Noyes R, Kletti R: Depersonalization in response to life-threatening danger. Compr Psychiatry 18:375–384, 1977

Noyes R Jr, Frye SJ, Slymen DJ, et al: Stressful life events and burn injuries. J Trauma 19:141–144, 1979

Orne MT: The nature of hypnosis: artifact and essence. Journal of Abnormal and Social Psychology 58:277–299, 1959

Putnam FW, Guroff JJ, Silberman EK, et al: The clinical phenomenology of multiple personality disorder: review of 100 recent cases. J Clin Psychiatry 47:285–293, 1986

Rose DS: "Worse than death": psychodynamics of rape victims and the need for psychotherapy. Am J Psychiatry 143:817–824, 1986

Scheff TJ: Catharsis in Healing, Ritual and Drama. Berkeley, CA, University of California Press, 1979

Siegel RK: Hostage hallucinations. J Nerv Ment Dis 172:264–272, 1984

Solomon Z, Mikulincer M, Bleich A: Characteristic expressions of combat-related post traumatic stress disorder in Israeli soldiers in the 1982 Lebanon war. Behavioral Medicine 14:171–178, 1988

Spiegel D: Multiple personality as a post traumatic stress disorder. Psychiatr Clin North Am 14:21–24, 1984

Spiegel D: Dissociating damage. Am J Clin Hypn 29:123–131, 1986

Spiegel D: Dissociation and hypnosis in post traumatic stress disorders. Journal of Traumatic Stress 1:17–33, 1988a

Spiegel D: Hypnosis, in American Psychiatric Press Textbook of Psychiatry. Edited by Talbott JA, Hales RE, Yudofsky SC. Washington, DC, American Psychiatric Press, 1988b, pp 907–928

Spiegel D: Hypnosis, dissociation and trauma: hidden and overt observers, in Repression and Dissociation: Defense Mechanisms and Personality Styles. Edited by Singer J. Chicago, IL, University of Chicago Press, 1990

Spiegel D, Bloom JR: Group therapy and hypnosis reduce metastatic breast carcinoma pain. Psychosom Med 45:333–339, 1983

Spiegel D, Hunt T, Dondershine H: Dissociation and hypnotizability in post traumatic stress disorder. Am J Psychiatry 145:301–305, 1988

Spiegel D, Frischholz EJ, Spiegel H, et al: Dissociation, hypnotizability and trauma. Paper presented at the 142nd annual meeting of the American Psychiatric Association, San Francisco, May 8, 1989

Spiegel H, Spiegel D: Trance and Treatment: Clinical Uses of Hypnosis. Washington, DC, American Psychiatric Press, 1978

Stutman RK, Bliss EL: Posttraumatic stress disorder, hypnotizability and imagery. Am J Psychiatry 142:741–743, 1985

Tart CT: States of Consciousness. New York, Dutton, 1975

Tellegen A: Practicing the two disciplines for relaxation and enlightenment: comment on "Role of the feedback signal in electromyograph biofeedback: The relevance of attention" by Qualls and Sheehan. J Exp Psychol [Gen] 110:217–226, 1981

Terr LC: Children of Chowchilla: a study of psychic trauma, in The Psychoanalytic Study of the Child. Edited by Solnit AJ, Eissler R, Freud A, et al. New Haven, CT, Yale University Press, 1979, pp 547–620

Watkins JG, Watkins HH: The management of malevolent ego states in multiple personality disorders. Dissociation 1:67–72, 1988

Wilkinson CB: Aftermath of a disaster: the collapse of the Hyatt Regency Hotel skywalks. Am J Psychiatry 140:1134–1139, 1983

Yalom ID: Existential Psychotherapy. New York, Basic Books, 1980

Chapter 3

The Resilience Hypothesis and Posttraumatic Stress Disorder

Frederic Flach, M.D.

The term *posttraumatic stress disorder* (PTSD) is of recent vintage. It applies to those individuals who have been subject to a period of intense stress and who, having responded with signs of profound anxiety and tension, enter a state of decompensation. According to DSM-III-R (American Psychiatric Association 1987), this phase is characterized by a fixation on the traumatic event that had provoked the patient's reaction, recurrent catastrophic dreams with elements of aggression and helplessness, irritability, startle patterns, a proclivity for aggressive and explosive emotional reactions, and a profound contraction of the general level of functioning.

Taken individually, each of these symptoms could occur at times in an otherwise healthy person. People do have nightmares. They may jump at sudden and unexpected noises. They may blow up angrily when tense. Certainly, there are occasions when everyone finds himself or herself operating below par.

Where, then, does an illness lurk?

ORIGIN OF THE STRESS CONCEPT

To answer this question, we must go back years to the origin of the concept of stress itself. We all know that Claude Bernard (1865) hypothesized the idea of the body being an internal milieu, within which a wide variety of events occurred. Years later, physiologist Walter Cannon (1939) devised the concept of homeostasis, namely that the body is organized in such a way as to maintain its own equilibrium, adjusting automatically in the healthy person to internal and external variations. It was Hans Selye (for a review, see Selye 1988) who first defined the so-called stress syndrome, indicating that "stress is the stereotyped part of the body's response to any demand. . . . It is associated with the wear and tear on the human machinery that accompanies any vital activity." He went on to describe what he termed the general adaptation syndrome, which evolves in three stages: 1) the "alarm reaction," during which defensive forces are mobilized; 2) the "stage of resistance," which reflects full adaptation to the stressor; and 3) the "stage of exhaustion," which inexorably follows as long as the stressor is severe enough and applied for a sufficient length of time, since the "adaptation energy" or adaptability of a living being is always finite.

Bernard (1865), Cannon (1939), and Selye (1988) addressed themselves primarily to the physiologic elements in homeostasis and stress. Karl Menninger (1963) may not have been the first to view human behavior within the context of homeostasis and its protection and preservation in the face of traumatic conditions, but he certainly developed these ideas brilliantly in his book *The Vital Balance*:

> Today in virtually every field of science the pattern of explanatory thinking is shifting from static, classificatory, single-cause analyses to dynamic, process-oriented genetic explanations.... In such terms we can define illness as being a certain state of existence which is uncomfortable to someone and for which medical science offers or is believed by the public to offer relief. The suffering may be in the afflicted person or in those around him or both, but a disturbance has occurred in the total economics of a personality.... The continuous internal and external adaptation to continuously changing internal and external conditions by an organism, which carries the triumphs and scars and hidden weaknesses of many similar prior efforts and failures, has been jolted by something which may take advantage of the consequences of previous battles and their residual scars.... A shift in balance occurs, with a lowering of the effective level of living. (p. 77)

However, Menninger stopped short of suggesting that a disruption in homeostasis was anything other than illness, thus allowing the age-old assumption that healthy human beings should more or less endure all without showing significant signs of emotional upheaval or exhaustion to remain unchallenged.

REDEFINING THE CONTEXT FOR ILLNESS

In the opening section of this chapter, I listed the traditional symptoms of PTSD. Since any one or all of these symptoms can occur in the healthiest of persons at one time or another, what then constitutes illness? To me, the key to the illness is centered in two issues: first, how the individual experiences the episode of disruption, and second, the persistence of the symptoms and the accompanying disability rather than the symptoms themselves.

For many years the main focus of my studies was depression, and I gradually began to redefine the nature of this illness. Rather than being in the structure of the depressed mood itself, it could be located at various stages in a natural cycle of disruption (depression) and reintegration (genuine recovery from the depressive episode), as a response to a significant loss or change (Flach 1986).

SPECIFIC OPPORTUNITIES FOR ILLNESS

There are three levels or opportunities for illness. The first such level can be seen in the failure to become depressed when such a response is called for, or in the denial or refusal (conscious or unconscious) to recognize and acknowledge the experience of depression. Over the years a variety of terms have been used to describe depression when depression is not overtly manifested in a patient's behavior or in his or her subjective emotional state, the most common one being *masked depression.* Instead of a mood change, such a patient may seem to remain emotionally intact, but may develop a variety of other complaints, such as headaches, gastrointestinal distress, or cardiovascular symptomatology. In the extreme, a condition known as alexithymia may exist, wherein the patient cannot even identify, much less verbalize, what emotions he or she is experiencing (Nemiah 1982). Or a patient may engage in a process of behavioral or psychopathologic substitution, throwing off signs of emotional distress that conceal and distract from the depressed mood, such as persistent or recurrent anxiety or phobic reactions. Or a patient may not react with either physical or psychological changes, continuing instead to feel and behave as if he or she has managed to survive stressful events unscathed, thus failing to experience the emotional dimensions of the experience, minimizing the chances to learn from it, and increasing vulnerability to the disruptive power of subsequent stressful events in the future.

The second opportunity for illness can be found in how the individual experiences depression. Certain behavioral changes can be considered common manifestations of normal depression, such as feelings of disappointment, discouragement, and even hopelessness. These changes also include insomnia, loss of appetite and weight, loss of sexual drive, impaired concentration, some level of anxiety and agitation, or conversely a mental and physical slowing up. The idea of a depressive reaction being pathologic enters when elements other than these are introduced.

For example, there should normally be an appropriateness between the events inducing depression and the depressive response itself. One can think "illness" when a depressive response is excessively strong in relation to the events that seem to have invoked it. Of course, to assess the appropriateness of the emotional response it is not enough to make that judgment by superimposing one's own values or even those of society onto another person. One must know what a particular person actually values, since it is the loss of something or someone valued that triggers depression, not just loss itself.

Quite clearly, the development of such psychopathologic symptoms as delusions and hallucinations in the context of depression cannot ordinarily be considered within normal limits. But even in patients with such serious psychopathology, the basic collapse of personality coherence itself may be viewed as a legitimate response to traumatic events, an observation that, when conveyed to patients as a right to be distressed, is often surprisingly reassuring.

The third opportunity for illness lies in the failure or inability of the patient to recover from depression spontaneously and in a reasonable period of time. Chronic depression is one of the most common conditions seen by physicians in all specialties. Although it is tempting to identify the depressed mood of such patients as the illness and develop a therapeutic regimen on that premise, I believe that such a viewpoint seriously misstates the case. It is obviously important to search out and identify those psychodynamic factors that may have contributed to the patient becoming depressed in the first place. However, it is no less important to acknowledge the patient's right to have become depressed and enable him or her to understand that the "illness" that the doctor intends to treat consists of those elements in the patient's personality, physiology, and environment that have conspired, so to speak, to thwart the patient in any effort at recovery. Personality rigidity, guilt, persistent resentment, lack of creativity, humiliation, and tenacious fear of and resistance to being out of control may not sound like signs of illness, but these may well be the cornerstone of an enduring disability.

The Resilience Hypothesis

My observations about depression led to the formulation of what I have come to call the *resilience hypothesis* (Flach 1977, 1988; Flach and Kaplan 1988). This is a theoretical structure that can be applied to the human response to stress and change well beyond mere depression. It casts a significantly different light on the nature of mental health and illness.

Psychobiological resilience is the efficient blending of psychological, biological, and environmental elements that permits human beings—and their families and, in fact, all humanly created organizations—to transit episodes of chaos necessarily associated with significant periods of stress and change successfully.

Consider that at any given moment in time each of us exists within a given homeostatic structure, within ourselves and in relation to the world around us. Such homeostasis is at once both physical and psychological. When physiologic homeostasis is attacked, the primary responsibility of our bodily defense mechanisms is to prevent the disruption from being fatal and to restore normal function as quickly and completely as possible to the homeostatic condition in which it existed before. However, psychological homeostasis follows a different law. When it is impacted by stress or change, resilience should provide the tools whereby the extent of the natural disruption that follows is kept within reasonable boundaries, if at all possible. This does not preclude the possibility, however, that if the stressful situations are of sufficient intensity and meaning, the consequent chaos may not assume dramatic proportions. When reintegration takes place, the homeostatic condition that is shaped should be to some degree different from that which existed prior to the events. Moreover, it should represent a higher, more complex, more adaptable level of organization. The adolescent should be more than the child, the adult more than the adolescent, the mature adult more than life's novice; the veteran soldier should be more than the green recruit. The new level of homeostasis should clearly not be at the point of maximum disability or even halfway toward successful reintegration, as is often the case among chronically ill psychiatric patients.

Hence, when one considers the reaction of soldiers to combat stress or that of ordinary people to any kind of traumatic event, perhaps the real question should not be, Why did some fall apart? but rather, Why on earth didn't they all fall apart; not in the middle of the crisis perhaps but why not afterward? Is it really healthy to spend years in battle or be involved in an airplane or automobile accident and emerge emotionally untouched? Did those millions of people who seem to have done so really achieve this phenomenal task? Or are many of them invisibly scarred, while others did quietly go through an appropriate phase of emotional disruption from which they have with equal discretion reintegrated themselves afterward? The fact is that we know much more about those who have become chronically disabled by traumatic stress than those who have not, because the former become our patients and are easily available for study.

ASSESSING RESILIENCE IN PATIENTS

When assessing patients with PTSD, an equally important question is why they have not been able to reintegrate successfully, with or without professional help, afterward. Or, to put the question differently, why has the new homeostasis that has been created settled at a level of partial or nearly complete dysfunction?

If resilience consists of those psychological, biological, and environmental forces that allow for successful disruption and promote subsequent reintegration, then the answer to these inquiries can be found by determining in what areas any particular patient lacks such resilience. There are various constituents of resilience.

Psychological Resilience

The first group of components are those with which we psychiatrists are most familiar—psychological strengths. Among these are:

Insight into oneself and others
A supple sense of self-esteem
The ability to learn from experience
A high tolerance for distress
A low tolerance for outrageous behavior

Openmindedness
Courage
Personal discipline
Creativity
Integrity
A keen sense of humor
A constructive philosophy of life that gives life meaning
A willingness to dream dreams that can inspire us all and give us genuine
   hope

This list of traits has been assembled from numerous sources. For example,
Arthur and McKenna (1989), who have worked directly with wartime survivors and reviewed the extensive literature on this subject, concluded that a
differential emphasis on the good, hope, the ability to engage in regressive
behavior from time to time, and a serious will to live enabled prisoners of war
literally to survive the most brutal and demeaning of conditions, although not
without lingering signs of depression or aggressive behavior. They also noted
that those who best handled severe trauma, such as airplane accidents, were
those with insight into the emotional impact of what they had just been
through and who were able to express their feelings to another immediately
following the event.

Biologic Resilience

The biological dimensions of resilience are not as well-known, although
certainly we deal with these inferentially whenever we administer a psychopharmacologic agent designed to reduce intense emotion or to enable a
patient to emerge gradually from a state of depression (Flach 1974). Thus
antidepressants can be viewed not only as mood-altering drugs but as agents
that restore and enhance biologic resilience.

Resilience-Enhancing Environments

The third dimension of resilience is environmental. Arthur and McKenna
(1989) also reported group morale and interaction as vital factors in enabling
prisoners of war to survive. Furthermore, the ability to share the emotional
impact of a disaster with another (empathetic) human being shortly after the
event was a critical route toward resolution of the troublesome feelings. Also,
studies of schizophrenic patients clearly indicate that training in social skills
and the presence of a supportive network of friends and family make a
considerable difference with regard to the maintenance of the recovered
state.

TREATMENT IMPLICATIONS

If, then, the stress that results from traumatic events, by its very nature, induces some degree of personality disruption, and if resilience is what enables the individual to pass through the period of distress and emerge to form a new integration afterward, what are the implications for treating patients thus affected?

First, it is important to ascertain whether a traumatic event has occurred at some time in the past in every psychiatric patient, regardless of diagnosis. Too often, important stressful events are overlooked in history taking or even in the course of ongoing psychotherapy. The patient fails to bring them up, and the therapist is not clued into asking about them.

Second, the importance of specific traumatic events in the life of the patient and usually in the evolution of the patient's psychopathology should be assessed. What is meaningful to one patient may not necessarily be so to another; events that may not seem meaningful on the surface may, on careful scrutiny, reveal a previously hidden significance.

Third, if the history and/or present evaluation of a patient who has been subject to extreme stress fail to reveal an appropriate emotional abreaction to the experience, and especially if the patient has stabilized at a level of significant dysfunction, it is conceivable that the therapeutic strategy may have to include the induction of disruption as preparation for subsequent reintegration at a healthier and more adaptational level. In classical psychoanalysis, regression most likely serves such a purpose, although it is not an appropriate treatment approach in most cases of PTSD. Over the years various other techniques have been used, including the induction of an altered state of consciousness with barbiturates to set the stage for emotional disruption and catharsis. The exploration of new, noninvasive techniques to create a temporary context of disruption would seem to be a legitimate area for future research, by no means restricted to patients with PTSD.

Fourth, traditional psychoanalysis operates on the premise that therapy peels away layers to expose core difficulties, bit by bit, but that somehow the patient should have the capacity to integrate the experience on his or her own during this process. An experienced analyst will carefully screen the patients for whom psychoanalysis is recommended. However, psychoanalytic techniques have been adopted by many therapists in settings that would hardly qualify as truly psychoanalytic; we are all familiar with patients who have been psychologically dissected, then left to stumble on their own for lack of this synthetic skill. It is often not enough to analyze, although the search for origins and their analysis have their place. By properly assessing the particular resilience strengths of each patient, the therapist would be prepared to provide the integration that the patient may lack.

Fifth, the circulation of psychological resilience should be a direct, purposeful goal of therapy, one that often cannot be achieved within the confines of psychotherapy alone. Carl Jung, for example, was noted for giving his patients exercises to perform on their own, not only to cultivate what he called active imagination—the ability to dream—but to enhance the patient's sense of self-reliance and to diminish the risk of forming an excessively dependent relationship with the therapist. Rehabilitation therapy, wherein the therapist focuses on specific ways in which the patient can learn occupational and social skills, for example, should be part of the treatment regimen for all patients who require such practical assistance in restructuring their lives after traumatic stress.

Finally, the patients' will to be well should be stimulated. This tactic not only includes an active effort to encourage patients to create future goals and motivate them to strive toward their goals, but also includes a need to reduce environmental influences that may interfere with their will to recover. Strong forces can encourage disability. Secondary gain is a concept much older than the field of psychiatry itself. One receives caring attention. One may receive financial compensation dependent on remaining disabled. One may also use disability to control family members and others. The need to engage life with all its risks does not have to be faced. When the clinician asks why a particular patient does not seem to be recovering despite the application of all logical treatment procedures, he or she must also ask whether the patient has become demoralized and lost the will to be better, and whether this indifference is fueled by environmental conditions. Restoring morale and reducing the influence of detrimental factors in the milieu, replacing them with factors that promote health, are essential steps in the treatment of all patients.

REFERENCES

American Psychiatric Association: Diagnostic and Statistical Manual of Mental Disorders, 3rd Edition, Revised. Washington, DC, American Psychiatric Association, 1987

Arthur RJ, McKenna GJ: Survival under conditions of extreme stress, in Stress and Its Management. Directions in Psychiatry Monograph Series, No 6. Edited by Flach F. New York, WW Norton, 1989

Bernard C: An Introduction to the Study of Experimental Medicine (1865). New York, Macmillan, 1927

Cannon WB: The Wisdom of the Body. New York, WW Norton, 1939

Flach F: Calcium metabolism in states of depression. Br J Psychiatry 110:588–593, 1974

Flach F: Choices. New York, JB Lippincott, 1977

Flach F: The Secret Strength of Depression, Revised Edition. New York, Bantam, 1986

Flach F: Resilience. New York, Fawcett Columbine, 1988

Flach F, Kaplan M: Visual Perceptual Rehabilitation in Psychiatric Patients in Psychobiology and Psychopharmacology. Directions in Psychiatry Monograph Series, No 2. Edited by Flach F. New York, WW Norton, 1988

McKenna GJ, Arthur RJ: Survival under adverse conditions, in Stress and Its Management. Directions in Psychiatry Monograph Series, No 6, Edited by Flach F. New York, WW Norton, 1989

Menninger K: The Vital Balance. New York, Viking Press, 1963

Nemiah J: Alexithymia and psychosomatic medicine, in Directions in Psychiatry, Vol 2. Edited by Flach F. New York, Heatherleigh, 1982, Lesson 27

Selye H: Creativity in basic research, in The Creative Mind. Edited by Flach F. Buffalo, NY, Bearly Press, 1988, pp 255–259

Phenomenology of
Posttraumatic Stress Disorder

Chapter 4

Diagnostic Validity of Posttraumatic Stress Disorder

Jessica Wolfe, Ph.D.
Terence M. Keane, Ph.D.

It is now commonly accepted that traumatic disorders can arise in response to a large variety of severe life stressors. Despite the diversity among these events, the concept of an extreme psychological reaction to catastrophic occurrences was first demonstrated exclusively in the context of war, specifically as a reaction to combat stress (Grinker and Spiegel 1945). The concept of a traumatic reaction dates back at least to the time of Homer's *Odyssey*, when warriors' diaries revealed grueling accounts of intense panic and disturbance both during and following battlefield encounters (Trimble 1985). Since that time, a number of individual reports of extreme agitation, fright, and disorientation have appeared following a variety of other military conflicts. These accounts eventually gave rise to a range of descriptors such as "shell shock," "combat neurosis," and "battle fatigue," all used to depict the severe, adverse emotional reactions of soldiers operating under life-threatening conditions.

Even within the limited realm of combat, little information was originally available to indicate how either individual or situational factors influenced the development of trauma syndromes. Consequently, the contribution of both types of factors remained poorly understood. A further consequence of this limitation in knowledge was reflected in a general lack of diagnostic clarity about posttraumatic stress disorder (PTSD). Most affected individuals were globally characterized and their disorders poorly distinguished from other types of common psychiatric disorders, such as adjustment syndromes and anxiety disorders. In fact, the concept of a valid, generic posttraumatic diagnosis was not seriously applied to civilians until much later.

The first formal criteria for the diagnosis of trauma-based disorders appeared with the publication of the standardized, diagnostic psychiatric text, the Diagnostic and Statistical Manual of Mental Disorders (DSM-I) (American Psychiatric Association 1952). This edition described these disorders as "traumatic neuroses," emphasizing the then popular Freudian belief that psychological disturbances were rooted in unresolved intrapsychic conflicts whose symptoms represented unconscious defensive workings. The DSM-I interpretation of acquired trauma syndromes had certain practical limitations—in particular, the failure to retain Freud's original belief that such "neuroses" were evidence of actual, rather than imagined, traumatic exposure. Nonetheless, the first DSM-I attempts at classification were valuable because they emphasized the need for professional attention to PTSD. This development set the stage for eventual scientific study into fundamental areas of the disorder, especially the validity, etiology, and phenomenology associated with posttraumatic stress.

DSM-II (American Psychiatric Association 1968) reexamined the earlier definition of posttraumatic syndromes and concluded that they should be less rigidly defined. As a result, the diagnostic labels of "transient situational disturbance" and "adjustment reaction" were applied to the disorder. This labeling appeared to reflect some basic unawareness of the disorder's debilitating symptom features and its frequently treatment-resistant course. Furthermore, the generality of the new categorization tended to discourage the growth of any widespread professional (and public) interest in this disturbance for at least another decade. As a consequence, few scientific advances took place during the 1970s in terms of appreciating the broad validity of PTSD or the complexity of factors associated with its formation.

Diagnosis

DSM-III (American Psychiatric Association 1980) endorsed the existence of a definitive posttraumatic syndrome. This event confirmed PTSD as a major diagnostic entity within the anxiety disorders. In addition, DSM-III outlined the disorder's primary and associated symptom features in some detail. Despite this advance, scientific controversy surfaced again, this time around issues such as the diagnostic "legitimacy" of the disorder, its true discriminability from other major (and potentially related) disturbances, and the accuracy of its symptom picture as portrayed at the time (Breslau and Davis 1987). One popular debate dealt with whether PTSD constituted a verifiable anxiety disorder or whether it should be alternatively recategorized as a variant or subset of other major syndromes, for example, major depression (Goodwin and Guze 1984), with which PTSD seemed to share many phenomenological features. In addition, both dissociative disorders and a newly proposed classification based on stressor-related characterological disturbance (Horowitz et al. 1987) received some preliminary consideration as alternative superordinate categorizations for PTSD.

Since that time, an increasing number of behavioral (Pallmeyer et al. 1986), phenomenological (Brett and Ostroff 1985; Silver and Iacono 1984), and assessment-based (Fairbank et al. 1983) studies have generated a substantial amount of factual data about PTSD and its distinctive symptomatology. This data base has been particularly successful in delineating the increasing number of diagnostic features uniquely associated with PTSD, thus helping to resolve some of the earlier doubts about diagnostic validity and taxonomy. For reasons involving both historical precedent and subject availability, the majority of these studies were originally carried out using male military or combat veteran populations. The studies, conducted from about 1979 to 1983, provided most of the earlier empirical support for the diagnostic validity of PTSD, and work continues to build on that foundation today. This body of research gained additional prominence when DSM-III-R

(American Psychiatric Association 1987) further refined existing theoretical and scientific hypotheses about the disorder.

One of the more important contributions of DSM-III-R was the provision of clear-cut and operationally based definitions for the stressor criterion in PTSD. In addition, DSM-III-R offered new information about the disorder's primary and secondary symptomatology as they were found in a wider range of populations, including for the first time traumatized children as well as adults. By gaining this type of diagnostic credibility, the field of PTSD was further stimulated in the early 1980s by the advent of new scientific and theoretical work, which subsequently contributed additional data about the validity of this disorder.

VALIDATIONAL PROCEDURES

Efforts to validate the diagnosis of PTSD are currently evolving rapidly. For the purposes of this chapter, these have been organized into four content areas: empirical efforts in diagnosis (based extensively on a variety of assessment procedures); model-building attempts (emphasizing phenomenology and conceptual formulations); focused biologic and physiologic approaches (reflecting the search for intrinsic biologic or centrally mediated markers); and epidemiologic approaches (examining disease distributions across populations). Each of these areas is reviewed below. The largest emphasis is on assessment and psychological test methodologies, which have, to date, provided much of the primary validational support for the diagnosis of PTSD.

Assessment Procedures

In the area of assessment and evaluation, commonly used diagnostic procedures incorporate descriptive (or case) interviews (Smith 1985), psychometric tests (Keane et al. 1988), and laboratory-based procedures (Blanchard et al. 1986; Malloy et al. 1983). Although historical and case report formats initially characterized the field of PTSD, the past 5 years have witnessed a rapid growth in the sophisticated use of other evaluative procedures for establishing this diagnosis, specifically standardized psychometric instruments such as the Minnesota Multiphasic Personality Inventory (MMPI) (Hathaway and McKinley 1951) subscales (Foy et al. 1984; Keane et al. 1984) and physiological paradigms measuring purported changes in autonomic system functioning (Blanchard et al. 1986; Malloy et al. 1983). With the recent availability of large sample sizes and the ability to assess homogeneously exposed groups (e.g., as in Vietnam War combatants), it has become increasingly possible to apply a comprehensive range of sophisticated statistical techniques to the information generated via the above methods (Keane et al. 1984; Ohlde et al. 1987; Silver and Iacono 1984). In addition, more precise measurement of exposure criteria—such as combat exposure scales (Keane et al. 1989)—has helped improve estimates of the contribution of the requisite stressor criteria.

One particular emphasis of the current test procedures relates to the use of a comprehensive, structured assessment "battery" (Keane et al. 1987). This approach is based on the theory that diagnostic acumen can be significantly enhanced by employing numerous and potentially convergent data bases. In fact, because these instruments tap diverse and pivotal parameters of functioning, they provide the opportunity to obtain consensual validation as well as an analysis of a range of behavioral skills. Since PTSD has long been challenged on the grounds of its seeming overlap with other diagnoses, this comprehensive approach to assessment clearly enhances diagnostic credibility by providing the opportunity for obtaining findings that deal with measurements of sensitivity and specificity.

The multidimensional, multimodal model also contributes to validation on a longer-term basis through its impact on treatment efforts. For example, the breadth of information obtained in these evaluations can readily be used to develop treatment goals in PTSD sufferers as well as to reevaluate their subsequent diagnostic status after treatment intervention.

A primary goal of the above evaluative approach has been the development of PTSD instrumentation that reliably characterizes the disorder and simultaneously distinguishes it from other serious, psychological disturbances, such as major unipolar affective disorder (Halbreich et al. 1988; Kudler et al. 1987). To accomplish this, the multifaceted assessment has been constructed according to several conceptual guidelines. First, the approach strictly emphasizes the combined use of objective and subjective data bases; this includes both quantifiable psychological inventories or tests and highly structured, clinician interview formats. Second, assessment measures focus on obtaining clear-cut estimates of past and current functional abilities in a wide range of skills felt to be impacted in the development of trauma disorders. These include a wide spectrum of cognitive, affective, behavioral, and physiologic capacities that have been theoretically and empirically shown to be affected in this disorder (Keane et al. 1985) as well as confirmed in the symptom reports of large numbers of traumatized patients. The multimodal evaluation of PTSD also strongly encourages the use of a systematic, chronologic format for gathering diagnostic information. This emphasis clearly recognizes the contribution of developmental phases to the acquisition of this type of disturbance. By encouraging clinicians to investigate all life periods of the patient, it becomes possible to examine not only recent precipitants but factors or variables throughout the life span that are likely to influence adjustment abilities as well as types of symptom formation (Foy et al. 1984; Green et al. 1988).

Many of the individual instruments used in these assessments are based on studies of combat-related PTSD. In fact, investigations of combatants have resulted in many of the existing reliable instruments for diagnosing and quantifying PTSD (Keane et al. 1987). Two of these measures—the Mississippi Scale for Combat-Related Posttraumatic Stress Disorder (Keane et al. 1988) and the PTSD subscale of the MMPI (Keane et al. 1984)—are currently in widespread use with veteran PTSD populations and are being increasingly regarded by other investigators as prototypes for the measurement of PTSD in their own nonmilitary, victim populations. Because few such instruments have existed until recently, the task still remains to evaluate their utility for civilian PTSD populations. If instruments of this type prove valid and reliable in a range of traumatized groups, multiple functions would be served, including justification for the broad-based validity of this disorder, the advancement of structured evaluative procedures in general, and the provision of information about stressor-specific symptom profiles that may uniquely characterize certain groups of survivors (Kosten et al. 1987).

Although an increasing number of traditional psychological tests are being examined and modified for their use in PTSD (e.g., Madakasira and O'Brien 1987), one other instrument in particular warrants mention—the Impact of Event Scale (IES) (Horowitz et al. 1979). This inventory has been used over the past 10 years in numerous traumatized civilian populations and has received considerable acceptance as one of the few available and widely applicable diagnostic instruments for furnishing data on DSM-III PTSD criteria. Although it was not originally developed in the context of current DSM-III criteria, the IES nonetheless provides data on two crucial PTSD symptoms—reexperiencing and numbing/avoidance phenomena—both regarded as hallmarks of the disorder. The IES has now been shown to have a reasonable degree of clinical and face validity (Schwarzwald et al. 1987); consequently, it represents an important method for integrating theoretical and empirical findings in PTSD.

Despite certain advances in psychometric instruments, there are, in fact, few standardized, examiner-administered interview formats for PTSD. Originally, validational efforts in this disorder were restricted by the use of traditional, unstructured interview methods. Although these interviews provided important descriptive, clinical information, they failed to evaluate existing DSM criteria in any systematic fashion; they also typically failed to differentiate a patient's particular clinical presentation from profiles found in more widely accepted disorders. Today, interview formats in general have improved with the addition of theoretical models and empirical findings in PTSD. Often, however, most are only variably oriented toward the specific measurement of defined PTSD criteria.

Overall, two types of interview formats exist for use in PTSD: generic psychiatric interviews and PTSD symptom-focused interviews. The more generic interviews serve the basic but important diagnostic purpose of inquiring about symptom criteria for *all* current DSM Axis I disorders. They thus allow examination of PTSD in conjunction with the possible presence of other syndromes. Recently, there has been increasing interest in the topic of comorbidity in PTSD (Rundell et al. 1989). As questions about comorbidity continue to increase, DSM-III-R interview formats will provide a valuable basis for assessing issues such as the incidence of comorbidity in this disorder as well as the clinical significance of associated disturbances (Keane and Wolfe, in press).

At present, the three most common psychiatric interview formats include the Structured Clinical Interview for DSM-III-R (SCID) (Spitzer and Williams 1985), the Schedule for Affective Disorders and Schizophrenia (SADS) (Endicott and Spitzer 1978), and the Diagnostic Interview Schedule (DIS) (Robins et al. 1981). Each interview comprehensively examines for the spectrum of major psychiatric disorders. However, their use in diagnostic validation is currently limited to some degree by the lack of comparative data sets that would substantiate rates of diagnostic sensitivity and specificity when using these instruments. The extensive use of the SCID in the National Vietnam Veterans Readjustment Study (NVVRS) (Kulka et al. 1988) helped provide some of the first scientific findings on the value of the SCID for discriminating PTSD. However, no widespread, comparative studies using diverse traumatized populations have been conducted to date that would permit comparisons of diagnostic sensitivity and accuracy.

In addition to the above reservations, each of the generic interview formats has methodological limitations for assessing PTSD. These include their derivation and structural organization according to phenomenological approaches, their imprecise quantification of most primary symptoms and overall disease severity, and a relatively limited emphasis on factors like disease course and developmental history. As a result, use of the DIS, for example, may yield a seemingly static picture of PTSD that belies the diversity of associated clinical features and underestimates the true incidence of the disorder (Keane and Penk 1988). These issues are of particular concern in diagnosing PTSD, where the interaction of numerous variables has now been recognized as a major factor in the evolution of the disorder (Foy et al. 1987).

On a positive note, the preceding interviews provide one of the few formats for the systematic comparison of PTSD symptom constellations with profiles indicative of other major mental disorders. As noted earlier, it is critical at preliminary stages of validation to assess PTSD in the context of possible other major psychological disturbances. This permits differentiation of the disorder from other diagnoses and allows eventual determinations of accompanying rates of comorbidity. In addition, because these interviews are in widespread use, they increase the likelihood that investigators working with various populations of PTSD will obtain diagnostic data in a systematic fashion, enabling comparisons within and among the full range of diagnostic possibilities.

In comparison to general interview formats, structured or focused interviews for PTSD specifically emphasize the assessment of current diagnostic criteria for the disorder. Of the few structured interview formats presently available, the most well-known have been developed largely in conjunction with combat populations. Both the Jackson Structured Interview for Combat-Related PTSD (Keane et al. 1985) and the Brecksville Interview for PTSD (Smith 1985), to name two, provide highly detailed information about the development, course, and typology of war-related PTSD as well as an extensive assessment of psychological functioning across all life periods. When used in conjunction with a variety of psychometric tests, especially those designed explicitly to measure the DSM symptoms of PTSD, these interviews have yielded a high rate of diagnostic accuracy and concordance. However, there is no comparative data available yet about the diagnostic utility of these interviews for other groups of trauma victims (e.g., rape survivors), where numerous and potentially disparate factors may be operational.

It is obvious that, aside from the assessment of certain basic historical and developmental factors along with well-established PTSD symptom criteria, some modifications will need to be made in both general and focused interview formats before they can be appropriately applied to victims suffering from the existing range of traumatic events (e.g., rape, criminal acts, natural disasters, sexual abuse). Ongoing work in the development of such interviews will directly increase success in diagnostic validity and will secondarily provide an improved understanding of the distinguishing versus shared components of trauma syndromes.

A few additional considerations of these formats are important. Since validational accomplishments in noncombat-related PTSD are at a relatively early stage, most investigators have tended to construct their own measurement protocols in accordance with their direct knowledge of their patients. As a result, there is considerable variability in the form and adequacy of some of these procedures. This variability often reflects an interaction between available methodological expertise and the differing amounts of knowledge that exist for any one category of trauma. In the area of criminology and victimization, organized and comprehensive assessment procedures have recently been developed that have begun to advance awareness of both the prevalence and range of pathology suffered by these victims (Kilpatrick et al. 1989). Similar approaches can be found in investigations of both natural disasters (Shore et al. 1986) and human-caused disasters (Green et al. 1983) and are starting to emerge in the field of rape trauma (Hartman and Burgess 1988; Herman 1988). At the present time, work in these areas has helped to establish empirically the widespread occurrence of PTSD, despite the fact that the distress of these victims has long been apparent to some practicing clinicians. Future investigations in these content areas will undoubtedly continue to consider diagnostic work in the field of combat-related PTSD and is correspondingly likely to add to the development of additional assessment methodologies targeted at distinctive components of stressor experiences.

Despite the above advances, widespread acceptance of the diagnostic category of PTSD is still not complete, and much work remains to be accomplished. For example, both the identification and implementation of planned assessments in a host of less well-recognized patient groups (e.g., survivors of traumatic medical procedures) still lag considerably. Often, researchers and clinicians in these areas have applied well-known, generic psychometric instruments—such as the Symptom Check List-90 (Derogatis et al. 1973)—in their efforts to evaluate and diagnose these patients. For the most part, however, these instruments have not been validated for use in PTSD. As a consequence, these assessments frequently yield measures of overall individual distress but are unable to document any accurate or reliable diagnosis of PTSD. Instead, such evaluations frequently produce diagnostic profiles characterized by broad-based descriptors indicating some form of behavioral or affective disturbance (e.g., depression, anxiety, panic, or somatization). Hence, although PTSD may be inferred, the diagnosis is often not adequately demonstrated. Considerable work is therefore required to develop assessment paradigms that can reliably detect the presence of PTSD and that can improve the validation of this disorder through the application of systematic and uniform diagnostic methodologies.

The attempt to conduct follow-up evaluations also presents a further limitation concerning the diagnostic validity of PTSD. One powerful route by which validity can be increased is through the use of reevaluation measures that demonstrate type and level of symptomatology after a specified period of time. In the case of a relatively new diagnostic category like PTSD, the body of existing validational data would be considerably strengthened by longitudinal findings that track the course of the disorder over time and evaluate the interaction of factors influencing its occurrence. At the current time, efforts of this type have been significantly limited in PTSD. In a majority of victim groups, patients are sufficiently distressed at the time of contact that they (or the evaluating clinician) are unwilling or unable to participate in comprehensive assessments. Consequently, there has been widespread variation in the chronology of administering various assessment procedures (e.g., on acute versus chronic bases). As a result, there is still little definitive knowledge about the course of this disorder as it relates to time of onset. While clinical needs must certainly guide research protocols, the careful documentation (and execution) of follow-up procedures would at least allow statistical consideration of these variables. Until that time, diagnostic knowledge remains limited concerning the impact of factors such as time elapsed since initial exposure and the significance of multiple intervening variables.

Models in PTSD

Several other factors need to be considered in reviewing approaches to diagnostic validity in PTSD. One of these relates to the development of conceptual models for this disorder and their subsequent impact on validation. The conceptual orientation of the investigator typically plays an important role in determining the direction of diagnostic studies in many disorders. In terms of PTSD, a "reductionistic" view of etiology was particularly popular in the earlier years of this field. This orientation was especially pronounced within combat-related PTSD, where the stressor of warfare appeared salient and quantifiable. Belief in the model led to the notion that a prominent evaluative focus should include the in-depth estimation of stressor severity and the accompanying degree of traumatic exposure. This view was based largely on original theories of PTSD, which had noted the adverse effects of stressor exposure on even well-adjusted individuals. The orientation was initially useful in highlighting the importance of measuring variables like situational parameters and threshold effects in trauma syndromes; however, the focus weighted earlier diagnostic investigations heavily toward a pronounced emphasis on external variables.

Since that time, subsequent research has made it clear that other factors are also widely influential in the development of PTSD (Pitman et al. 1987; van der Kolk and Greenberg 1987). Consequently, many clinical and social scientists now regard the development and diagnosis of this disorder from a more multifaceted point of view, emphasizing a particular need for understanding the interactional effects of dispositional, personality, background, and contextual factors (Solomon and Mikulincer 1987). As conceptual models of PTSD have broadened, diagnostic procedures have also been modified to reflect the consideration of multiple, interactive variables. These modifications will have a practical effect on validational studies in that the interactive model is likely to contain greater ecological validity (Kolb 1987).

In terms of other impacts by models of PTSD, a final issue deals with the topic of intergrating diagnostic data on survivors from varying victim classes. Since PTSD is no longer seen as restricted to the experiences of heavily exposed combat veterans, it is logical to expand diagnostic and validational approaches toward the development of instrumentation that is tied to more global PTSD criteria. At the same time, it is essential that evaluative techniques be sufficiently specific that they reflect the diverse experiences and reactions of individuals surviving different forms of trauma. Like developments in the field of combat-related PTSD, researchers in sexual abuse, victimization, and disaster survival in particular are now showing increased concern for the need to develop precise instrumentation. These diagnostic techniques require certain a priori decisions about which etiologic and experiential factors may be population-specific and which phenomena may be applicable across classes. As these efforts proceed, critical advances in identifying individual, categorical, and generic aspects of trauma syndromes can be expected.

Biologic-Physiologic Approaches

At the other end of the diagnostic spectrum, a number of investigators consider it important to investigate PTSD along more focused lines of inquiry. Their efforts represent valuable attempts to determine whether diagnostic "markers" exist for this disorder, and in what ways these may be specific or idiosyncratic to individuals developing PTSD. While certain investigations have stressed the role of biologic, biochemical, and neuroendocrine mechanisms in trauma syndromes (Kosten et al. 1987; Krystal et al., in press), other pursuits reflect attempts to define specific physiologic alterations (e.g., heart rate reactivity) in patients with PTSD (Blanchard et al. 1986; Malloy et al. 1983). Such markers, if they exist, could potentially be used to strengthen diagnostic acumen and to develop improved measurement capabilities for assessing treatment outcomes in PTSD.

At this time, investigations into the autonomic system functioning of trauma patients have yielded some of the most compelling diagnostic information on PTSD. A number of investigators (Blanchard et al. 1982; Malloy et al. 1983; Pitman et al. 1987) have demonstrated the presence of heart rate reactivity in certain PTSD patients that significantly distinguishes these individuals from both well-adjusted controls and patients with other severe psychological disorders. By comparison, definitive evidence for biochemical and neuroendocrine alterations, as well as patterns of pharmacologic responsivity (suggesting biochemical mediation), are sufficiently preliminary that these investigations are limited in their current contribution to validational efforts in PTSD. Despite this, work in the preceding areas is important for its strong reliance on homogeneous subject groupings and its active pursuit of diagnostic subtypes. Like ongoing examinations in physiologic reactivity, these related fields of work are likely to gain additional evaluative import when they are combined with a range of multidimensional assessment techniques.

Epidemiologic Contributions

The last topic on validation and diagnosis relates to recent epidemiologic efforts in PTSD. Recently, several studies have been completed that have attempted to document the incidence of PTSD in both the general population and in American veterans from the Vietnam War (Centers for Disease Control 1988; Kulka et al. 1988). In one study examining the prevalence of PTSD in the general United States population (Helzer et al. 1987), a rate of 1% was established for this disorder. Although seemingly low, this percentage is in fact comparable to the incidence of schizophrenia in this nation; it therefore highlights the degree to which PTSD may constitute a real public health concern for the country at large. In a separate study investigating the incidence of combat-related PTSD from the Vietnam War (Centers for Disease Control 1988), the rate of current PTSD in Vietnam veterans was found to be 2%. This rate compares curiously to a morbidity rate of 15% for this disorder, which was reported by the NVVRS (Kulka et al. 1988), a subsequent, nationally representative study of Vietnam veterans.

Despite the clinical importance of all of these findings, discrepancies among them raise diagnostic questions. Reviews of the individual investigations reveal, in fact, that they contain noteworthy methodological differences that are likely to have contributed substantially to the reported differences, at least within those using veteran populations (Kulka et al. 1988). For example, one basis for the reported discrepancies is a difference in measurement methodology. Currently, a number of scientists feel that the multiple measures format used in the NVVRS (Kulka et al. 1988) results in the most specific and sensitive method for diagnosing PTSD. Although these issues are not fully resolved, the projects have succeeded in providing some of the first epidemiologic data available for the field of PTSD. Furthermore, the rates of this disorder strongly suggest that epidemiologic exploration is a critical diagnostic tool, and one that offers the opportunity to conduct investigations across multiple categories of PTSD sufferers. Epidemiologic protocols, in planned combination with other diagnostic procedures, therefore warrant extension to a broader range of trauma populations for use as important and basic validational techniques (Goodwin and Guze 1984).

FUTURE DIRECTIONS

In concluding this review, it appears logical that one particular area for future development in the validation of PTSD involves the application of the multifaceted assessment approach to other victim groups. This would yield information capable of influencing development of both conceptual models and clinical applications in PTSD. A potential confound to this approach is the fact that very limited knowledge is currently available about the degree to which disparate victim classes are similar in their development and manifestation of trauma symptomatology. Hence, despite the theoretical utility of a standardized assessment approach, it is likely that considerably more needs to be learned about the disorder's representation across stressor events and victim groups. Eventually, it seems likely that an even greater degree of specificity and discriminability in diagnostic techniques will be required as development of this field proceeds (cf. Wolfe, in press).

Awareness of the potentially diverse factors associated with trauma disorders also raises the need to consider new factors in evaluating PTSD. Despite the fact that considerable validational work is now occurring, there has been only minimal attention paid to variables other than those that explicitly depict negative sequelae of the stressor. Evaluations of the contributions of more common developmental variables, such as gender, age, psychosocial stage, and family composition (which may serve as distinct mediators and contributors to patterns of traumatic response), all warrant investigation. Similarly, surprisingly little is understood about the adjustment of the numerous individuals who have been exposed to definitive life traumas but do not subsequently develop PTSD. A critical issue here will involve attempts to understand what factors contribute to more favorable patterns of adjustment, allowing these individuals to escape relatively unscathed from potential traumatization.

References

American Psychiatric Association: Diagnostic and Statistical Manual of Mental Disorders. Washington, DC, American Psychiatric Association, 1952

American Psychiatric Association: Diagnostic and Statistical Manual of Mental Disorders, 2nd Edition. Washington, DC, American Psychiatric Association, 1968

American Psychiatric Association: Diagnostic and Statistical Manual of Mental Disorders, 3rd Edition. Washington, DC, American Psychiatric Association, 1980

American Psychiatric Association: Diagnostic and Statistical Manual of Mental Disorders, 3rd Edition, Revised. Washington, DC, American Psychiatric Association, 1987

Blanchard E, Kolb L, Pallmeyer T, et al: The development of a psychophysiological assessment procedure for post-traumatic stress disorder in Vietnam veterans. Psychiatr Q 54:220–229, 1982

Blanchard E, Kolb L, Gerardi RJ, et al: Cardiac response to relevant stimuli as an adjunctive tool for diagnosing post-traumatic stress disorder in Vietnam veterans. Behavior Therapy 17:592–606, 1986

Breslau N, Davis G: Post-traumatic stress disorder: the stressor criterion. J Nerv Ment Dis 175:255–264, 1987

Brett E, Ostroff R: Imagery and post-traumatic stress disorder: an overview. Am J Psychiatry 142:417–424, 1985

Centers for Disease Control: Health status of Vietnam veterans. JAMA 259:2701–2724, 1988

Derogatis L, Lipman R, Covi L: SCL-90: an outpatient psychiatric rating scale—preliminary report. Psychopharmacol Bull 9:13–25, 1973

Endicott J, Spitzer R: A diagnostic interview: Schedule for Affective Disorders and Schizophrenia. Arch Gen Psychiatry 35:837–844, 1978

Fairbank J, Keane T, Malloy P: Some preliminary data on the psychological characteristics of Vietnam veterans with PTSD. J Consult Clin Psychol 51:912–919, 1983

Foy D, Sipprelle R, Rueger D, et al: Etiology of PTSD in Vietnam veterans: analysis of premilitary, military and combat exposure influences. J Consult Clin Psychol 52:79–81, 1984

Foy D, Carroll E, Donahoe C.: Etiological factors in the development of PTSD in clinical samples of Vietnam combat veterans. J Clin Psychol 43:17–27, 1987

Goodwin D, Guze S: Psychiatric Diagnosis. New York, Oxford University Press, 1984

Green B, Grace M, Lindy J, et al: Levels of functional impairment following a civilian disaster: the Beverly Hills Supper Club fire. J Consult Clin Psychol 51:573–580, 1983

Green B, Lindy J, Grace M: Long-term coping with combat stress. Journal of Traumatic Stress 1:399–412, 1988

Grinker R, Spiegel J: Men Under Stress. Philadelphia, PA, Blakiston, 1945

Halbreich U, Olympia J, Glogowski J, et al: The importance of past psychological trauma and pathophysiological process as determinants of current biologic abnormalities. Arch Gen Psychiatry 45:293–294, 1988

Hartman C, Burgess A: Rape trauma and treatment of the victim, in Post-traumatic Therapy and Victims of Violence. Edited by Ochberg F. New York, Brunner/Mazel, 1988

Hathaway SR, McKinley JL: Minnesota Multiphasic Personality Inventory: Manual for Administration and Scoring. Minneapolis, MN, University of Minnesota Press, 1951

Helzer J, Robins L, McEvoy L: Post-traumatic stress disorder in the general population. N Engl J Med 317:1630–1634, 1987

Herman J: Father-daughter incest, in Post-traumatic Therapy and Victims of Violence. Edited by Ochberg F. New York, Brunner/Mazel, 1988, pp 175–195

Horowitz M, Wilner N, Alvarez W: Impact of Event Scale: a measure of subjective distress. Psychosom Med 41:209–218, 1979

Horowitz M, Weiss D, Marmar C: Diagnosis of post-traumatic stress disorder: commentary. J Nerv Ment Dis 175:267–268, 1987

Keane T, Penk W: The prevalence of post-traumatic stress disorder: letter to the editor. N Engl J Med 318:1690–1691, 1988

Keane T, Wolfe W: Comorbidity in post-traumatic stress disorder: an analysis of community and clinical studies. Journal of Applied Social Psychology (in press)

Keane T, Malloy P, Fairbank J: The empirical development of an MMPI subscale for the assessment of combat-related post-traumatic stress disorders. J Consult Clin Psychol 52:888–891, 1984

Keane T, Zimering R, Caddell J: A behavioral formulation of PTSD in Vietnam veterans. Behavior Therapy 8:9–12, 1985

Keane T, Wolfe J, Taylor K: Post-traumatic stress disorder: evidence for diagnostic validity and methods of psychological assessment. J Clin Psychol 43:32–43, 1987

Keane T, Caddell J, Taylor K: Mississippi Scale for Combat-Related Post-Traumatic Stress Disorder: three studies in reliability and validity. J Consult Clin Psychol 56:85–90, 1988

Keane T, Fairbank J, Caddell J, et al: Clinical evaluation of a measure to assess combat exposure. J Consult Clin Psychol 1:53–55, 1989

Kilpatrick D, Saunders B, Amick-McMullen A, et al: Victim and crime factors associated with the development of crime-related post-traumatic stress disorder. Behavior Therapy 20:199–214, 1989

Kolb L: A neuropsychological hypothesis explaining post-traumatic stress disorders. Am J Psychiatry 144:989–995, 1987

Kosten T, Mason J, Giller E, et al: Sustained urinary norepinephrine and epinephrine elevation in post-traumatic stress disorder. Psychoneuroendocrinology 12:13–20, 1987

Krystal J, Kosten T, Perry B, et al: Neurobiological aspects of PTSD: review of clinical and preclinical studies. Behavior Therapy (in press)

Kudler J, Davidson J, Meador K, et al: The DST and posttraumatic stress disorder. Am J Psychiatry 144:1068–1071, 1987

Kulka R, Schlenger W, Fairbank J, et al: National Vietnam Veterans Readjustment Study (NVVRS) Report: description, current status, and initial PTSD prevalence estimates. Washington, DC, Veterans Administration, 1988

Madakasira S, O'Brien K: Acute posttraumatic stress disorder in victims of a natural disaster. J Nerv Ment Dis 175:286–290, 1987

Malloy P, Fairbank J, Keane T: Validation of a multimethod assessment of posttraumatic stress disorders in Vietnam veterans. J Consult Clin Psychol 51:488–494, 1983

Ohlde CD, Shauer AH, Garfield NJ, et al: Preliminary steps in the development of a screening instrument to assess post-traumatic stress disorder. Journal of Counseling and Development 66:104–106, 1987

Pallmeyer T, Blanchard E, Kolb L: The psychophysiology of combat-induced post-traumatic stress disorder in Vietnam veterans. Behav Res Ther 24:645–652, 1986

Pitman R, Orr S, Forgul D, et al: Psychophysiologic assessment of post-traumatic stress disorder imagery in Vietnam combat veterans. Arch Gen Psychiatry 44:970–975, 1987

Robins L, Helzer J, Croughan J, et al: National Institute of Mental Health Diagnostic Interview Schedule: its history, characteristics, and validity. Arch Gen Psychiatry 38:381–389, 1981

Rundell J, Ursano R, Holloway H, et al: Psychiatric response to trauma. Hosp Community Psychiatry 40:68–74, 1989

Schwarzwald J, Solomon Z, Weisenberg M, et al: Validation of the Impact of Event Scale for psychological sequelae of combat. J Consult Clin Psychol 55:251–256, 1987

Shore J, Tatum E, Vollmer W: Psychiatric reactions to disaster: the Mount St. Helens experience. Am J Psychiatry 143:590–595, 1986

Silver S, Iacono C: Factor analytic support for DSM-III's post-traumatic stress disorder for Vietnam veterans. J Clin Psychol 40:5–14, 1984

Smith J: Sealing over and integration: modes of resolution in the post-traumatic stress recovery program, in Trauma and Its Wake. Edited by Figley C. New York, Brunner/Mazel, 1985

Solomon Z, Mikulincer M: Combat stress reactions, post-traumatic stress disorder, and social adjustment: a study of Israeli veterans. J Nerv Ment Dis 175:277–285, 1987

Spitzer R, Williams J: Structured Clinical Interview for DSM-III-R, Patient Version. New York, Biometrics Research Department, New York State Psychiatric Institute, 1985

Trimble M: Post-traumatic stress disorder: history of a concept, in Trauma and Its Wake. Edited by Figley C. New York, Brunner/Mazel, 1985, pp 5–14

van der Kolk B, Greenberg M: The psychobiology of the trauma response: hyperarousal, constriction, and addiction to traumatic reexposure, in Psychological Trauma. Edited by van der Kolk B. Washington, DC, American Psychiatric Press, 1987, pp 63–87

Wolfe J: Women veterans and PTSD: new frontier, in Against All Odds: The Alienation and Isolation of Women Veterans. Edited by Perri M, Perez J. Urbana, IL, University of Illinois Press (in press).

Chapter 5

Personality Disorders and Posttraumatic Stress Disorder

James H. Reich, M.D., M.P.H.

This chapter will focus on the relationship of personality disorder to posttraumatic stress disorder (PTSD). It will examine the subject mainly from a psychiatrist's perspective (i.e., looking at personality disorders as a syndrome), although some work using dimensional personality measures will also be cited. Given space limitations, I will not review every article on the subject, but will try to focus on the most pertinent and well designed. I shall briefly describe and cite previous review articles so that those interested in pursuing the issue further will have an appropriate starting point. Table 5-1 summarizes important aspects of some key empirical articles, which will be discussed.

Research on personality and PTSD can be divided into two broad areas. The first is whether personality pathology is associated with PTSD after the onset of PTSD or concurrently with PTSD. This is an area where there is fairly good agreement, with most researchers feeling that such an association is present. The second area is whether personality or personality disorder can predispose to the development of PTSD. Seldom in the psychiatric literature has a question resulted in such polarized and strongly held positions. Whereas some academicians take the position that there is absolutely no personality predisposition to the development of PTSD, others feel such a predisposition is key to the development of this condition.

A look at the methodological difficulties in researching this area may reveal why there is such disagreement. Not all research designs are equally powerful. Cross-sectional protocols, where all data are gathered at one point in time, are useful in discovering associations between variables, but cannot determine whether one or the other came first or predisposed toward the second. Prospective studies that follow subjects forward through time are capable of making etiologic inferences. Case control designs where a group of subjects is identified in the present and where past records are reviewed are subject to biases of sample selection and early information gathering. Their efficacy is somewhere between cross-sectional and prospective. Since PTSD by definition involves the subject experiencing trauma beyond the normal realm of experience, prospective studies of PTSD cannot be planned but must wait for chance to place a qualified investigator in a position to examine the impact of a natural catastrophe. Of course, this is a rare event.

Another methodological problem is that of sample selection. Subjects who come to the attention of clinicians and researchers are usually patients. Patients are a subset of people found in the community. The pressures of situations making "patienthood" tend to make this group unrepresentative of persons found in the community at large. In fact, it is not possible to start from a patient population and draw correct inferences about the nature or

Table 5-1. Selected summary of major empirical studies on personality and posttraumatic stress disorder (PTSD)

Authors	N	Type of population	Design of study	Combat measure	PTSD measure	Diagnostic system	Previous psychiatric history examined	Psychiatric family history examined	Comorbidities found	Conclusions on predisposing factors
Penk et al. (1981)	207	Drug and alcohol abusers	Retrospective	Vietnam Veterans Survey	Vietnam Veterans Survey	DSM-III	No	No	Not reported	Degree of combat found to be a significant predictor of later stress problems
Helzer et al. (1987)	2,493	Community survey	Prospective	Interview questionnaire	Interview	DSM-III	Yes	No	Obsessive-compulsive disorder, dysthymic disorder, manic-depressive disorder, panic disorder, antisocial personality, phobias, drug abuse, alcohol abuse	PTSD predicted by behavioral characteristics before age 15, also by combat and trauma
Card (1983)	1,500	Vietnam veterans and controls	Prospective follow up	Retrospective interview questionnaire	Retrospectively derived scale	DSM-III	Yes	No	Not available	Author's conclusion was that combat exposure was the overriding etiologic variable
Wilson and Krauss (1982)	114	Combat veterans	Retrospective	Vietnam Era Stress Inventory	Vietnam Era Stress Inventory	Unclear	Premorbid personality	No	Not available	1. Combat role 2. Specific Vietnam stressors 3. Homecoming support

		Sample	Design	Trauma assessment	PTSD measure	Diagnosis		4. Premorbid personality		Results
Horowitz et al. (1980)	66	Patients referred to a stress disorder clinic (non-personality disordered)	Cross-sectional	Measured traumatic life events instead	Impact of Event Scale	DSM-III	—	—	Anxiety, depression	DSM-III PTSD appeared valid in those exposed to overwhelming stress; those with personality disorders had worse symptoms
Davidson et al. (1985)	36	Chronic PTSD study	Family history study	—	Interview	DSM-III	Yes	Yes	Alcohol abuse, unipolar depression, bipolar illness, generalized anxiety, substance abuse	Family history of PTSD most similar to that of anxiety disorders
Foy et al. (1984)	43	Vietnam veterans seeking psychological counseling	Retrospective	Combat exposure scale	PTSD diagnostic scale	DSM-III	Premilitary adjustment	No	Not available	Both combat exposure and military adjustment were predictors; premilitary adjustment did not predict

PTSD: Etiology, Phenomenology, and Treatment

Table 5-1. Selected summary of major empirical studies on personality and posttraumatic stress disorder (PTSD) *(continued)*

Authors	N	Type of population	Design of study	Combat measure	PTSD measure	Diagnostic system	Previous psychiatric history examined	Psychiatric family history examined	Comorbidities found	Conclusions on predisposing factors
Brill and Beebe (1951)	955	Enlisted personnel treated for psychoneuroses during World War II	Cohort follow-up	Not specified; charts & questionnaires used	Not specified; charts & questionnaires used	Not specified	Yes	No	Not available	48% of treated patients had emotional difficulty prior to the service, 20% had "pathologic personalities," 14.6% "overt neuroses"; preservice personality related to postservice disability; combat a nonprognostic factor; disability was related to severity of illness during the service
McFarlane (1988a)	45	Previously healthy subjects recently exposed to severe trauma; community sample	Cohort follow-up	Not applicable	Questionnaire rating	DSM-III	Yes	Yes	Reported subsequently	Neuroticism, introversion, and family history of psychiatric disorder were predictors

| McFarlane (1988b, 1988c) | 469 | Community sample exposed to stressors | Follow-up | Not applicable | General Health Question-naire | DSM-III | Yes | No | Panic disorder, major depression | Predictors of chronic course were as follows: 1. Adverse life events before the disorder 2. Neuroticism 3. A history of treated psychological disorder 4. Tendency to avoid thinking about the experience; difficulty in concentrating was the best predictor of delayed PTSD; severity of stressor may be a biased measure in PTSD patients |

prevalence of a disease in the community. Most studies of PTSD have been in patient populations.

In reviewing the empirical studies relevant to personality predisposing to PTSD, I shall start with the cross-sectional studies, move to the community survey, and finally to prospective studies, focusing in more detail on the latter two designs. Before proceeding, it might be well to mention also the nonmethodological reasons why personality as a possible predisposition to PTSD is so controversial. Those who feel strongly about personality not being implicated as a predisposing PTSD factor may feel that to claim otherwise is "blaming the victim" and that, for example, those men who fought in combat deserve to be treated more honorably. Those who feel the other way may think that many people who would have had emotional problems anyway use PTSD as a means of blaming society for their difficulties. Regardless of political position, PTSD must be acknowledged as a legitimate disease to be treated. If personality is a predisposing factor, it is important to understand it because it might help us develop appropriate treatment. If personality is not a predisposing factor, it is also valuable to know this. In that case, research and treatment efforts could be redirected in other directions.

Previous Relevant Reviews

Several reviews and relevant related papers suggest that previously present emotional disorders (which could be related to personality factors) predispose to the development of PTSD. Andreasen and Noyes (1972) made this observation in their study of severely burned patients. After a review of PTSD combat literature, Worthington (1978) concluded that those who had adjustment difficulties after combat are the same group suffering adjustment difficulties prior to combat. The review of Ettedgui and Bridges (1985) also concluded that preexisting emotional illness may predispose to PTSD. Scrignar's (1984) position is that anxiety-related personality traits may predispose to PTSD. In their review, Wilson and Krauss (1982) feel that personality may be a contributing factor to PTSD. McFarlane (1986, 1987), whose work will be described in greater detail later, also indicated that personality may well be an important predisposing variable. Silverman (1986) noted that many PTSD patients have no identifiable indications of poor emotional health prior to the stressor. However, he suggested that preexisting emotional disorders and coping styles could interact with stressors in potentially negative ways.

Several articles represent the psychoanalytic position. Sudak et al. (1984) hypothesized that those who fall prey to the syndrome may have suffered specific deprivations as children. Christenson et al. (1981) postulated that severe stress may reactivate early development traumas and present them as PTSD. Horowitz (1983, 1986) advanced a psychoanalytically based interaction model between personality and PTSD; he feels that the meaning of the traumatic event to an individual is an important determinant to outcome. Personality is often the key to an individual's attribution of meaning. Similar positions are taken by others (Hendin 1984; Hendin et al. 1983; van der Kolk 1987).

Scurfield's (1985) review is valuable in discussing the methodological factors that make it difficult to reach definitive conclusions about the etiology of PTSD. However, he did not appear to attribute much significance to personality as a predisposing factor. Card (1983), who will also be reviewed in greater detail later, feels that personality variables are, at best, negligible contributors to the development of PTSD.

LITERATURE RELEVANT TO THE CO-OCCURRENCE OF PTSD AND PERSONALITY PATHOLOGY

The conclusion that patients who already have PTSD have negative personality changes is one of the few areas of general agreement in the PTSD personality literature. Cavenar and Nash (1976) described and presented case examples of these changes. Erlinger (1983) discussed these personality problems from a legal point of view. Lindy and Titchener (1983) described personality changes found after the Buffalo Creek disaster, as did Titchener and Kapp (1976). There are several reports of the occurrence of PTSD and antisocial personality disorder (Behar 1984; Sierles et al. 1983). Bailey (1985) reviewed this latter area.

The exact nature of the changes described vary. At one extreme there is some form of a paranoid adjustment to life, whereas at the other are those who appear to have made a normal adjustment, but whose dealing with recurrent thoughts or images reduces the energy they have available for work and relationships. If there is a common denominator, it appears that many of the subjects with PTSD have had their image of the fairness or stability of the world so disrupted that they are forced to devote time and energy to adjust to the emotional disturbance this causes. It is this adaptation that probably is responsible for the reported personality changes occurring after the onset of PTSD.

EMPIRICAL LITERATURE RELEVANT TO PERSONALITY PREDISPOSING TO PTSD

Cross-Sectional Studies

One report (Koranyi 1969) that did not use specific PTSD symptoms, measures of personality, or outcome deserves mention. After personally examining more than 1,000 survivor syndrome patients, Koranyi's clinical impression was that preexisting personality had no effect on the development of PTSD. Although weak methodologically, this work does represent a great deal of clinical experience.

Penk et al. (1981) designed a study to test Figley's hypothesis that combat and degree of combat exposure predict symptoms that have been described as related to PTSD. The population studied included 87 combat and 120 noncombat veterans seeking drug abuse treatment. This was an unusual sample in that it was homogeneous for drug abusers. However, it was not homogeneous for type of drug abuse; it included opiate, polydrug, and alcohol abusers. As different types of drug abusers are most likely different, it is unclear exactly to whom this sample generalizes. A fairly comprehensive test battery was given, including intelligence testing, the Minnesota Multiphasic Personality Inventory (MMPI) (Hathaway and McKinley 1943), a measure of adjustment in their family or origin and current family, and the five-section Vietnam Veteran Survey. This survey deals with demographic information, military service information, combat experience in Vietnam, and problems encountered and treatment services sought out after leaving the military. Statistical examination of the data included covariance and multivariate analyses. Symptoms hypothesized to be related to PTSD were the major outcome variables. The hypothesis that PTSD-related symptoms would be predicted by combat history was confirmed; the MMPI and measures of family adjustment did not, however, predict PTSD symptoms. This surprised the authors, who speculated that the MMPI and other tests used may be appropriate to the measurement of PTSD symptoms. It would appear that the authors have hit on a valid point. The MMPI is not designed to measure personality; it is primarily a symptom measure. Similarly, many premorbid adjustment measures may just not be "cut right" to measure pertinent areas. It would also seem that what should be estimated premorbidly is evidence of DSM-III (American Psychiatric Association 1980) Axis I and Axis II disorders.

Brill and Beebe (1951) conducted a follow-up study of 955 cases of enlisted men treated for psychoneurosis during World War II. Although this may not be a perfect sample since it is a heterogeneous population, hard to diagnose retrospectively by present-day standards, the findings of this study are of considerable interest; 48% of those treated had significant emotional difficulty prior to entry into the service, 20% were diagnosed as "pathologic personalities," and 15% had "overt neuroses." Brill and Beebe do note that these latter two diagnoses were not always associated with severe impairment. Of those well integrated prior to the service, 8% were at least moderately disabled, while the percentages for overt neuroses and pathologic personality disorders were 39% and 51%, respectively. This could indicate that personality disorders did predispose to PTSD.

Horowitz et al. (1980) made very careful measurement of symptoms of people who had PTSD symptoms after being exposed to overwhelming stress. An attempt was made in this study to eliminate those with personality disorders. This makes it a hard study to generalize from for personality variables. However, they reported that those subjects who did have symptoms of personality disorders appeared to have more severe symptoms.

Foy et al. (1984) performed a well-designed retrospective study of Vietnam veterans seeking psychological treatment. They excluded psychotic and primary drug abuse patients from the study. Of their 43 subjects, 21 were rated as PTSD positive. The goal of the study was to determine whether the variables of premilitary adjustment, military adjustment, and combat exposure predicted the outcome variables of PTSD and postmilitary adjustment. All subjects underwent an extensive structured interview that included specific adjustment indices, a combat exposure scale, a problem checklist, and a PTSD scale. The three predictor variables were used in a multiple regression format to try to predict the two outcome measures. The results were that both military adjustment and combat exposure significantly predicted both PTSD and postmilitary adjustment, whereas premilitary adjustment predicted neither. The strengths of this study are its careful and systematic measurements and assessments and its appropriate statistical analysis. However, it also presents two weaknesses. First, the specific sample may not be highly generalizable. Second, one wonders if they asked the correct questions for premilitary adjustment. Common sense would lead one to expect that premilitary and military adjustment would be related. It may be that more questions on previous psychopathology, family history, or personality would have been more useful. It is possible that the military adjustment variable could have been a proxy for some personality variables.

Wilson and Krauss (1982) performed an interesting retrospective analysis attempting to predict which veterans would be at risk for PTSD. Using a self-report instrument called the Vietnam Era Stress Inventory as measurement instrument and factoring it into various subscales, they tested four hypotheses: 1) that the number of combat roles would be related to PTSD scores, 2) that the frequency of exposure to specific stressors would increase PTSD scores, 3) that lack of support during homecoming would be positively associated with PTSD symptoms, and 4) that premorbid personality would not be related to PTSD symptoms. They found support for their first three hypotheses. Also, to their surprise, they found some connection between their premorbid personality measures and PTSD symptoms. This is significant as they did not even sample the entire range of DSM-III personality disorders. Their assessment was that narcissism was the primary personality variable of importance. The strengths of the study include its carefully designed questionnaire and analysis, well-structured hypotheses, and inclusion of DSM-III personality measurements. Weaknesses include the retrospective nature of the data, lack of a control group, and failure to gather data on a wider range of personality pathology. The personality findings are especially interesting, as they ran counter to their premises.

A study by Davidson et al. (1985) is unquestionably an important one. They took 36 consecutive admissions for treatment to a PTSD ward. Using DSM-III criteria, the authors were able to document the significant psychiatric comorbidity found in PTSD. They found alcohol abuse in 41%, nonbipolar depression in 41%, bipolar disease in 25%, anxiety disorder in 19%, substance abuse in 16%, and schizophrenia in 6%. However, what makes the study special is that the investigators took a comprehensive family history on their patients. They found that 66% of the probands gave a positive family history; 60% reported drug or alcohol abuse, 22% various types of anxiety, 20% depression, 20% other disorders, 11% unspecified psychosis, and 6% PTSD.

By comparing this profile with retrospectively constructed depression and generalized anxiety disorder samples, they came to the conclusion that the PTSD family history was most similar to that of generalized anxiety. They concluded that PTSD could be an anxiety disorder variant. Family history of personality disorder was not measured in this report. However, as some personality disorders do run in families and are often associated with anxiety disorders and substance abuse, the possibility of a familial personality predisposition is raised by the study and should be pursued by future research.

Community Surveys

Helzer et al. (1987) conducted a high-quality psychiatric community epidemiologic survey that included PTSD. They did this by including PTSD questions in their site (St. Louis) of the Epidemiologic Catchment Area study. Surveyed were 2,493 community residents. Prevalence rates of PTSD of 1% in the general population, 3.5% in civilians exposed to physical attack and in Vietnam veterans who were not wounded, and 20% in wounded Vietnam veterans, were found.

Of considerable interest was the ability of behavioral problems before age 15 to predict PTSD. The behavioral problems assessed were stealing, lying, truancy, vandalism, running away from home, fighting, misbehaving at school, early sexual experience, substance abuse, school expulsion or suspension, academic underachievement, and delinquency. Having four or more of these symptoms predicted PTSD (6% versus 1%). For those exposed to combat, early behavioral problems predicted a greater likelihood of having PTSD (64% versus 40%, $P > .01$). Helzer et al. (1987) concluded that "behavioral characteristics that antedate exposure to a traumatic event influence a person's response to that event" (p. 1633). This is a well-designed community epidemiologic study yielding specific relationships between early behavioral characteristics and development of PTSD. The only DSM-III personality disorder measured by the ECA study, however, was antisocial conduct, and it is quite possible that other personality traits or disorders could also predispose to PTSD outcome.

Prospective Studies

Before discussing the two major prospective studies on PTSD (Card 1983; McFarlane 1988a, 1988b, 1988c), I shall briefly discuss another prospective study by Vaillant and Vaillant (1981), even though it is not on PTSD. The reason for this is that many clinicians and researchers are skeptical that personality or developmental characteristics early in life can be associated with significant later life events. In a well-designed study of 456 inner-city men, these authors were able to show that capacity to work in early adolescence predicted successes in adult life and was a more potent predictor than social class, membership in a family with multiproblems, and other adolescent variables in predicting adult mental health. This should raise the possibility that personality variables would interact with environmental events to affect the course of illnesses.

Moving to studies specific to PTSD, the work of Card (1983) is of interest due to its prospective nature and careful design. It used 1,500 age-matched males who had been part of a study of high school students. One-third of the sample had been in Vietnam, one-third had been in the military and seen no combat, and one-third had not been in the military. Initial ratings were taken at age 15, and the follow-up was at age 36. Card's PTSD scale was retrospectively derived from other questions. By this measure, 19% of the Vietnam veterans in her study had PTSD, whereas only 12% of her comparison groups had this condition. It is likely that this measure overdiagnosed PTSD and may also be different in various ways from what a clinician diagnoses as PTSD. She found that combat was far and away the largest predictor of PTSD symptoms. Card also found that self-confidence at age 15, as measured by a standardized personality measure, and drinking problems in the military were also predictive. She felt, however, that these were only relatively minor findings.

The first comment that should be made on Card's (1983) study is that any personality measure that can predict outcome 21 years later is relatively powerful. The second is that only if the proper variables were tested for will there be appropriate results. The original personality testing was performed examining normal personality variants and not pathological ones. It would seem that drinking problems in the military and self-confidence at age 15 could represent proxies for important personality variables. However, the failure to measure pathological personality variables, combined with the

retrospective nature of the PTSD scale (which gives higher PTSD preva-
lences than expected), may obscure the findings.

McFarlane (1986, 1987, 1988a, 1988b, 1988c) has made a major contribution to the understanding of PTSD. This author was in the proximity of
a major natural disaster (a fire) and quickly designed a prospective study to
observe the development of PTSD and other psychiatric symptoms. He did
this in several ways. First, he gathered information on a group of persons
asking for psychiatric treatment. Next, he prospectively followed 469 community-volunteer fire fighters over 3 years using self-report measures: a life
events scale, the General Health Questionnaire, the Maudsley Personality
Inventory, and others. In addition, a subsample of 50 patients who appeared
by self-report scores to be at risk for PTSD were interviewed at 8 months.
The importance of the community-volunteer fire-fighting sample cannot be
overestimated. They represented, in effect, a community sample of above-
average functioning who were all exposed to the same traumatic stressor and
followed prospectively. This makes this data set unique.

In his initial examination of patients presenting for psychiatric treatment, McFarlane (1986) found that exposure and losses sustained in the
disaster were inadequate predictors of psychiatric disorder. Many of these
patients (especially those who presented early) were patients with preexisting psychiatric disorder that had been exacerbated by recent stress.
McFarlane felt constitutional personality and social factors would be important predictors of who would seek treatment. In his analysis of the fire-
fighting sample, McFarlane (1987) examined the specific effects of the
disaster and life events on the outcome of psychiatric symptoms. He found
that although life events and disaster events could separately contribute to
morbidity, they together accounted for only 9% of the General Health Questionnaire variance. He concluded that vulnerability was a more important
factor in breakdown than degree of stress experienced. At 8 months,
McFarlane interviewed 50 of these fire fighters who appeared to be at risk
for PTSD by their self-report scores; 11 had PTSD at interview. Those
having PTSD, as compared to those who did not, had significantly higher
Maudsley Personality Inventory neuroticism scores and significantly lower
Maudsley Personality Inventory extroversion scores. He concluded that a
complex relationship may exist between exposure, other factors (such as
personality), and the development of PTSD. At 29-month follow-up of the
entire 469 member group, neuroticism (as measured by the Maudsley
Personality Inventory) in the group with chronic persistent PTSD was significantly higher than in those groups where there was no PTSD or where the
symptoms had resolved.

An important area of bias investigated by McFarlane (1988b) was that
involved in reporting of frequency of injury from the disasters. In those with
chronic PTSD, this frequency remained unchanged over 7 months, whereas

in the non-PTSD group, it decreased 57% over the same time period. This indicates that studies that do not perform their measures relatively soon after the incident may overestimate the influence of exposure and, as a consequence, underestimate the relative importance of other factors such as personality.

DISCUSSION

One observation seems fairly clear. Patients who suffer from PTSD, especially if it is chronic, will have some tendency toward deleterious personality change. The nature of this change, although not completely clear, may have a relationship to the meaning placed on the traumatic event by the individual, although some could also be the deleterious effects of chronic illness. The further delineation of these changes is an area of necessary future research. Should this research be successful, it might pave the way toward the development of more specific psychotherapy treatment (perhaps a cognitive psychotherapy approach).

The issue of personality traits predisposing toward PTSD is an emotionally charged one due to the stigma attached to mental illness. It does not necessarily have to be that way. There is a familial disposition toward heart disease. However, this does not mean that someone with a positive family history is any worse a person or that his or her family is "tainted." Also, even though there is such a predisposition, many people without such a predisposition also develop heart disease. At best, a predisposition to cardiac illness should be taken as a legitimate indication to take certain preventive life-style measures. Ideally, should a personality predisposition toward PTSD be verified, it should be treated the same way.

The evidence for personality to predispose toward PTSD is fragmentary, but certainly shows a trend in a positive direction. Skilled clinicians point out that the meaning of a traumatic event is certainly involved in the pathogenesis of PTSD, and it is hard to believe that personality would not interact with the attribution of meaning. Although cross-sectional studies do not always show a link between PTSD and personality, the best-designed studies reviewed here (Card, Helzer et al., and McFarlane's work) all show some association. Future studies will have to focus on better delineation of preexisting Axis I disorders, Axis II disorders, and other relevant personality traits to further elucidate the specific relationship.

REFERENCES

American Psychiatric Association: Diagnostic and Statistical Manual of Mental Disorders, 3rd Edition. Washington, DC, American Psychiatric Association, 1980

Andreasen NC, Noyes R: Factors influencing adjustment of burn patients during hospitalization. Psychosom Med 34:517–525, 1972

Bailey JE: Differential diagnosis of posttraumatic stress and antisocial personality disorders. Hosp Community Psychiatry 36:881–883, 1985

Behar D: Confirmation of concurrent illnesses in posttraumatic stress disorder. Am J Psychiatry 141:1310–1311, 1984

Brill NQ, Beebe GW: Follow-up study of psychoneuroses. Am J Psychiatry 108:417–425, 1951

Card JJ: Lives After Vietnam. Lexington, MA, Lexington Books, 1983, pp 93–114

Cavenar JO, Nash JL: The effects of combat on the normal personality. Compr Psychiatry 17:647–653, 1976

Christenson RM, Walker JI, Ross DR, et al: Reactivation of traumatic conflicts. Am J Psychiatry 138:984–985, 1981

Davidson J, Swartz M, Storck M, et al: A diagnostic and family study of posttraumatic stress disorder. Am J Psychiatry 142:90–93, 1985

Erlinger CP: Post-traumatic stress disorders, Vietnam veterans and the law. Behavioral Sciences and the Law 1:25–50, 1983

Ettedgui E, Bridges B: Posttraumatic stress disorder. Psychiatr Clin North Am 8:89–103, 1985

Foy DW, Sipprelle R, Ruegger DB, et al: Etiology of postraumatic stress disorder in Vietnam veterans: analysis of premilitary, military and combat exposure influences. J Consult Clin Psychol 1:79–87, 1984

Hathaway SR, McKinley JC: Minnesota Multiphasic Personality Inventory. Minneapolis, MN, University of Minnesota Press, 1943

Helzer JE, Robins LN, McEvoy L: Posttraumatic stress disorder in the general population. N Engl J Med 317:1630–1634, 1987

Hendin H: Combat never ends: the paranoid adaptation to posttraumatic stress. Am J Psychother 38:121–131, 1984

Hendin H, Haas AP, Singer P, et al: The influence of precombat personality on posttraumatic stress disorder. Compr Psychiatry 24:530–534, 1983

Horowitz MJ: Post-traumatic stress disorders. Behavioral Sciences and the Law 1:9–23, 1983

Horowitz MJ: Stress-response syndromes: a review of posttraumatic and adjustment disorders. Hosp Community Psychiatry 37:241–249, 1986

Horowitz MJ, Wilner N, Kaltreider N, et al: Signs and symptoms of posttraumatic stress disorder. Arch Gen Psychiatry 37:85–92, 1980

Koranyi EK: A theoretical review of the survivor syndrome. Diseases of the Nervous System (Suppl) 30:115–118, 1968

Lindy JD, Titchener J: "Acts of God and Man": character change in survivors of disasters and the law. Behavioral Sciences and the Law 1:85–96, 1983

McFarlane AC: Posttraumatic morbidity of a disaster. J Nerv Ment Dis 174:4–14, 1986

McFarlane AC: Life events and psychiatric disorder: the role of a national disaster. Br J Psychiatry 151:362–367, 1987

McFarlane AC: The aetiology of posttraumatic stress disorders following a natural disaster. Br J Psychiatry 152:116–121, 1988a

McFarlane AC: The longitudinal course of posttraumatic morbidity. J Nerv Ment Dis 176:30–40, 1988b

McFarlane AC: The phenomemology of posttraumatic stress disorders following a natural disaster. J Nerv Ment Dis 176:22–29, 1988c

Penk WE, Robinowitz R, Roberts WR, et al: Adjustment differences among male substance abusers varying in degree of combat experience in Vietnam. J Consult Clin Psychol 49:426–437, 1981

Scrignar CB: Post-traumatic Stress Disorder. New York, Praeger, 1984, pp 39–56

Scurfield RM: Post-trauma stress assessment and treatment: overview and formulations, in Trauma and Its Wake. Edited by Figley C. New York, Brunner/Mazel, 1985, pp 219–256

Sierles FS, Jang-June C, McFarland RE, et al: Posttraumatic stress disorder and concurrent psychiatric illness: a preliminary report. Am J Psychiatry 140:1177–1179, 1983

Silverman JJ: Post-traumatic stress disorder. Adv Psychosom Med 16:115–140, 1986

Sudak HS, Martin RS, Corradi RB, et al: Antecedent personality factors and the post Vietnam syndrome. Milit Med 149:550–554, 1984

Titchener JL, Kapp FT: Family and character change at Buffalo Creek. Am J Psychiatry 133:295–299, 1976

Vaillant GE, Vaillant CO: Natural history of male psychological health: work as a predictor of positive mental health. Am J Psychiatry 138:1433–1440, 1981

van der Kolk BA: Psychological Trauma. Washington, DC, American Psychiatric Press, 1987

Wilson JP, Krauss GE: Predicting post-traumatic stress disorders among Vietnam veterans, in Post-traumatic Stress Disorder and the War Veteran Patient. Edited by Kelley WE. New York, Brunner/Mazel, 1982, pp 102–147

Worthington RE: Demographic and preservice variables as predictors of post-military service adjustment, in Stress Disorders Among Vietnam Veterans. Edited by Figley CR. New York, Brunner/Mazel, 1978, pp 173–187

Chapter 6

Are All Vietnam Veterans
Like John Rambo?

Bruce Boman, M.B.B.S., F.R.A.N.Z.C.P., Ph.D.

The typical image of the Vietnam veteran, reinforced by a spate of movies and television dramas, is that of an impulsive, poorly controlled, walking time bomb addicted to narcotics and alcohol, who, more often than not, has a criminal and prison record. One needs only to think of *Rambo*, *Taxi Driver*, *The Stone Killers*, "Police Story," and "Kojak" in this regard, not to mention the character of Colonel Kurtz in *Apocalypse Now*, a man so overwhelmed and deranged by his exposure to the senseless slaughter of the Vietnam War that he has thrown off the last vestiges of civilized restraint and has regressed back to a state of primitive, amoral savagery.

The wide publicity given to isolated incidents of seemingly inexplicable, explosive, and impulsive homicide committed by Vietnam veterans, such as the McDonald's massacre, has certainly cemented this image. Other examples of this recurrent journalistic theme include the celebrated Jon Nordheimer May 25, 1971, article in the *New York Times* documenting the events leading up to the death, while committing armed robbery, of Dwight Johnson, an ex-army sergeant, combat hero, and Medal of Honor recipient; an article in the June 30, 1975, edition of *Newsweek*, which asserted that many of the pilots ferrying illicit drugs into the country were unemployed Vietnam veterans; and in a May 27, 1975, article in, again, the *New York Times*, which asserted that half a million Vietnam veterans had attempted suicide.

Increasingly, attorneys in the United States are considering psychiatric disorders alleged to be associated with Vietnam service as a defense in criminal trials. Thus, in April 1980, in Birmingham, Alabama, the lawyers for Charles Head, a Vietnam veteran who had murdered his brother-in-law, claimed that his combat-induced mental disequilibrium had so impaired his ability to distinguish right from wrong that he could not be held responsible for the slaying. The jury concurred and Head was acquitted. In April 1979, a Boston jury acquitted a former helicopter pilot on drug-running charges after they had been told in psychiatric evidence that his Vietnam experiences had turned him into an "action junkie" and that smuggling drugs was his way of reliving the thrills of war.

The 96th Congress U.S. House Committee on Veterans' Affairs (1979) disclosed in a presidential review memorandum on Vietnam-era veterans that 29,000 of this group were incarcerated in state or federal jails, 37,500 were on parole, 250,000 were on probation, and 87,000 were awaiting trial, and that Vietnam-era veterans comprised 55% of the 13,000 ex-servicemen receiving outpatient care from the Veterans Administration for drug abuse.

There is also a marked degree of consistency in the clinical literature describing the kinds of psychopathology demonstrated by Vietnam veterans

81

receiving psychiatric attention with an almost stereotyped syndrome of anti-authoritarianism, impulsive violence, alcoholism, drug abuse, parasuicidal behaviors, broken marriages, child abuse, chaotic interpersonal relationships, a surly chip on the shoulder resentment, and repeated criminal offending (Boman 1985b). Shatan's (1978) post-Vietnam syndrome includes the diagnostic feature of rage and other violent impulses directed against indiscriminate targets (Horowitz and Solomon 1978). In their book on Vietnam veterans, Brende and Parson (1985) spoke of them having become "neurologically wired" to respond to low-intensity stimuli with irritability and violence, remaining within these individuals "a residual of the killer-self ready to make an appearance with the slightest provocation."

However, even before the conclusion of the Vietnam War, this stereotype was beginning to be built up by reports both in the popular press and in the psychiatric literature of the massacre at My Lai, the "fragging" of superior officers by their troops, and the epidemic of heroin abuse among the United States military stationed in South Vietnam. Fisher (1972), a United States military psychiatrist, spoke of a situation of anarchy and lawlessness among the troops in Vietnam, and of 1,000 cases referred to him for assessment, 960 were diagnosed as having an antisocial personality disorder associated with a desire to escape military duties and responsibilities. All were returned to their units for disciplinary action. Between 1969 and 1972 there were almost 800 recorded incidents of the use of explosive devices against superior officers (Bond 1976). In 1971, 43% of United States servicemen departing Vietnam had used heroin, 25% amphetamines, and 23% barbiturates during their tour of duty (Robins et al. 1975).

When DSM-III (American Psychiatric Association 1980) introduced the diagnostic category of posttraumatic stress disorder (PTSD), aspects of such antisocial behaviors were included as associated diagnostic features—that is, "sporadic and unpredictable explosions of aggressive behavior, [occurring] upon even minimal or no provocation" (p. 237). In DSM-III-R (American Psychiatric Association 1987), this has been watered down to "irritability or outbursts of anger" (p. 250). The question remains, however, what hard evidence is there to support the hypotheses that Vietnam veterans are more likely to indulge in such antisocial behaviors and that their PTSD is associated with explosive violence, substance abuse, or suicidal behaviors. A number of points have to be made right from the start, emphasizing the need for controlled studies in which socioeconomic and background variables are taken into account.

First, from 1960 to 1970 there had occurred a dramatic increase in recorded crime among young people in general in the United States and not just among Vietnam veterans. Thus, among those 18 years and younger over this 10-year period, there had been a 226% increase in homicide and non-negligent manslaughter charges, a 98% increase in forcible rape, a 234%

increase in charges of robbery, a 158% increase in aggravated assault charges, an 87% increase in charges over the carrying and possession of weapons, a 125% increase in charges for drunkenness, and a 3,205% increase in charges of breaking narcotic laws (Federal Bureau of Investigation 1971).

Second, the crisis of morale and discipline in the United States military in the late 1960s and early 1970s was not confined to troops stationed in Vietnam, but occurred on a very widespread basis. Indeed, the highest desertion and AWOL (away-without-leave) rates on record in the Marine Corps were registered in 1975, 2 years after the conclusion of United States military involvement in Indochina.

Third, the most common form of psychopathology observed in young adult males, whether or not they have been to war, has been reported to be a cluster of impulsive, violent, rebellious, and antisocial behaviors, and young adult males comprise the majority of prison populations (Akers 1973; Mazer 1972).

Fourth, the very factors that increased the risk of young men serving in Vietnam (especially in the lower ranks and in combat units) are exactly those that increase the risk of the above deviant behaviors: having less education, coming from deprived socioeconomic strata, and belonging to minority racial groupings (Akers 1973; Pilisuk 1975). As the United States became more heavily committed to Vietnam, rising labor supply demands led to a lowering in the standard of men drafted, especially as higher qualified young men from the middle classes not infrequently obtained draft deferments to attend college or were more successful in being able to enlist in the National Guard. With the introduction of "Project 100,000," draftees were inducted with even lower standards of intelligence and education, and it is now evident that such young men were quite ill-suited for the exacting demands of counterinsurgency warfare and had disciplinary problems and court-martial conviction rates about double that of their comrades (Pilisuk 1975).

IS THERE ANY EVIDENCE LINKING ANTISOCIAL BEHAVIOR AND NARCOTIC USE WITH VIETNAM VETERAN STATUS?

When considering the antisocial and disciplinary problems exhibited by troops in Vietnam, an important issue to be addressed is whether such behaviors were, in fact, a continuation of premilitary patterns of deviance. A consistent observation made on men who had participated in the "fragging" of their superior officers was that such behavior was very often a continuation of preservice impulsive violence and, reflecting this propensity for aggression, many had actually enlisted with the aim of volunteering for combat duty in Vietnam (Gilhooly and Bond 1976). Thus one study of soldiers convicted of "fragging" demonstrated high levels of developmental pathology, including parental separations and brutality, poor school performance, preservice antisocial behavior, and chaotic interpersonal relationships. All of the subjects had displayed, pre-Vietnam, a characterological impulsivity and lack of frustration tolerance, and many had volunteered for the army to escape domestic problems or to try to resolve insecurities in the areas of their masculinity or independence (Bond 1976).

Likewise, another study of men who had indulged in excessive and militarily unnecessary violence and killing while on active service found a higher incidence of arrests prior to military service and that the subjects more often came from lower socioeconomic groupings and deprived ethnic minorities and more frequently had developmental histories characterized by enuresis, fire setting, fights, arrests, and dropping out of school (Yager 1976). Their parents had also often displayed high levels of impulsive violence, and, like the servicemen who had indulged in "fragging," these men were more often volunteers. The most frequent explanations for wanting to go to Vietnam were "to prove myself as a man" and "to see if I could take it," again suggesting that vulnerabilities in the areas of independence, self-esteem, and masculinity may have been behind their determination to see active service. Providing evidence that such acts of excessive violence were not especially related to combat stress, being wounded, or losing comrades in action were variables independent of such antisocial conduct (Yager 1976). The free availability of inexpensive, high-grade heroin, the 1960s youth-centered drug culture, and the lack of commitment and poor morale among United States troops in Vietnam after the Tet offensive were probably more the factors behind the widely observed explosive outbreak of narcotic use than any individual psychopathology (Baker 1971; Zinberg 1972), and it has already been pointed out that a similar epidemic of drug abuse occurred in the United States over this same period (Zinberg 1972).

Suggesting the relative absence of marked individual psychopathology among troops using heroin in Vietnam, it has been shown that their use of drugs prior to military service had not been more frequent than or heavy as that of their comrades who did not use drugs in Vietnam, that they did not have raised levels of premilitary antisocial behaviors, that they did not display any excess of adverse early experiential environments, and that their Minnesota Multiphasic Personality Inventory (MMPI) (Hathaway and McKinley 1943) responses were considerably less pathologic than those of civilian drug addicts (Nace and Meyers 1974; Nace et al. 1978; Robins et al. 1975). In one large epidemiologic survey, only 1% of a group of United States servicemen who used heroin while in Vietnam had actually been addicted to it before enlistment (Robins et al. 1975). Providing evidence that combat stress was not an important factor predisposing to heroin use, it was found that its use was equally prevalent among support and frontline troops (Hollow 1974). Indeed, in studies of Australian servicemen in Vietnam, it was found that deviant behavior, overall, tended to be concentrated among support troops, with the incidence of personality disorders manifested as behavioral disturbances being about 18 times as frequent among support compared with frontline troops, and the incidence of alcoholism approximately 4 times as great (Boman 1982). Similar observations were also made on United States servicemen (Borus 1974; Jones and Johnson 1975). The prevalence of alcohol abuse by soldiers in Vietnam was put at 7% as alcoholics and 5% as borderline alcoholics (Greden et al. 1975). These figures are congruent with those reported from among United States military personnel in America and Europe (Allen and Mazzuchi 1985; Cahalan et al. 1972). Troops who drank heavily in South Vietnam tended to have had many preservice difficulties, including parental heavy drinking, criminal convictions before enlistment, and a less advanced level of educational achievement. A significant percentage had enlisted to avoid a jail sentence, but then went on to have a high level of administrative punishments and court-martials (Greden et al. 1975).

In summary, there is considerable evidence that men who "fragged" their superior officers, indulged in militarily unnecessary violence, or drank heavily while in Vietnam had displayed high levels of similar psychopathology prior to military induction; that they often came from deprived families and socioeconomic backgrounds; and indeed, that their motives for enlisting not infrequently were associated with a desire to escape domestic, marital, or legal difficulties or were an attempt to resolve insecurities in the spheres of masculinity and independence. On the other hand, heroin use in Vietnam did not seem to be linked to social deviance or personal psychopathology, but rather was a reflection of the drug's ready availability, the high level of anomie felt by troops in the latter stages of the Vietnam War, and the drug-centered youth culture of that period. There is little evidence that combat stress in itself was associated with any of the above behaviors.

Contrary to widespread fears in the United States that military personnel who had used narcotics and other drugs in Vietnam would bring their addictions back home with them, causing a major public health problem, it quickly became apparent that their rate of heroin dependence had virtually dropped back to preenlistment levels some 12 months after repatriation (Robins et al. 1975). Indeed, the best predictor of drug abuse among Vietnam veterans was a premilitary history of drug abuse and antisocial behavior (Helzer et al. 1975; Robins et al. 1974, 1975). Some of the factors associated with continued narcotic use in veterans include coming from a home broken by death, desertion, or divorce before the age of 16; a parental history of alcoholism or arrests; an adolescence characterized by fighting, truancy, heroin use, dropping out of school, legal trouble, and drunkenness; and a voluntary enlistment into the military (Robins et al. 1974, 1975). Importantly, heroin use in Vietnam was not predictive of postservice criminal behavior or violence (Nace et al. 1978). If then drug use in Vietnam is not a factor strongly linked with post-repatriation addiction, are Vietnam veterans any more likely to abuse drugs than their peers?

In seven studies in which Vietnam veterans were compared with matched controls (Baker 1971; Ewalt 1981; Figley and Southerly 1980; Pearce et al. 1985; Silver and Iacono 1984; Strange 1974; Yager et al. 1984), no difference emerged on this variable; in one of them (Yager et al. 1984), the use of marijuana, cocaine, amphetamines, and barbiturates was actually less among the Vietnam veterans than a control group who had never been in the military. Similarly, a mortality survey among Vietnam-era draft-eligible men from California and Pennsylvania failed to show any increase in death rates from narcotic overdose over that which would have been expected (Hearst et al. 1986). It appears that even heavy combat exposure in Vietnam may not be strongly linked to later drug use among veterans; three studies (Boman 1985a; Pearce et al. 1985; Yager et al. 1984) found no correlation, another study (Ewalt 1981) found a statistically nonsignificant trend for greater heroin use among heavy combat veterans, and another study (Atkinson et al. 1984) found that Vietnam veterans with PTSD actually had a lower rate of substance abuse than those free of PTSD. It has also been reported that participation in atrocities while in Vietnam and later heroin addiction were related only for black veterans but not for white veterans (Yager et al. 1984).

IS THERE ANY EVIDENCE LINKING ALCOHOLISM WITH VIETNAM VETERAN STATUS?

Alcoholism forms another facet of the popular stereotype of the Vietnam veteran. Once again, there have been numerous reports of its abuse among Vietnam veterans in psychiatric treatment. However, it should be pointed out that among United States ex-servicemen overall, when background variables are taken into account, there is no association between veteran status and alcoholism (Boscarino 1980). Four studies specifically focusing on Vietnam veterans have also found an absence of association (Braatz and Lumry 1969; Ewalt 1981; Pearce et al. 1985; Silver and Iacono 1984). Indeed, in another study, service in Vietnam was actually negatively correlated with problem drinking (Yager et al. 1984). Once again, level of combat exposure failed to emerge as a predictive factor (Pearce et al. 1985), and even men who had experienced a major traumatic event on active service, like seeing a friend horribly mutilated by a grenade, did not differ on a problem-drinking scale from veterans who had been posted to secure rear areas (Yager et al. 1984). This latter study also found that participation in abusive violence while in Vietnam had a negative correlation with later consumption of alcohol and no statistically significant correlation with problem drinking. It has also been determined that Vietnam veterans are probably drinking no

more than World War II veterans at a comparative time after their repatriation (Braatz et al. 1971) and possibly even less than ex-servicemen from the
Korean campaign.

Two surveys of problem drinking among United States Vietnam veterans have reported a prevalence of alcoholism of 8% (Goodwin et al. 1975;
Hunter 1978), a rate almost identical to that seen among young American
males overall (Allen and Mazzuchi 1985). A follow-up study of military
personnel treated for drug addiction in Vietnam found that, 2 years post-
repatriation, even this group had an alcoholism rate of no more than 16%
(Nace et al. 1978).

As with heroin use, preservice factors are predictive of problem drinking among returnees. These include parental alcoholism, early age of drinking, early onset of polydrug use, a low educational level, poor scholastic
achievement, truancy, and expulsion from school (Goodwin et al. 1975; Nace
et al. 1977). A consistent pattern emerges of adolescent problem drinking, a
continuation of this behavior into the military and during service in Vietnam,
and then its persistence back to civilian life. Very often, in fact, these men
had tended partially to replace alcohol with heroin in Indochina, only to give
this up and return to alcohol on their repatriation (Goodwin et al. 1975). A
large mortality survey of Australian Vietnam veterans found that their death
rates from such alcohol-related causes as motor vehicle accidents, homicide,
and suicide were significantly lower than expected and that even deaths from
liver cirrhosis were no higher than anticipated (Fett et al. 1984). A United
States mortality survey also provided evidence that eligibility for military
service during the Vietnam War was associated with a subsequent lower-
than-expected death rate from cirrhosis (Hearst et al. 1986). In the Australian mortality survey, when the Vietnam veterans were compared with a
matched group of ex-servicemen who had not been out of the country, a small
but statistically significant elevated death rate from cirrhosis did emerge,
suggesting that Vietnam service may have pushed up alcohol consumption
levels, but still not to a degree to make it greater than the average for young
adult males of the same age and background (Fett et al. 1984).

IS THERE ANY EVIDENCE LINKING VIOLENCE AND INCREASED MORTALITY RATES FROM HOMICIDE AND SUICIDE WITH VIETNAM VETERAN STATUS?

Once again, when the question of violence, criminality, and suicide is addressed, controlled studies have dispelled the prevailing image of the antisocial Vietnam veteran with a hair-trigger control over his explosively violent
impulses. In one study of criminal behavior among a population of 202
Vietnam veterans, there was demonstrated no excess of such conduct over
that which would have been predicted from premilitary variables (Nace et

al. 1978). Research conducted by Ralph Nader's Center for the Study of Responsive Law, likewise, reached the conclusion that there was no significant evidence indicating widespread violence among Vietnam veterans, and indeed their level of violence was probably no more than that manifested by young, working-class American males (Starr 1973).

Two other controlled studies on Vietnam returnees have found that their potential for violent aggression was no greater than servicemen with no Vietnam experience (Boman 1958a; Strange and Brown 1970). Supporting these observations, Petrik et al. (1983) could find no correlation between combat history and marital violence; Roberts et al. (1982) found that PTSD and non-PTSD groups of veterans scored similarly on the aggression items of the Horowitz Inventory (Horowitz and Solomon 1978) as well as on a hostility scale of the MMPI; and Van Kampen et al. (1986) found that neither rage nor low frustration tolerance was correlated with combat history or the presence of PTSD symptoms. Likewise, Atkinson et al. (1984) found that Vietnam veterans with PTSD were no more likely to be violent or impulsive or to be incarcerated than their comrades free of PTSD, an observation made similarly among Australian Vietnam veterans (Boman 1985a). Another MMPI study found that scales measuring resentment and aggression also failed to differentiate between a group of United States veterans with combat-related emotional problems and another free of such difficulties (Burke and Mayer 1985).

In a widely quoted study by Borus (1974), which involved 577 Vietnam veterans, it was found that their rate of disciplinary and legal maladjustment was no greater than that manifested by 172 service personnel who had not seen any overseas service, a finding also reported by Braatz and Lumry (1969). Published data from the Center for Policy Research in New York indicated that the arrest and conviction rate for Vietnam returnees was no higher than that seen in veterans who had concurrently served in the military, but had not been out of the United States (Yager et al. 1984); when background variables were accounted for, Vietnam service actually was negatively correlated with arrest and conviction rates. Furthermore, while greater levels of combat exposure in Vietnam tended to be associated with an increased chance of a veteran being convicted, this linkage held only for crimes of a nonviolent nature.

Like alcoholism and drug abuse, it has been found that premilitary variables were predictive of later violence among Vietnam returnees. These variables included coming from a minority racial group or the lower socioeconomic classes; being exposed to parental violence and brutality; having a history of arrests, fights, and gang affiliation in adolescence; enlisting in the military while on probation or parole; and volunteering for a posting in Vietnam (Yager 1976). Veterans manifesting violent behavior were more likely to have indulged in acts of extreme violence while on active service and to have volunteered for a second tour of duty in Vietnam (Yager 1976; Yager et al. 1984).

As has been mentioned, the Australian mortality study (Fett et al. 1984) found that the death rate among Vietnam veterans from violent causes (suicide, homicide, and motor vehicle accidents) was significantly lower than that anticipated for men in their age group and that there was no statistically significant difference in rates, for any of these causes, between Vietnam veterans and men who had served in the military in Australia at the same time. A survey by the Australian Department of Veterans' Affairs of suicide among the 10,000 Vietnam veterans resident in the state of Victoria also found a lower-than-anticipated suicide rate (Spragg, unpublished report, 1981). After an extensive review of the available information, the Australian Senate Standing Committee on Science and the Environment (1982) ventured the opinion that there was no evidence indicating an increase in mortality from violent causes among Australian Vietnam veterans. On the other hand, data on the death rates of United States Vietnam veterans from violent causes are more pessimistic; there are now four studies indicating that these individuals have a greater chance of dying from suicide or a motor vehicle accident (Hearst et al. 1986; Kogan and Clapp 1985; Lawrence et al. 1985; 96th Congress U.S. House Committee on Veterans' Affairs 1979).

IS THERE ANY EVIDENCE LINKING UNEMPLOYMENT WITH VIETNAM VETERANS' STATUS?

Another measure among Vietnam veterans that deserves examination is their employment rate, which, despite claims to the contrary, is probably congruent with that reported for males from the same socioeconomic and geographic backgrounds (Kohen et al. 1977). Indeed, a significant number of Vietnam returnees have reported that their armed forces experience had been beneficial to their later careers and that this benefit may have been particularly so for the young black ex-serviceman (Kohen and Shields 1980). In a survey of Vietnam veterans living in Salt Lake County, there was no difference on measures of social adjustment, self-concept, and anomie between them and veterans who had not served in Indochina (Worthington 1976). Figley and Southerly (1980) reached the same conclusions after interviewing almost 1,000 Vietnam veterans:

> An important finding of the study was that the majority of the veterans adjusted very well to military service in general and the transition back to civilian life in particular. Even though a considerable number of the draftees were angry initially, most did not regret the experience. In fact two-thirds of the sample believed that their years in the military helped them to know themselves better.

Conclusions

There is, consequently, quite a substantial body of evidence suggesting that the popular, Ramboesque image of the Vietnam veteran is far from justified. Indeed, as a group, it seems they are at least as law-abiding as their contemporaries who saw no active service. There is, however, a spectrum of behavioral deviance within the population of Vietnam returnees, with those personnel who had been exposed to heavy combat probably being at greater risk for alcoholism, drug abuse, and convictions for nonviolent offenses. What has definitely emerged from other psychiatric research is a close and consistent association between combat exposure and the development of PTSD (Frye and Stockton 1982; Silver and Iacono 1984; Wilson and Krauss 1985; Yager et al. 1984), a condition that, in the main, is disabling in a quiet, unobtrusive way and can often lead to considerable impairment in the sufferer's level of psychosocial functioning (Frye and Stockton 1982).

In addition, research has found that some 40% of seemingly well-functioning United States Vietnam veterans may suffer from this condition and that there is a negative relationship between its presence and the availability of social support, possibly because of its alienating effect on the veteran's family and friends (Frye and Stockton 1982; Keane et al. 1985; Wilson and Krauss 1985). Hence, by focusing on the behavioral deviance and antisocial behaviors of what may well be a relatively small and highly atypical group of Vietnam veterans, there is the risk that the psychosocial problems of the "silent majority" will be overlooked.

It must also be noted again that the very factors that increased the likelihood of young men serving in Vietnam, especially in the lower ranks and combat units, were those that augmented the risk of antisocial behavior, such as little education, coming from deprived socioeconomic strata, belonging to minority racial groups, and having high levels of developmental pathology.

References

Akers RL: Deviance and conformity, in Society Today. Edited by Stark R. Del Mar, CA, CRM Books, 1973

Allen J, Mazzuchi J: Alcohol and drug abuse among American military personnel; prevalence and policy implications. Milit Med 150:250–255, 1985

American Psychiatric Association: Diagnostic and Statistical Manual of Mental Disorders, 3rd Edition. Washington, DC, American Psychiatric Association, 1980

American Psychiatric Association: Diagnostic and Statistical Manual of Mental Disorders, 3rd Edition, Revised. Washington, DC, American Psychiatric Association, 1987

Atkinson RM, Sparr LF, Sheff AG, et al: Diagnoses of post traumatic stress disorder in Vietnam veterans: preliminary findings. Am J Psychiatry 141:694–694, 1984

Baker SL: Drug abuse in the United States Army. Bull NY Acad Med 47:541–549, 1971

Boman B: The Vietnam veteran ten years on. Aust N Z J Psychiatry 16:107–127, 1982

Boman B: Post-traumatic stress disorder (traumatic war neurosis) and concurrent psychiatric illness among Australian Vietnam veterans: a controlled study. J R Army Med Corps 131:128–131, 1985a

Boman B: Psychiatric disturbances among Australian Vietnam veterans. Milit Med 150:77–79, 1985b

Bond TC: The why of fragging. Am J Psychiatry 133:1328–1331, 1976

Borus JF: Incidence of maladjustment in Vietnam returnees. Arch Gen Psychiatry 30:554–557, 1974

Boscarino J: Drinking by veterans and non-veterans: a national comparison. J Stud Alcohol 41:854–859, 1980

Braatz GA, Lumry GK: The young veteran as a psychiatric patient. Milit Med 134:1434–1439, 1969

Braatz GA, Lumry GK, Wright MS: The young veteran as a psychiatric patient in three areas of conflict. Milit Med 136:455–457, 1971

Brende JP, Parson ER: Vietnam Veterans: The Road to Recovery. New York, Plenum, 1985

Burke HR, Mayer S: The MMPI and the post-traumatic stress syndrome in Vietnam-era veterans. J Clin Psychol 41:152–156, 1985

Cahalan D, Cisin IA, Gardner G: Drinking patterns and problems in the US Army, 1972 (Report 73–6 for Deputy Chief of Staff). Arlington, VA, Department of the Army, Personnel Headquarters, 1972

Ewalt JR: What about the Vietnam veteran? Milit Med 146:165–167, 1981

Federal Bureau of Investigation: Crime in the United States, Uniform Crime Reports: 1970. Washington, DC, U.S. Government Printing Office, 1971

Fett MJ, Dunn M, Adena MA, et al: Australian Veterans—Health Studied: the Mortality Report (Part 1). Canberra, Australia, Australian Government Publishing Service, 1984

Figley CR, Southerly WT: Psychosocial adjustment of recently returned veterans, in Strangers at Home. Edited by Figley CR, Leventman S. New York, Praeger Publications, 1980

Fisher HW: Vietnam psychiatry. Portrait of anarchy. Minn Med 55:1165–1167, 1972

Frye JS, Stockton RA: Discriminant analysis of post traumatic stress disorder among a group of Vietnam veterans. Am J Psychiatry 139:52–56, 1982

Gilhooly D, Bond T: Assaults with explosive devices on superiors. Milit Med 141:700–703, 1976

Goodwin DW, Davis DH, Robins LN: Drinking amid abundant illicit drugs. Arch Gen Psychiatry 32:230–233, 1975

Greden JF, Frenkel SI, Morgan DW: Alcohol use in the army: patterns, associated behavior. Am J Psychiatry 132:11–16, 1975

Hathaway SR, McKinley JC: Minnesota Multiphasic Personality Inventory: Manual for Administration and Scoring. Minneapolis, MN, University of Minnesota, 1943

Hearst N, Newman TB, Hulley SB: Delayed effects of the military draft on mortality: a randomized natural experiment. N Engl J Med 314:620–624, 1986

Helzer E, Robins LN, Davis DH: Antecedents of narcotic use and addiction: study of 898 Vietnam veterans. Drug Alcohol Depend 1:183–190, 1975

Hollow HC: Epidemiology of heroin dependence among soldiers in Vietnam. Milit Med 139:108–113, 1974

Horowitz MJ, Solomon GF: Delayed stress response syndromes in Vietnam veterans, in Stress Disorders Among Vietnam Veterans. Edited by Figley CR. New York, Brunner/Mazel, 1978, pp 268–280

Hunter EJ: The Vietnam POW veteran: immediate and long term effects of captivity, in Stress Disorders Among Vietnam Veterans. Edited by Figley CR. New York, Brunner/Mazel, 1978, pp 188–206

Jones FD, Johnson AW: Medical and psychiatric policy and practice in Vietnam. Journal of Social Issues 31:49–65, 1975

Keane TM, Scott WO, Chavoya EA, et al: Social support in Vietnam veterans with post-traumatic stress disorder: a comparative analysis. Journal of Consulting and Clinical Psychology 53:95–102, 1985

Kogan MD, Clapp RW: Mortality Among Vietnam Veterans in Massachusetts, 1972–1983. Boston, MA, Department of Public Health, 1985

Kohen AI, Shields PM: Reaping the spoils of defeat: labor market experiences of Vietnam-era veterans, in Strangers at Home. Edited by Figley CR, Leventman S. New York, Praeger Publications, 1980

Kohen AI, Grasso JT, Myers SC, et al: Career Thresholds, Vol 6 (U.S. Department of Labor Research and Development Monograph No 16). Washington, DC, U.S. Government Printing Office, 1977

Lawrence CE, Reilly AA, Quickenton P, et al: Mortality patterns of New York State Vietnam veterans. Am J Public Health 75:277–279, 1985

Mazer M: Two ways of expressing psychological disorder: the experience of a demarcated population. Am J Psychiatry 128:933–937, 1972

Nace EP, Meyers AL: The prognosis for addicted returnees: a comparison with civilian addicts. Compr Psychiatry 15:49–56, 1974

Nace EP, O'Brien CP, Mintz J, et al: Drinking problems among Vietnam veterans, in Currents in Alcoholism, Vol 2. Edited by Seixas FA. New York, Grune & Stratton, 1977

Nace EP, O'Brien CP, Mintz J, et al: Adjustment among Vietnam veteran drug users two years post service, in Stress Disorders Among Vietnam Veterans. Edited by Figley CR. New York, Brunner/Mazel, 1978, pp 71–128

96th Congress U.S. House Committee on Veterans' Affairs: Presidential review memorandum on Vietnam-era veterans (House Committee Print No. 38). Washington, DC, U.S. Government Printing Office, 1979

Pearce KA, Schauer AH, Garfield NJ, et al: A study of post-traumatic stress disorder in Vietnam veterans. J Clin Psychol 41:9–14, 1985

Petrik N, Rosenberg AM, Watson CG: Combat experience and youth: influences on reported violence against women. Prof Psychol Res Pract 14:895–899, 1983

Pilisuk M: The legacy of the Vietnam veteran. J Soc Issues 31:3–12, 1975

Roberts WR, Penk WE, Gering ML, et al: Interpersonal problems of Vietnam veterans with symptoms of post-traumatic stress disorder. J Abnorm Psychol 91:444–450, 1982

Robins LN, Davis DH, Goodwin DW: Drug use by US Army enlisted men in Vietnam: a follow-up on their return home. Am J Epidemiol 99:235–249, 1974

Robins LN, Helzer JE, Davis D: Narcotic use in Southeast Asia and afterward. Arch Gen Psychiatry 32:955–961, 1975

Senate Standing Committee on Science and the Environment: Psychiatric morbidity among Vietnam veterans and veteran mortality, in Pesticides and the Health of Australian Vietnam Veterans: First Report. Canberra, Australia, Australian Government Publishing Service, 1982

Shatan CF: Stress disorders among Vietnam veterans: the emotional content of combat continues, in Stress Disorders Among Vietnam Veterans. Edited by Figley CR. New York, Brunner/Mazel, 1978, pp 43–52

Silver SM, Iacono CU: Factor-analytic support for DSM-III's post-traumatic stress disorder for Vietnam veterans. J Clin Psychol 40:5–14, 1984

Starr P: The Discarded Army: Veterans After Vietnam. New York, Charterhouse, 1973

Strange RE: Psychiatric perspectives of the Vietnam veteran. Milit Med 139:96–98, 1974

Strange RE, Brown DE: Home from the war: a study of psychiatric problems in Vietnam returnees. Am J Psychiatry 127:488–492, 1970

Van Kampen M, Watson CG, Tilleskjor C, et al: Adolescent vulnerability to post traumatic stress disorder. J Nerv Ment Dis 174:137–144, 1986

Wilson JP, Krauss GE: Predicting post-traumatic stress disorder among Vietnam veterans, in Post-traumatic Stress Disorder and the War Veteran Patient. Edited by Kelly WE. New York, Brunner/Mazel, 1985, pp 102–147

Worthington ER: The Vietnam era veteran, anomie and adjustment. Milit Med 141:169–170, 1976

Yager J: Post combat violent behavior in psychiatrically maladjusting soldiers. Arch Gen Psychiatry 33:1332–1335, 1976

Yager J, Laufer R, Gallops M: Some problems associated with war experiences in men of the Vietnam generation. Arch Gen Psychiatry 41:327–334, 1984

Zinberg NE: Heroin use in Vietnam and the United States. Arch Gen Psychiatry 26:486–488, 1972

Chapter 7

Psychosomatic Manifestations of Chronic Posttraumatic Stress Disorder

Wolter S. de Loos, M.D., Ph.D.

M edical illnesses of survivors of the massacres and terrors of World War II bear a clearly psychosomatic character. Any physician who becomes involved in caring for these subjects has to consider the biopsychosocial complexity of human nature to analyze the patient's complaint, evaluate its psychological and medical significance, and provide appropriate treatment, whether surgical, medical, or psychotherapeutic. This process proves to be time consuming, particularly since patients had traumatic experiences more than 40 years ago and have now reached middle or old age. For many of these victims, the war still has not ended and will never do so.

This clinical experience throws a heavy shadow on the prospects of full recuperation of younger survivors of more recent human violence. Experience with subjects who were traumatized during World War II has demonstrated that the clinical recognition of a traumatic stress syndrome may, in fact, be delayed for decades, even for more than 40 years (Krell 1988; Van Dyke et al. 1985).

In retrospect, clinical recognition was often preceded by more subtle signs of impending decompensation. These are usually described as "nonspecific" when the underlying cause is either not recognized or investigated by an empathic clinician. Such nonspecific complaints often prove to be of a physical character and may persist after the manifestation of frank posttraumatic stress disorder (PTSD).

Usually, when survivors of trauma apply for help, either to their family doctors, to emergency rooms, or to different physician specialists, they accentuate their physical complaints. Survivors rarely mention a traumatic war history in their initial medical contacts unless they have already been identified as victims.

The histories of survivors of all kinds of severe war experience have demonstrated that many of these individuals did not understand the underlying cause of their problems until a syndrome of nightmares and intrusive recollections provided thematic material necessary for recognition. It has also been the case that subjects keep the material hidden even from their direct environment, seeking help only for their physically disturbing symptoms.

Apart from severe psychological trauma, many World War II victims were also subjected to extreme exhaustion, malnutrition, emaciating diseases, and physical abuse. This combination of deleterious circumstances eventually led to death, other than by execution or extermination, in a very high percentage of subjects. In the survivors it may have caused conse-

95

quences with which the medical sciences are not familiar. The clinical picture of premature aging after concentration camp imprisonment drew interest in the form of numerous retrospective studies (Herberg 1961; Schenck 1977; Thygesen et al. 1970) and experimental research in animals (Ebbesen 1980). Although tropical nutritional amblyopia ("camp eyes") had already been described in civilian circumstances (Moore 1937), this condition still remained an enigma in survivors of Japanese camps (Dekking 1947; Schnitker et al. 1951). Furthermore, its deterioration after a decade of normal civilian life (Baird and MacDonald 1956) and its association with "concentration camp vertigo" (Kuilman 1946) and conjunctival, oral, and skin lesions (Jacobs 1951) have remained obscure. The same must be said for many other medical sequelae in World War II survivors, such as neuropsychological disturbances in concentration camp inmates (Thygesen et al. 1970) and merchant fleet personnel of convoys (Askevold 1980). As a whole, this has left us with many intriguing and unresolved questions.

PSYCHOSOMATIC ASPECTS OF CHRONIC PTSD

It has proven useful for everyday clinical practice to analyze the psychosomatic aspects of chronic PTSD along the following main categories: 1) psychosocial disturbances, 2) somatoform reactions, 3) psychophysiologic symptoms, 4) somatic diseases, and 5) behavioral-somatic interactions.

Psychosocial Disturbances

At the psychosocial level, disturbances are basically related to fear of death, concomitant chronic arousal, and conditioning to trauma-related stimuli. At a later stage, chronic persistence of the syndrome is often accompanied by depression and exhaustion., In clinical practice, and especially in departments of medicine, the diagnosis of anxiety may be missed. Patients will often complain of the following: "My breath is taken away." "Something is coming toward me." "I must go out immediately." "I can act immediately if necessary, but if I can't do anything, I feel terrible." "I feel like stiffening." "I feel tight."

Somatoform Reactions

Somatoform reactions may precede or accompany the diagnosis of PTSD. Their significance can often be understood with the knowledge of the patient's specific traumatic history. Conversion, hypochondriasis, and psychogenic pain occur with considerable frequency. At times it can be helpful to explain to the patient that *the body can remember the pain and emaciation of the past*. Masking of physical ailments may be a problem in these individuals, and they may be worried more by their somatoform complaints than by bona fide concomitant chronic illnesses.

Psychophysiological Symptoms

Psychophysiological effects of arousal and anxiety are core symptoms of all posttraumatic reactions. They often precede the psychiatric diagnosis of PTSD, presenting as "functional complaints" or with descriptions like DaCosta's syndrome of irritable heart, hyperkinetic heart syndrome, effort syndrome, cardiac neurosis, neurocirculatory asthenia, autonomous dysfunction, hyperventilation, panic attacks, "multiple doctor syndrome," and the "fat folder syndrome" (Paul 1987). At a close examination many cases of irritable bowel syndrome also show nonbowel symptoms belonging to the same symptom complex (McKell and Sullivan 1947). Other syndromes that are not that generally recognized as belonging to the same entity include fibromyalgia, "allergic to everything," "sugar intolerance," "reactive hypoglycemia," weakly proven cases of lactose intolerance, the mitral valve prolapse syndrome, and also probably "Syndrome X" (1987).

The most effective way of understanding the biological significance of the psychophysiological anxiety syndrome is probably to describe it in terms of the defense reaction (Abrahams and Hilton 1958; Hess and Brugger 1943). This has been described by Cannon (1953) as "the organic preparations for action . . . in flight or conflict—either one requiring perhaps the utmost struggle." It is characterized by increased breathing, pupillodilation, piloerection, heart rate increase, and blood pressure increase with redistribution of blood flow to the voluntary muscles at the expense of the splanchnic region, kidneys, and skin. The tone of postural muscles increases, and behavioral arousal may be accompanied by fighting, rage, or flight reactions. Neurophysiological studies have elucidated a central nervous system substrate in which the cell bodies with an organizational and initiating function are located in the periaqueductal gray (Hilton and Redfern 1986) and in the mediobasal and central amygdaloid nucleus (Hilton and Zbrozyna 1963; Iwata et al. 1987; Stock et al. 1978), whose stimulation can elicit both the behavioral and the physiological components of the defense reaction.

Earlier, this effect had been investigated in detail in the ventromedial hypothalamus of the rat (Yardley and Hilton 1986), the cat (Eliasson et al. 1953), and primates (Smith et al. 1980). Subsequently, the defense reaction was shown to be susceptible to classical and instrumental conditioning in dogs (Federici et al. 1985) and various primates (DeVito and Smith 1982; Smith et al. 1979, 1980), in which it was designated by Stebbins and Smith (1964) as the "conditioned emotional response." The same terminology was chosen by Kolb (1984) for the strong autonomous responses in war veterans after conditional stimuli related to their wartime experiences. These considerations suggest that DaCosta's syndrome, Kolb's conditioned emotional responses, and other synonymous syndromes represent, in fact, chronically repeated defense reactions elicited by conditional stimuli derived from traumatic experiences. Van der Kolk (1987) has drawn attention to the phenomenon of kindling of the amygdala as a possible substrate for behavioral sensitization. This might well explain the seemingly spontaneous and epileptiform outbursts of vegetative and neuromuscular activity exhibited by many of these patients. It is an interesting hypothesis that there might be some mechanism of long-term potentiation, possibly mediated by vasopressin, which is known for its consolidating activity in conditioned behavior (Kovacs et al. 1987) and its neurophysiological activity (Urban 1987).

A list of signs and symptoms of the psychophysiological anxiety syndrome is shown in Table 7-1. This has proven useful for a thorough history taking and for recognition of anxiety. In addition, the clinician must inquire for classic PTSD symptoms.

Vegetative and psychomotor symptoms of exhaustion and/or depression frequently occur in chronic PTSD, superimposed on the anxiety symptoms. The physiological symptoms of depression, such as those listed in Table 7-2, have not been thoroughly studied. Seligman's model of learned helplessness

Table 7-1. Signs and symptoms of the psychophysiological anxiety syndrome

Neuropsychological	*Neuromuscular*	*Respiratory*
Dizziness	Paresthesia	Breathlessness
Change of consciousness	Tremor	Irregular breathing
Depersonalization	Tetany	Sighs
Derealization	Bruxism	Breath-holding spells
Blurred vision	Temporomandibular pain	Hyperventilation
Pupillodilation	Tension headache	
	Fibromyalgia	*Various*
Circulatory	Intercostal muscle pains	Urge to urinate
Pounding heart	Sudden exhaustion	Erections, ejaculations
Irregular beats	Muscle weakness	Piloerection
Tachycardia		Perspiration
Angina of the chest	*Digestive*	Skin exanthema
Pallor	Difficulty swallowing	Acute fever
	Esophageal spasms	
	Bloating and belching	*On examination*
	Nausea/vomiting	Fearful eyes
	Abdominal pains	Sharp blood pressure
	Acute diarrhea	changes
		Ischemic electrocardio-
		graphic changes
		Leucocytosis
		Hypokalemia

Table 7-2. Physiological and subjective bodily changes associated with depression

Change of circadian rhythm with early awakening
Decreased motor performance
Coldness
Pain
Disturbed food intake and body weight regulation
Loss of libido; impotence, anorgasmia
Dry mouth
Anhydrosis, asteatosis of the skin
Constipation
Low blood pressure and orthostatic hypotension

(Seligman 1975) may be a way of understanding in biologic terms depression in PTSD, although its psychological interpretation has elicited some controversy (Glazer and Weiss 1976). It is not clear either whether the syndrome of exhaustion in chronic PTSD is biologically identical to the vital depression in the older psychiatric nomenclature.

Somatic Diseases

Diseases with evident organic damage are of major concern in the medical treatment of World War II survivors, including "classic" psychosomatic diseases, chronic degenerative diseases, infections and their aftermath, and the neoplasms, as listed in Table 7-3. It has proven extremely difficult to analyze the influence of wartime factors on physical morbidity and mortality. Selection of the fittest in order to survive the extreme terrors and hardships of political and ideologic persecution has influenced the outcome noted in epidemiologic surveys. The problems with such studies are illustrated by investigations addressing the delayed effects of the military draft on mortality (Hearst et al. 1986). The Norwegian study by Ettinger and Strom (1981) clearly showed increased morbidity in all main diagnostic categories and increased mortality in a distinct number of diseases, some of them unexpected by their nature or by the latency time elapsed to manifest themselves.

Behavioral-Somatic Interactions

Interactions between behavioral and organic factors constitute a very important source of complications. With regard to psychological problems, patients with PTSD often have major difficulties in adhering to advice concerning diet, life-style, and medications. The availability of food often has a profound emotional significance for them. This may impair metabolic control in diabetes, or it may facilitate obesity, although anorexia is also occa-

Table 7-3. Frequently occurring somatic diseases in World War II survivors

Circulatory	*Various*
Hypertension	Polyneuropathy
Arteriosclerosis	Diffuse brain damage
Myocardial infarction	Tropical nutritional amblyopia
Aortic aneurysm	Degenerative joint disease
Cerebrovascular accidents	Osteoporosis
Cardiomyopathy	Parasitic infections: strongyloidiasis
Skin	*Gastrointestinal*
Pruritus	Peptic ulcer
Dyshydrotic eczema	Diverticular disease
Urticaria	Polyps and carcinoma
Neurodermatitis	Alcoholic liver disease
Psoriasis	Pancreatitis
Lichen planus	
Alopecia	
Pulmonary	
Tuberculosis	
Pneumonia	
Chronic obstructive lung disease	
Emphysema	
Bronchial carcinoma	

sionally seen. Drug therapy constitutes a problem of its own. Abuse or refusal or antianxiety or antidepressive medication is common, and it should be noted that sometimes the same happens with medical therapy. A number of patients seem to be emotionally dependent on drugs prescribed years before, which may have become useless because of side effects or have become outdated or even counterproductive. To persuade such patients to accept a change of treatment requires considerable psychological skills on the part of the physician. Placebo use of vitamins, homeopathics, or drugs of disputed pharmacologic activity is a common occurrence. The above-mentioned difficulties warrant great caution in the use of medications, which furthermore reinforce somatization of emotional problems and make patients less amenable for other appropriate therapies, whether medical or psychological.

Heavy smoking and drinking are well-known problems in PTSD patients. Alcohol is often used as self-medication against anxiety. It frequently results in episodical drinking, which occasionally may be treated successfully with psychopharmacologic therapy. Persistent chronic alcoholism also occurs and is at least as difficult to treat as in any other patient. The medical consequences of alcohol and tobacco addiction are well known and are an extensive source of medical care in chronic PTSD patients. Addiction to psychoactive drugs appears to be related to cultural factors; heroin or cocaine abuse are rare in World War II victims, but they are frequently reported in Vietnam veterans.

Accident proneness and suicidal behavior also influence medical and surgical morbidity and mortality. The same is true for hypochondriasis as well as other somatoform problems and the psychophysiological anxiety syndrome. These occasionally lead to unjustified operations giving rise to iatrogenic morbidity or also to doctors' delay in making correct diagnoses of intercurrent medical illness. On the other hand, PTSD patients' mistrust of doctors or their self-reproach and survival guilt may also cause postponement in their seeking of medical treatment.

PATIENT MANAGEMENT

A common feature of people who have been subjected to trauma caused by others is their strongly increased level of suspicion. When they apply for help, the medical situation itself induces feelings of anxiety and helplessness. It is important, therefore, to anticipate these reactions by changing the way patients are received and handled in the doctor's office or hospital. Patients should be given the feeling that they are in control of their situation. During physical examinations, avoid small rooms and do not shut the door when leaving the patient alone. Be aware in diagnostic procedures of their sensitivity to needles, electrodes, or the computed tomography scan tunnel. Admission to hospital wards may provoke acute anxiety and even flashbacks and nightmares as patients may be reminded of the hospital barracks of concentration camps, where they were at the mercy of Nazi doctors murdering patients with experimental injections and other procedures. Also, operations and general anesthesia may induce loss of control, acute anxiety, and even delirium with aggressive motor behavior. Acting-out or obsessive-compulsive behavior may challenge a doctor's ability to help because of negative countertransference even in situations of serious somatic disease. Countertransference reactions are often based on feelings of inadequacy to respond to the underlying existential cry for help and to heal the incurable psychic wounds. Also, the implicit or overt reference to past severe traumatization by Nazi doctors may generate some defensive behavior in the physician.

These phenomena require substantial adaptations in patient management in terms of psychological training and support of medical staff. There is an above-average need of time per patient, empathy, and frustration tolerance. Historical and cultural knowledge are also valuable to understand the meaning of the thematic references made by the victims. Understanding of these psychosomatic aspects is necessary to comprehend the complex clinical presentation of survivors of war and violence.

References

Abrahams, VC Hilton SM: Active muscle vasodilation and its relation to the "flight and fight reactions" in the conscious animal. Proc Physiol Soc, Nov 1957. J Physiol (Lond) 140:16P–17P, 1958

Askevold F: The war sailor syndrome. Dan Med Bull 27:220–223, 1980

Baird JT, MacDonald D: Survey of optic atrophy in Hong Kong prisoners of war after ten years. Canadian Service Medical Journal 12:185–193, 1956

Cannon WB: Bodily Changes in Pain, Hunger, Fear and Rage: An Account of Recent Researches Into the Function of Emotional Excitement, 2nd Edition. Boston, MA, Charles T Branford Co, 1953

Dekking HM: Tropical nutritional amblyopia ("camp eyes"). Ophthalmology 113:65–92, 1947

DeVito JL, Smith OA: Afferent projections to the hypothalamic area controlling emotional responses (HACER). Brain Res 252:213–226, 1982

Ebbesen P: Experimental studies of premature aging. Dan Med Bull 27:248–250, 1980

Eliasson S, Folkow B, Lindgren P, et al: Activation of sympathetic vasodilator nerves to the skeletal muscles in the cat by hypothalamic stimulation. Acta Physiol Scand 27:18–37, 1953

Ettinger L, Strom A: New investigations on the mortality and morbidity of Norwegian ex-concentration camp prisoners. Isr J Psychiatry Relat Sci 18:173–195, 1981

Federici A, Rizzo A, Cevese A: Role of the autonomic nervous system in the control of heart rate and blood pressure in the defense reaction in conscious dogs. J Auton Nerv Syst 12:333–345, 1985

Glazer HI, Weiss JM: Long-term interference effect: an alternative to "learned helplessness." J Exp Psychol [Anim Behav] 2:202–213, 1976

Hearst N, Newman TB, Hulley SB: Delayed effects of the military draft on mortality: a randomized natural experiment. N Engl J Med 314:620–624, 1986

Herberg HJ: Premature senility in former prisoners of war, in Later Effects of Imprisonment and Deportation (international conference organized by the World Veterans Federation). The Hague, The Netherlands, 1961, pp 113–114

Hess WR, Brugger M: Das subkortikale Zentrum der affektiven Abwehrreaktion. Helvetica Physiologica and Pharmacologia Acta 1:33–52, 1943

Hilton SM, Redfern WS: A search for brain stem cell groups integrating the defense reaction in the rat. J Physiol (Lond) 378:213–228, 1986

Hilton, SM, Zbrozyna AW: Amygdaloid region for defense reactions and its efferent pathway to the brain stem. J Physiol (Lond) 1165:160–173, 1963

Iwata J, Chida K, LeDoux JE: Cardiovascular responses elicited by stimulation of neurons in the central amygdaloid nucleus in awake but not anesthetized rats resemble conditioned emotional responses. Brain Res 418:183–188, 1987

Jacobs EC: Oculo-oro-genital syndrome: a deficiency disease. Ann Intern Med 35:1049–1054, 1951

Kolb LC: The post traumatic stress disorders of combat: a subgroup with a conditioned emotional response. Milit Med 149:237–243, 1984

Kovacs GL, Szabo G, Sarnyai Z, et al: Neurohypophyseal hormones and behavior. Prog Brain Res 72:109–118, 1987

Krell R: Survivors of childhood experiences in Japanese concentration camps (letter). Am J Psychiatry 145:383–384, 1988

Kuilman J: Kampduizeligheid. [Concentration camp vertigo]. Ned Tijdschr Geneeskd 90:1000–1003, 1946

McKell TE, Sullivan AJ: The hyperventilation syndrome in gastroenterology. Gastroenterology 9:6–16, 1947

Moore DF: Nutritional retrobulbar neuritis followed by partial optic atrophy. Lancet 2:1225–1227, 1937

Paul O: DaCosta's syndrome or neurocirculatory asthenia. Br Heart J 58:306–315, 1987

Schenck EG: Voralterung als Folge exogener Einflusse auf eine endogene Bereitschaft. Therapie der Gegenwart 116:446–470, 1977

Schnitker MA, Mattmann PE, Bliss TL, et al: A clinical study of malnutrition in Japanese prisoners of war. Ann Intern Med 35:69–98, 1951

Seligman MEP: Helplessness: On Depression Development and Death. San Francisco, WH Freeman, 1975

Smith OA, Hohimer AR, Astley CA, et al: Renal and hindlimb vascular control during acute emotion in the baboon. Am J Physiol 236:R198–205, 1979

Smith OA, Astley CA, DeVito JL, et al: Functional analysis of hypothalamic control of the cardiovascular responses accompanying emotional behavior. Federation Proceedings 39:2487–2494, 1980

Stebbins WC, Smith OA: Cardiovascular concomitants of the conditioned emotional response in the monkey. Science 144:881–883, 1964

Stock G, Schlor KH, Heidt H, et al: Psychomotor behavior and cardiovascular patterns during stimulation of the amygdala. Pflugers Arch 376:177–184, 1978

Syndrome X (editorial). Lancet 2:1247–1248, 1987

Thygesen P, Hermann K, Willanger R: Concentration camp survivors in Denmark: persecution, disease, disability, compensation: a 23-year follow-up: a survey of the long-term effects of severe environmental stress. Dan Med Bull 17:65–108, 1970

Urban IJA: Brain vasopressin: from electrophysiological effects to neurophysiological function. Prog Brain Res 72:163–172, 1987

van der Kolk BA: Psychological Trauma. Washington, DC, American Psychiatric Press, 1987

Van Dyke C, Zilberg NJ, McKinnon JA: Posttraumatic stress disorder: a thirty year delay in a World War II veteran. Am J Psychiatry 142:1070–1073, 1985

Yardley CP, Hilton SM: The hypothalamic and brainstem areas from which the cardiovascular and behavioural components of the defence reaction are elicited in the rat. J Auton Nerv Syst 15:227–244, 1986

Chapter 8

Headache and Posttraumatic Stress Disorder

Seymour Diamond, M.D.
Michael Maliszewski, Ph.D.

P osttraumatic stress disorder (PTSD) is a formal psychiatric diagnostic category that has generated much interest in recent years. Generally defined, this disorder consists of a set of symptoms that emerge from an event or set of events that are on a level that exceeds the normal range of human experience. Examples of such events might include rape, assault, disasters (natural or caused by humans), or military combat experience. Responses to such experiences would include terror, fear, and marked helplessness. The individual who has undergone such trauma generally reexperiences the event in the form of recurrent, intensive recollections or dreams that are vividly relived as if they were occurring at that time. A quality of numbness may be experienced after the trauma. This may lead to a sense of estrangement from other people, "emotional blunting," and lack of interest in previously rewarding activities. Associated features noted in the literature include anxiety, depression, instability, vertigo, headaches, concentration difficulties, phobic reactions, poor memory, and poor sleep patterns.

At the present time, several criticisms have been raised concerning this diagnostic category (Brett and Ostroff 1985; Green et al. 1985; Horowitz et al. 1987), with the role of the stressor event in the disorder being one of several concerns raised (Breslau and Davis 1987; Lindy et al. 1987). Regarding the latter point, the issue of stressor and diagnostic specificity (i.e., linking the stressor event to a unique clinical syndrome) is an important point. Much data evaluating psychopathological and psychophysiological responses to trauma or disaster were collected prior to the formal concept of PTSD as a psychiatric disorder (Lindy et al. 1987). Furthermore, there is much overlap of PTSD diagnosis with other psychiatric disorders, such as depressive, anxiety, panic, and substance abuse disorders (Behar 1984; Burstein 1984; Sierles et al. 1986). Differential diagnosis of these conditions has not been adequately elucidated, nor has the impact of trauma (and its repetitive "psychic" reenactment) sufficiently been investigated. To this end, literature exploring the relationship of PTSD to chronic pain syndromes (Benedikt and Kolb 1986; Muse 1985) reveals the need for careful diagnosis and a detailed medical and social history to overcome the lack of recognition of PTSD in pain patients who have not responded to traditional treatment regimens. Given our earlier identification of headache as one symptomatic feature of PTSD, it is important to place the relation of PTSD to headache in proper perspective, identifying specific diagnostic considerations as well as treatment strategies observed to alleviate PTSD-related headache disorders. To explore this topic, several areas will be reviewed, including 1) a brief conceptualization of headache disorders, 2) the relationship of pain and headache to PTSD, and 3) PTSD and headache classification: diagnosis and treatment considerations. It will be noted from the beginning that a high proportion of PTSD patients present pain complaints; however, at pain centers, headache associated with PTSD is rare.

CURRENT CONCEPTUALIZATION OF HEADACHE DISORDERS

Formal classification of headache disorders dates back to 1962 with the outline prepared by the National Institute of Neurological Disease and Blindness (Ad Hoc Committee on Classification of Headache 1962). Over the years, a number of revisions have followed, with the most recent taxonomy developed by the Headache Classification Committee of the International Headache Society (HCCIHC) (1988). While an outline of some 13 distinct categories of headache classifications is included, migraine, tension-type, and cluster headaches are the most common of these pain disorders. Migraine is an idiopathic, recurring headache disorder that is unilateral or bilateral in location, of moderate to severe intensity, generally aggravated by physical exertion, and has accompanying features such as nausea, photosensitivity, and sonophobia. Tension-type headache (more commonly known as muscle contraction or "tension" headache) is a recurrent episodic headache, often bilateral in location, of mild to moderate intensity, experienced as constricting or tightening in quality and devoid of nausea and vomiting. Cluster headache consists of unilateral throbbing pain, lasting 15 minutes to 3 hours in duration, often occurring several times daily, generally located behind or around the eye, appearing abruptly with no forewarning and more frequently observed to occur among men.

It should be noted that all of these three headache conditions may be associated with physical and/or psychological trauma, although a distinct and separate designation of headache associated with head trauma appears in the International Headache Society classification. To this end, the three major types of headaches may be observed to develop as posttraumatic headaches in close temporal relation to a specific head trauma and receive a diagnosis that is "posttraumatic" in nature (e.g., meet criteria for posttraumatic headache and present as a migraine headache), although symptoms associated with cluster headache are a relatively rare occurrence. In such cases, the trauma has generally been viewed by headache specialists as primarily physical in nature. Psychological sequelae stemming from such injury may include the following: impaired memory, reduced attention span, heightened distractability, inattentiveness, decreased ability to concentrate, forgetfulness, difficulty in turning from one subject to another, deterioration of synthetic thinking, inability to grasp new or abstract concepts, lack of spontaneity accompanied by apathy and loss of initiative, reduced motivation, decreased libido, irritability, emotional response, mood swings, anxiety, depression, and frustration (Speed 1986). However, likely as a result of the essentially strict medical classification of headache disorder, psychological features and causes of headache pain have been less rigorously investigated than physical symptoms and characteristics.

PAIN, HEADACHE, AND POSTTRAUMATIC STRESS DISORDER

Paralleling the secondary role accorded to psychological aspects of headache disorders, formal inclusion of PTSD diagnosis within pain syndromes has been a relatively recent development (Benedikt and Kolb 1986; Muse 1985; Rapaport 1987). Although the prevalence of this syndrome among the chronic pain population may be quite significant (Muse 1985), only two studies have been conducted thus far that specifically explore the pain-PTSD relationship.

A study conducted by Benedikt and Kolb (1986) found that 22 (10%) of 225 male patients referred to a Veterans Administration pain clinic for treatment of chronic pain were later diagnosed as having PTSD. Prior to their admission to this setting, none of the patients had ever received a diagnosis of PTSD. The pain in all cases was localized at the site of a former injury, primarily at the extremities (45%) and back (41%). The pain had begun at the time of the injury, persisting until treatment was received at the pain center. According to the authors, prior treatments for the pain at other settings (inclusive of medication, surgery, and electrical stimulation) were unsuccessful due to a failure of patients to recognize the psychological aspects of their pain complaints. Psychiatric features were also observed to comprise these patients' medical histories: 38% had a previous history of alcohol abuse, 13% had a history of drug abuse, 27% had attempted suicide (23% having an ongoing history of suicidal ideation), 14% had received antipsychotic medication, and 40% had received anxiolytic medication.

A study by Wolf et al. (1988) explored the presence of pain in 22 Vietnam veteran inpatients who had received a diagnosis of PTSD. Seventeen patients (77%) presented some form of pain, including backache, headache, pain at site of injuries received in Vietnam, neck pain, and pain in joints of upper and lower extremities. Of those men experiencing headache pain, the majority had tension headaches. A few patients presented migraine headaches. No cluster headaches were observed. It might be added that a variety of dermatologic complaints (45%) and allergy-related symptoms (36%) were also reported. The authors noted that treatment approaches to PTSD of these men necessitated addressing not only the somatic complaints and trauma of Vietnam, but also those psychological aspects that preceded their wartime experiences.

Thus chronic pain, including headache, appears to be a frequent complaint among PTSD patients. On the other hand, data on the frequency of PTSD-headache syndromes at specialized, medically oriented (as opposed to psychiatric) settings are not presently available, but it may be speculated that the occurrence is either quite rare or has, hitherto, been unrecognized among the large number of individuals who receive treatment annually for headaches nationwide (estimated at more than 42,000,000) (Diamond and Furlong 1977). We can say that, at the Diamond Clinic, the PTSD-headache syndrome is actually quite rare. We present below one case that will serve to illustrate treatment approaches.

Case History

Mr. G, a 40-year-old married Caucasian male, was admitted to our inpatient headache unit presenting a 10-year history of headache pain. A diagnosis of this disorder revealed the presence of migraine without aura and tension-type headaches. The migraine headache was reported as occurring bilaterally in the frontal and temporal regions and could radiate to the top of the head. It could occur once or twice a week, lasting for 1 to 12 hours. Associated symptoms included nausea, vomiting, photophobia, tearing of the left eye, and numbness/tingling on the left side of the face. The tension-type headache could occur in the occipital region and was accompanied by a constant tightness in the musculature of the neck. The pain was described as a sharp, throbbing pain. Onset of the headache was reported to have occurred in 1978 without any precipitating factors, although whiplash was sustained in a motor vehicle accident in 1980, which further aggravated his condition. Pain was also observed to increase during periods of hard exercise or cold weather. A history of headache was reported in the family, including the mother, two aunts, an uncle, and a sister.

Mr. G was a Vietnam veteran who had experienced the trauma of the war in 1966 and 1967. He had been admitted to a Veterans Administration hospital in his home state for treatment of PTSD in 1977. Symptoms that he had exhibited at this time included recurrent nightmares of traumatic events, depression, irritability, instability, emotional lability, memory difficulties, low frustration tolerance, sleeping difficulties, and occasional headaches. Although he had not been placed on any medications, he was involved in a variety of group therapy treatment programs involving counseling and visual media presentations to adjust to unresolved issues related to combat activities. Mr. G reported he had benefited from treatment at this facility and was presently involved in helping other Vietnam veterans deal with the emotional problems stemming from the war. However, while some of his symptoms tended to decrease (e.g., recurrent nightmares), other features such as headache, depression, low frustration tolerance, and irritability had increased.

On admission to our inpatient headache unit, a variety of medical tests were performed, including skull X-ray, electroencephalogram with and without sedation, complete blood count, sequential multichannel autoanalyzer chemistry (SMAC), urinalysis, thyroid testing, and electrocardiogram. All findings were within normal limits except for cholesterol of 262. A chest X-ray was negative except for discoid atelectasis. A magnetic resonance image of the brain revealed mild asymmetry of the lateral ventricles, which was diagnosed as probably representing a normal variation. Treatment was initiated with propranolol 80 mg/day and amitriptyline 50 hs and a single injection of dexamethasone 16 mg. Promazine HCl 100 mg im was provided every 4 to 6 hours prn during the first 48 hours of hospitalization. Because the patient complained of persistent severe headache and insomnia, the propranolol and amitriptyline dosages were slowly increased, and stabilized at 160 mg and 100 mg, respectively. Mr. G was instructed on the indications, usage, and possible side effects of the medications. While medications were being administered, the patient also received physical therapy consisting of deep heat and massage to the neck and shoulders, daily biofeedback (electromyogram and temperature training), and exposure to stress management and relaxation techniques. He was also placed on a tyramine-free diet.

A psychological evaluation of this patient revealed a number of personality features commonly found among migraine/tension-type headache sufferers, such as being emotional, perfectionistic, and conscientious; encapsulating feelings; having a strong need for control; and concentrating at tasks for long periods of time through to completion without interruption. Specific stressors identified by the patient included work in the field of engineering in a high-pressure environment, a 16-year-old daughter having adjustment problems in the home setting, a father who was dying of a kidney ailment, and a sister who was undergoing a number of operations for medical problems. Alcoholism was described as present on the paternal side of the family, including the father and several uncles and cousins. The patient had been married for 22 years. He reported that the strain of managing his headache pain had been severe and had so interfered with his relationship with his wife that he had recently separated from the family. In addition to prescribing medication to cope with the pain, psychological intervention strategies focused on providing Mr. G with nonpharmacologic treatment approaches to assist with pain management (breathing exercises, monitoring of arousal levels, visualization techniques), stress management techniques in the work setting, improving communication skills at home with his wife and daughter, providing the patient with specific information on psychological factors contributing to his headache (e.g., traumatic memories of Vietnam War experience), and increasing his awareness of earlier life experiences that likely played an influential role in contributing to the onset and course of his headache pain. Mr. G was discharged from the hospital in improved condition. Outpatient therapy for pain and stress management, continuation of the tyramine-free diet, and a set of progressive relaxation exercises to be practiced daily were also prescribed.

Posttraumatic Stress Disorder and Headache Classifications

We have presented a case illustrating a multidimensional approach to the treatment of headache disorders with a PTSD component. Historically, "posttraumatic" disorders in the fields of medicine and psychiatry and in the area of headache have been examined from different directions. Headache specialists have largely concentrated on the aftermath of physical injury, whereas functional symptoms have dominated psychiatric nosology. Our case example has presented features associated with both components. To this end, in their review of this topic, Adler et al. (1987) noted that many symptoms of postphysical trauma can appear as either psychological or organic in nature. Such symptoms include: headache; lightheadedness or dizziness; trouble concentrating and maintaining vigilance; fatigue; insomnia; memory and attention problems; anxiety; emotional lability; trouble with crisp, novel, or creative thought; decreased sensitivity to social norms; and occasional tearfulness or depression. Headache researchers have recognized for some time the psychological aftermath of suffering from physical posttraumatic headaches, despite formal classification accentuating the medical components. However, they have yet to elucidate clearly the apparent continuum of headache-PTSD disorder, discerning diagnostically when a PTSD diagnosis is warranted for a headache disorder (particularly those stemming from head trauma where physical trauma is evident). We have attempted a first step in this direction and wish to stress the importance of treating the patient as a unique individual. Complying with a strict medical diagnosis of the headache and treatment of the condition in a traditional medical and purely pharmacologic fashion or addressing the problem as purely a psychological disorder is not sufficient or clinically appropriate.

We hope that future studies along this multidimensional approach to the headache patient may provide a better understanding of the origins of the pain and its holistic treatment.

References

Ad Hoc Committee on Classification of Headache: Classification of headache. JAMA 179:717–718, 1962

Adler CS, Adler SM, Packard RC: Psychiatric Aspects of Headache. Baltimore, MD, Williams & Wilkins, 1987

Behar D: Confirmation of concurrent illnesses in post-traumatic stress disorders (letter). Am J Psychiatry 141:310, 1984

Benedikt RA, Kolb LC: Preliminary findings on chronic pain and post-traumatic stress disorder. Am J Psychiatry 143:908–910, 1986

Breslau N, Davis GC: Post-traumatic stress disorder: the stressor criterion. J Nerv Ment Dis 175:255–264, 1987

Brett EA, Ostroff R: Imaging and post-traumatic stress disorder: an overview. Am J Psychiatry 142:417–424, 1985

Burstein A: Post-traumatic stress disorder found in general hospital psychiatric consultations. Am J Psychiatry 141:723–724, 1984

Diamond S, Furlong WB: More Than Two Aspirin. New York, Avon, 1977

Green BL, Lindy JD, Grace MC: Post-traumatic stress disorder: toward DSM-IV. J Nerv Ment Dis 173:406–411, 1985

Headache Classification Committee of the International Headache Society: Classification and diagnostic criteria for headache disorder, cranial neuralgias and facial pain. Cephalalgia 8 (suppl 7):9–96, 1988

Horowitz MJ, Weiss DS, Marmar C: Commentary: diagnosis of post-traumatic stress disorder. J Nerv Ment Dis 175:267–268, 1987

Lindy JD, Green BL, Grace MC: Commentary: the stressor criteria and post-traumatic stress disorder. J Nerv Ment Dis 175:269–272, 1987

Muse M: Stress-related post-traumatic chronic pain syndrome: criteria for diagnosis and preliminary report on prevalence. Pain 23:295–300, 1985

Rapaport MH: Chronic pain and post-traumatic stress disorder (letter). Am J Psychiatry 144:120, 1987

Sierles FS, Chen JJ, Messing ML, et al: Concurrent psychiatric illness in non-Hispanic outpatients diagnosed as having post-traumatic stress disorder. J Nerv Ment Dis 174:171–173, 1986

Speed WG: Post-traumatic headache, in The Practicing Physician's Approach to Headache. Edited by Diamond S. Baltimore, MD, Williams & Wilkins, 1986, pp 113–119

Wolf ME, Alavi A, Mosnaim AD: Pain, dermatological and allergic conditions in post-traumatic stress disorder. Research Communications in Psychology, Psychiatry and Behavior 13:237–240, 1988

Chapter 9

Back to the Front: Recurrent Exposure to Combat Stress and Reactivation of Posttraumatic Stress Disorder

Zahava Solomon, Ph.D.

Combat stress has long been implicated in the genesis of psychiatric disorders (Grinker and Spiegel 1945; Stauffer et al. 1949; Titchner and Ross 1974). During battle, the most common consequence of exposure to combat stress is labeled combat stress reaction (CSR), also known as battle shock, combat exhaustion, or war neurosis. CSR occurs when a soldier is unable to marshal effective coping mechanisms to deal with threatening stimuli in combat. It encompasses a variety of labile and polymorphous, behavioral, cognitive, and affective manifestations that result in impaired functioning. CSR manifestations include restlessness, psychomotoric deficiencies, withdrawal, increased sympathetic activity, stuttering, confusion, nausea, vomiting, and paranoid responses (Grinker and Spiegel 1945). The critical feature is that the soldier ceases to function militarily and acts in a manner that endangers both himself and his fellow combatants (Kormos 1978). CSR, now viewed as an acute form of posttraumatic stress disorder (PTSD), is a highly prevalent disturbance among combatants; however, not everyone who is exposed to combat stress develops CSR. To date, the search for risk factors has encompassed a host of personality, social, and environmental variables (Cooperman 1973; Glass 1957; Levav et al. 1977).

Combat-related posttraumatic reactions can have implications for a person's functioning, in both military life and civilian life. Militarily, the injury can impair a person's physical and mental fitness, reduce motivation, and undermine reliability in security assignments and ability to participate in future wars. In civilian life, posttraumatic reactions may be expressed in functional disturbances in the family and at work (Solomon 1988). Posttraumatic reactions also have somatic components. By exacerbating subclinical disease processes, they can trigger the clinical onset of such disorders as diabetes, ulcer, and hypertension. By disrupting biologic homeostasis and weakening the immune system, posttraumatic reactions can also impair the body's natural immunity to organic diseases (Titchner 1987). According to DSM-III (American Psychiatric Association 1980), PTSD can also take the form of a chronic or delayed onset psychiatric entity. The present report focuses on a unique variety of this disorder: reactivated combat-related PTSD. Here, a previous PTSD episode is reexperienced following renewed exposure to similar combat stress.

Reactivation of a stress disorder may occur following a variety of stressful life events. In an extensive review, Silver and Wortman (1980) contend that traumatic experiences often render the afflicted individual vulnerable in the face of future adversity. Even in situations where the person appears to have overcome the trauma, heightened vulnerability may ensue. Lindeman (1944) noted that a previous unresolved grief reaction may be reactivated when the bereaved is reminded of his or her loss. The precipitating factor for the delayed reaction may be a deliberate recall of circumstances surrounding the death, or it may be a spontaneous occurrence in the patient's life. Similar observations were made by Weiner et al. (1975) regarding recurrent anniversary grief reactions that were generated by stimuli reminiscent of the original loss.

Whereas the phenomenon of reactivated traumatic reaction has been documented in both the military and civilian realms, empirical research concerning recurrent combat-related PTSD is rather limited. Christenson et al. (1981) suggested that losses associated with the aging process, including parental loss, children leaving home, impending retirement, and increased medical illnesses, serve as triggers that can reactivate and unmask latent war-related PTSDs. They found latent PTSD symptoms, such as nightmares about World War II, that were dormant in their patients for many years. This observation is in line with an earlier 20-year follow-up study of World War II veterans in which war-related PTSD symptoms became evident during the aging process (Archibald and Tuddenham 1965).

To our knowledge, reactivation of combat-related posttraumatic stress reactions following exposure to a new combat experience is a clinical subgroup that has not been systematically studied. The unfortunate reality of Israel's military situation, where armed conflicts with neighboring countries result in the same soldiers fighting in war after war, presents a unique opportunity for the study of reactivated combat-related PTSD. Even when spared the rigors of actual combat, Israeli men are regularly exposed to military stimuli that serve as continuous reminders of their combat experience.

In this chapter, I examine a number of aspects related to the reactivation of combat-related PTSD following participation in war. First, I focus on a preliminary issue concerning the effects of recurrent exposure to combat stress and examine whether and how the exposure to prior combat stress influences the likelihood of acute PTSD (CSR episode) in a new war. Second, I examine the clinical aspects of reactivated combat-related PTSD. Third, I attempt to compare the long-term clinical features of reactivated PTSD with those of a single combat-related acute PTSD episode and to identify correlates of reactivation.

RECURRENT EXPOSURE TO BATTLE STRESS

The role of recurrent exposure to combat in the development of a CSR episode (acute PTSD) has received little attention, but intuitively it would seem to be an important factor. Studies of psychological and somatic responses to stress offer a number of competing, often contradictory, views on the effects of repeated exposure to stress.

According to the vulnerability perspective, repeated exposure to stressful life events is a risk factor. With each stressful life event, available coping resources may decrease, thereby increasing vulnerability to physical and emotional disturbances (Coleman et al. 1980; McGrath 1970; Selye 1976; Vinokur and Selzer 1975).

The stress inoculation perspective considers repeated stress to have a positive effect on health and coping, since it operates as an "immunizer." According to this view, multiple stressful experiences contribute to the development of useful coping styles. Each similar stressful episode increases familiarity, leading to a decrease in the amount of perceived stress and thereby enabling more successful adaptation (Epstein 1983; Janis 1971; Keinan 1979).

The stress resolution perspective suggests that it is the outcome of the earlier stressful experience, and not the mere exposure to stressful events, that determines its impact on subsequent coping and health. According to Block and Zautra (1981), successful resolution of a stressful episode promotes a feeling of well-being and improved coping resources, whereas an unsuccessful outcome leads to increased distress and a decrease in coping resources. This view is well documented by research on the sense of mastery and learned helplessness. This body of research indicates that mastery develops when individuals are exposed to stressful events that they succeed in overcoming by their own reactions (Bandura 1977), and that helplessness is aroused when the opposite occurs and repeated attempts at coping result in failure (Maier and Seligman 1976).

To assess the various implications of prior combat experience on mental health during war, we conducted a study (Solomon et al. 1987b) of Israeli soldiers who participated in the 1982 Lebanon War. The sample consisted of two groups. The first group, the CSR group, encompassed 382 frontline Israeli soldiers who fought in the Lebanon War and were diagnosed as having CSRs. These soldiers showed neither indication of serious physical injury nor existence of other combat-related disorders, such as brief reactive psychosis or factitious disorder.

The second group, the control group, consisted of 334 soldiers who had participated in the same frontline combat units as the CSR soldiers, but had not shown symptoms of CSR. For each CSR casualty, a matched control subject was randomly selected from among eligible soldiers who had similar sociodemographic features, including age, education, military rank, and assignment.

The results of this study on CSR rates as a function of prior combat experience and previous CSR reveal that CSR rates in the 1982 Lebanon War were highest among soldiers with prior CSR episode (66%), lowest among soldiers without prior CSR (44%), and in between (57%) for soldiers without prior combat experience. These findings clearly indicate that prior exposure to combat may be either detrimental or beneficial for dealing with future combat-related stress, depending on the earlier psychological outcome. This implies that the apparently contradictory vulnerability and stress inoculation perspectives may both be valid and integrated in the stress resolution hypothesis. The findings that soldiers without prior CSR are less vulnerable to subsequent combat stress than soldiers with no prior combat experience support the stress inoculation hypothesis. At the same time, these results also indicate that soldiers with a prior CSR episode are more vulnerable to subsequent combat stress than their peers who had no combat experience, and this can be interpreted as supporting the vulnerability hypothesis.

Several explanations may account for the predominance of the stress resolution hypothesis in predicting future reactions in battle. Bandura's (1977) explanation is that stressful experiences help a person to define his or her expectations of subsequent adversities. Such expectations have consistently been documented as influencing future behavior by creating an ongoing and self-perpetuating process. Bandura's suggestions thus lead to two possible scenarios. In the first, an individual who coped well in a previous situation involving a particular stressor develops a sense of mastery and enhanced self-efficacy, and believes that he or she is well equipped to deal with subsequent similar stressors. In the second scenario, a person who dealt unsuccessfully with a stressful situation may come to doubt his or her ability to cope with subsequent similar stressors, which increases vulnerability.

In additional studies of rates of reactivated CSR and number of previous combat experiences, it was found that the risk for reactivated CSR increased linearly with the number of previous war experiences: 57% in subjects who participated in one war, 67% in soldiers who participated in two wars, and 83% in those who fought in three wars.

CLINICAL TYPOLOGY OF REACTIVATED COMBAT-RELATED PTSD

Having demonstrated that prior CSR episodes reduce soldiers' resilience to combat stress and increase the likelihood of a recurrent CSR episode in a new war, we proceeded to analyze the particular clinical nature and course of these reactivated episodes. For this purpose, we focused only on CSR casualties of the Lebanon War who had a prior CSR episode, sampling 35 soldiers. Four groups of combat-related reactivated PTSD were identified: uncomplicated reactivation, specific sensitivity, moderate generalized sensitivity, and severe generalized sensitivity.

The uncomplicated reactivation group consisted of 23% of the sample. Individuals in this category demonstrated the highest degree of functioning, after having suffered earlier CSR; they consisted of psychiatric casualties of the 1973 Yom Kippur War who had either been diagnosed as CSR or had suffered from immediate CSR that was undiagnosed. These soldiers subsequently appeared to be fully recovered from the effects of their traumatic experiences and were symptom free during the interval between the 1973 Yom Kippur War and the 1982 Lebanon War. However, when these men were called up for the 1982 Lebanon War, and were once again exposed to battle, they developed full-blown PTSD.

The specific sensitivity group, comprising 50% of the sample, consisted of soldiers who, despite persistent minor and diffuse symptoms resulting from the 1973 war, succeeded in their overall professional and social functioning in the period between 1973 and 1982. They even did well on their occasional uneventful periods of reserve duty despite a rise in their tension level. However, these men displayed a selective sensitization in that specific stimuli reminiscent of the original trauma retained the power to reactivate the disorder. When these men encountered stimuli directly related to the original trauma, there was an increase in the intensity of their PTSD symptomatology. Specifically, during these individuals' reserve services, stress-related symptoms such as hypersensitivity to noise and weapons, reduced appetite, diarrhea, and increased anxiety were often exhibited.

These distressing symptoms, however, did not severely impede performance. These soldiers had invested much effort in coping, predominantly employing the mechanisms of denial and repression to enable adequate functioning. The heightened sensitivity to specific military stimuli, however, became more apparent when war broke out in 1982. Most of the soldiers in this group reacted with high anticipatory anxiety on receiving the order to report for active service. After they were mobilized and entered the military domain, exacerbation of stress residuals occurred in response to relatively minor events that reminded the soldiers of their earlier traumatic experiences. In many of these instances, reactivation of a residual or subclinical PTSD to a full-blown PTSD syndrome occurred without any intense combat exposure.

The moderate generalized sensitivity group included 9% of the sample. During the 1973–1982 interim period, the soldiers in this group had recurrent acute stress reactions to stimuli that were only remotely related or apparently unrelated to the original trauma. As a consequence, they experienced intense suffering, which permeated many areas of their lives. PTSD symptomatology was apparent in civilian settings, and it increased in military life. These men reported sleep disturbances, nightmares, anxiety, irritability, and uncontrollable outbursts of anger during the 1973–1982 period.

Soldiers in this group tried in various ways to avoid dealing with situations that aroused acute anxiety, but were not successful in reducing their distress. To attain mastery, some of them used phobic avoidance mechanisms; others reported using alcohol and drugs. Yet despite their failure to reduce anxiety and distress, these men continued to serve in the reserves.

When the orders for the 1982 Lebanon War were issued, intense anticipatory anxiety was present, severely hindering their capacity as combatants. Some of them reacted with a full-blown syndrome following minor military stimuli and were discharged prior to entering the battlefield.

The severe generalized sensitivity group comprised 18% of the sample. The soldiers in this group were still listed on the army active roster, despite their total inability to function in any setting. They were called up for combat, but did not actually take part in the 1982 Lebanon War. The arrival of the call-up note in the mail worsened their condition to such an extent that they experienced more or less immediate, severe, paralyzing anticipatory anxiety.

In general, our findings show that exacerbation of residual PTSD symptoms ensued in the majority (77%) of the psychiatric casualties. This finding is consistent with earlier clinical evidence suggesting that traumatic experiences scar the traumatized individuals, weakening their resilience to future stress (Silver and Wortman 1980).

Our findings also suggest that repeated sporadic exposure to military stimuli, and especially periods of service in the reserves, tend to reactivate latent memories of traumatic war experiences, delaying recovery from PTSD. It may be that the damages of early traumatic experiences were not adequately treated. More than half of the subjects in the sample who were in treatment dropped out. In the majority of the cases, there was evidence that soldiers went to great lengths to keep their mental state from their commanders, comrades, friends, and even close family. Their symptoms were accompanied by feelings of shame, guilt, and lowered self-esteem. In the Israeli reality, where the army is highly valued as a necessary means for survival, male identity is strongly linked to military functioning. It seems that social norms and the resultant reluctance to admit problems and seek professional help may be possible intervening variables that increase the risk for reactivation of combat-related PTSD among Israeli soldiers.

COURSE AND CORRELATES OF REACTIVATED PTSD

The current section presents findings of studies that examine the clinical picture and various correlates of reactivated PTSD (Solomon and Mikulincer 1987; Solomon et al. 1987a, 1987c).

The Clinical Picture of Reactivated PTSD

To assess whether there is a distinct clinical picture that differentiates first-time PTSD from reactivated PTSD, we compared two different groups of Israeli soldiers 3 years after the 1982 Lebanon War. The first-time PTSD group consisted of 39 soldiers who had sustained acute PTSD episodes during the Lebanon War and who had also served in the army during the Yom Kippur War without having been identified as experiencing an episode of PTSD at that time. The second group, labeled reactivated PTSD, consisted of 55 soldiers who had suffered from acute PTSD during the Lebanon War and had previously experienced a PTSD episode during the Yom Kippur War.

The comparisons between first-time PTSD and reactivated PTSD indicate that the victims of the latter are distinguished from those of the former by their more severe pathology, which manifests itself in a significantly higher rate of intrusive war-related thoughts and imagery, a higher overall level of psychiatric distress, and a diminished level of social functioning. With regard to cognitive aspects, the reactivation group revealed a significantly different attitude toward PTSD when compared to the one-time PTSD group: the former tended to regard PTSD casualties as victims of circumstances beyond their control, to a greater extent than the latter group. As a result, the reactivation cases advocated a more lenient and generous approach on the part of army authorities toward PTSD casualties. Milgram (1986) reported that external attribution of responsibility for PTSD is functional; it absolves the soldiers of guilt and inferiority feelings, which tend to impede recovery. It was also noted that the reactivation group reported feeling significantly more anticipatory anxiety with regard to participation in another war, and their expectation of being able to cope positively was lower.

Correlates of Reactivated PTSD

It is of considerable importance to determine which variable can predict reactivation of PTSD. Despite the importance of this matter, the existing research, which is based on retrospective reporting by the soldiers themselves, does not allow the drawing of firm conclusions. Furthermore, difficulties are encountered, since measures used to investigate these issues may be outcome variables rather than predictor items.

Two groups of soldiers were studied: 55 soldiers who experienced PTSD in 1973 and 1982, the reactivated PTSD group, and 30 soldiers who experienced PTSD in 1973 and participated in the 1982 war without experiencing another PTSD episode, the Yom Kippur PTSD group. The two groups were compared on four sets of variables. The first set included sociodemographic characteristics of each group, such as age, marital status, economic status, educational level, and living conditions. Results yielded no significant differences between the reactivated PTSD group and the Yom Kippur PTSD group.

The second set of variables included measures related to the soldiers' assessment of their experiences during the Lebanon War. Subjects received a questionnaire tapping thoughts about possible errors made by officials during the war, the justness of the war, opinions about the efficacy of the Israel Defense Forces and readiness and competence of the unit, and feelings of loneliness, guilt, loss, and threat in combat. Results showed that soldiers in the reactivated PTSD group reported more loneliness, guilt, and threat during battle, and reported having thought that the unit was less prepared for the war than did soldiers in the Yom Kippur PTSD group.

The third set of variables included some measures related to personality traits. Results yielded no significant differences between the two groups of soldiers in the personality measures analyzed.

The fourth set of measures included three questionnaires related to social resources. Results showed that subjects in the reactivated PTSD group felt more lonely, perceived less social support, and viewed their family as less cohesive and expressive and more conflictive than did soldiers in the Yom Kippur PTSD group. The picture that emerges is that the sociodemographic and personality variables that were analyzed did not differentiate the groups, whereas the soldiers' feelings during the war and their social resources differed. This would suggest that soldiers who experienced a second episode of PTSD are blaming not themselves for the PTSD, but the situation in which they found themselves, and their social and familial network. This can be seen as an amplification of the tendency of PTSD casualties to attribute their problems to external factors (Mikulincer and Solomon 1988).

Conclusions

The conclusion that emerges from the current work is that individuals who have experienced an episode of PTSD are at significantly greater risk for another episode of PTSD than are individuals who participated in battle without any observed psychological breakdown. Furthermore, it appears that soldiers who experience a reactivated episode of PTSD manifest a more severe clinical syndrome than soldiers who experience a single episode. Even though some soldiers may participate in battle after a PTSD episode without further breakdown, the debilitating effects of the early episode are still detectable a decade later. We thus conclude that exposure to trauma has very long-term consequences, symptoms being persistent and prolonged. We hope we can live in a world in which we all are at peace with one another.

References

American Psychiatric Association: Diagnostic and Statistical Manual of Mental Disorders, 3rd Edition. Washington, DC, American Psychiatric Association, 1980

Archibald HC, Tuddenham RD: Persistent stress reaction after combat. Arch Gen Psychiatry 12:475–481, 1965

Bandura A: Self efficacy: toward a unifying theory of behavioral change. Psychol Rev 84:191–215, 1977

Block M, Zautra A: Satisfaction and distress in a community: a test of the effects of life events. Am J Community Psychol 9:165–180, 1981

Christenson RM, Walker JL, Ross DR: Reactivation of traumatic conflict. Am J Psychiatry 138:984–985, 1981

Coleman JC, Butcher JN, Carson RC: Abnormal Psychology and Modern Life. Glenview, IL, Scott Foresman, 1980

Cooperman RR: Adjustment in the military (technical report). Jerusalem, Department of Behavioral Science, Israel Defense Forces, 1973

Epstein S: Natural healing processes of the mind: graded stress inoculation as an inherent coping mechanism, in Stress Reduction and Prevention. Edited by Meichenbaum D, Yarenko ME. New York, Plenum, 1983

Glass AJ: Observations upon the epidemiology of mental illness in troops during warfare. Abstract of paper presented at the Symposium of Preventive and Social Psychiatry, Washington, DC, Walter Reed Army Institute of Research, 1957

Grinker RR, Spiegel JP: Men Under Stress. Philadelphia, PA, Blakiston, 1945

Janis IL: Stress and Frustration. New York, Harcourt Brace Jovanovich, 1971

Keinan G: The effects of personality and training variables on the experiences of stress and quality of performance in situations where physical integrity is threatened. Unpublished doctoral dissertation, Tel Aviv University, Tel Aviv, Israel, 1979

Kormos HR: The nature of combat stress, in Stress Disorders Among Vietnam Veterans. Edited by Figley CP. New York, Brunner/Mazel, 1978, pp 3–22

Levav I, Greenfeld H, Baruch E: Psychiatric combat reactions during the Yom-Kippur War. Am J Psychiatry 136:637–641, 1977

Lindeman E: Symptomatology and management of acute grief. Am J Psychiatry 101:141–148, 1944

Maier SF, Seligman ME: Learned helplessness: theory and evidence. J Exp Psychol [Gen] 105:3–46, 1976

McGrath JE: Setting measures and theses: an integrative review of some research of social and psychological factors in stress, in Social and Psychological Factors in Stress. Edited by McGrath JE. New York, Holt Rinehart & Winston, 1970

Mikulincer M, Solomon Z: Attributional style and combat-related PTSD: a prospective study. J Abnorm Psychol 97:308–313, 1988

Milgram N: An attributional analysis of war-related stress: modes of coping and helping, in Stress and Coping in Time of War: Generalizations from the Israeli Experience. Edited by Milgram N. New York, Brunner/Mazel, 1986

Selye H: The Stress of Life. New York, McGraw-Hill, 1976

Silver RL, Wortman CB: Coping with undesirable life events, in Human Helplessness. Edited by Garber J, Seligman ME. New York, Academic, 1980, pp 279–340

Solomon Z: The effect of combat related post-traumatic stress disorder on the family. Psychiatry 51:323–329, 1988

Solomon Z, Mikulincer M: Combat stress reaction, PTSD and social adjustment: a study of Israeli veterans. J Nerv Ment Dis 175:277–285, 1987

Solomon Z, Garb R, Bleich A, et al: Reactivation of combat-related post traumatic stress disorder. Am J Psychiatry 144:51–55, 1987a

Solomon Z, Mikulincer M, Jakob BR: Exposure to recurrent stress: combat stress reaction among Israeli soldiers in the 1982 Lebanon War. Psychol Med 17:433–440, 1987b

Solomon Z, Oppenheimer D, Mikulincer J, et al: Course and correlates of reactivated combat stress reaction, in Reactivation of Combat Stress Reaction (Technical Report). Edited by Solomon Z. Medical Corps, Research Branch, Department of Mental Health, Israel Defense Forces, 1987c

Solomon Z, Weisenberg M, Schwarzwald J, et al: Posttraumatic stress disorder among frontline soldiers with combat stress reactions: the 1982 Israeli experience. Am J Psychiatry 144:448–454, 1987d

Stauffer SA, Lumsdaine AA, Lumsdaine MH, et al: The American Soldier, Vol 3: Combat and Its Aftermath. Princeton, NJ, Princeton University Press, 1949

Titchner JL: Post-traumatic decline: a consequence of unresolved destructive drives, in Trauma and Its Wake, Vol 2. Edited by Figley CR. New York, Brunner/Mazel, 1987

Titchner JL, Ross WO: Acute or chronic stress as determinant of behavior, character, and neurosis, in Adult Clinical Psychiatry: American Handbook of Psychiatry, 2nd Edition. Edited by Arieti S, Brody EB. New York, Basic Books, 1974

Vinokur A, Selzer M: Desirable versus undesirable life events: their relationship to stress and mental distress. J Pers Soc Psychol 32:329–337, 1975

Weiner A, Gerber I, Battim D, et al: The process and phenomenology of bereavement, in Bereavement: Its Psychological Aspects. Edited by Schoenberg B, New York, Columbia University Press, 1975

Chapter 10

Individual and Community Responses to an Aircraft Disaster

Kathleen Wright, Ph.D.
Robert J. Ursano, M.D.
Larry Ingraham, Ph.D.
Paul Bartone, Ph.D.

After refueling at Gander, Newfoundland, on December 12, 1985, a chartered airliner crashed on takeoff, exploding on impact. The snowy crash site cut a long swath of burned and broken trees and debris, with bodies, equipment, and personal possessions strewn over a wide area. The crash killed 248 United States Army soldiers who were members of the elite 101st Airborne Division stationed at Ft. Campbell, Kentucky. The soldiers were returning home after 6 months of United Nations peace-keeping duty in the Sinai desert. The families of these soldiers awaited their homecoming in a festive mood, anticipating the Christmas holidays.

Word of the tragedy reached the headquarters at Ft. Campbell shortly after the crash. During the next frantic hours, the flight manifest was confirmed, and families were told to assemble at the brigade gymnasium for an announcement. In the meantime, Department of Defense personnel worked with Canadian officials to recover the bodies at Gander. The crash site was gridded and searched, and bodies, equipment, and possessions collected. The remains were initially stored in an airport hangar at Gander awaiting transport to Dover Air Force Base, Delaware. Over the next 2 months, Dover became the site of an extensive mortuary and body identification operation.

The Army dead represented one-third of the battalion deployed to the Sinai. Approximately one-third of those who died were married and maintained their homes at Ft. Campbell, a tightly knit military community straddling the border of Kentucky and Tennessee. The crash shattered the community, leaving 36 children without fathers. It was the United States Army's deadliest single-incident tragedy in peacetime and the worst aviation disaster ever to occur on Canadian soil. Individuals and groups affected by the Gander air crash extended far beyond the borders of Ft. Campbell. This extensive community included bereaved families, survivors in the affected military units, Gander crash site workers, Dover Air Force Base mortuary personnel, and a multitude of service providers, both professional and volunteer, who came in contact with the dead and the bereaved.

In the immediate aftermath of the tragedy, a small research team was sent to Ft. Campbell and Dover Air Force Base to observe and document responses of affected individuals and groups (Wright et al. 1987). This participant observation study continued over the 6-month period following the air crash. This chapter is a condensation of team observations made during that period. It provides an overview of responses observed in several groups of primary participants in the aftermath of the disaster.

BODY HANDLERS

The literature indicates that those engaged in body handling and recovery are at increased risk of posttraumatic stress disorder (PTSD) during the 6 months following exposure (Frazer and Taylor 1982; Harris 1986; Hersheiser and Quarantelli 1976; Jones 1985; Raphael 1984; Ursano et al. 1988). Some reports indicated as high as 40% of body handlers experienced signs and symptoms of distress. The lack of immediate, acute reactions cannot be interpreted as "all is well," however, because chronic and delayed stress reactions have also been reported. The overall conclusion is that those participating in body recovery and identification should have their level of exposure monitored and be followed to identify any medical and/or psychiatric complications that may result from such exposure.

The Gander body identification, a complicated process because of the destruction and burning in the crash, occurred at Dover Air Force Base, the largest port mortuary in the Department of Defense. The final identification was made 9.5 weeks after the air crash. More than 1,000 individuals participated directly in the process. These included approximately 120 professionals, primarily from the Armed Forces Institute of Pathology, augmented by medical and graves registration personnel from various Army installations and by logistical support experts from different Air Force bases. More than 400 individuals from Dover Air Force Base assisted in the identification process, many as body handlers. The majority of these were enlisted male volunteers. Their job was to help move the remains from one station to another in the mortuary identification process. The body handler served as an escort for the dead, ensuring that records, personal effects, and body parts were not lost as the identification proceeded.

The majority of the dead were airlifted from the Gander crash site to Dover during a 3-day period, although body parts continued to be recovered and transported over the initial weeks following the crash. The sheer number of bodies and their mutilated and burned condition resulted in an extremely complex and lengthy identification process requiring intense hours of work over the course of months by those at the mortuary. Only the first few bodies arrived intact; the rest arrived as body parts, complicating the identification process. The condition of the bodies also contributed significantly to the stress, especially for the volunteer participants. Some went into the mortuary, took one look, and left. Others lasted several days. The majority were able to escort a body through the entire identification process.

The mortuary was organized into a series of stations. At the initial stations, personal effects retrieved at the crash site were carefully sorted and tagged for return to the dead soldier's family. Work areas in this location were congested and hectic. In the adjacent and enormous inner room of the mortuary, bodies and body parts waited in long rows prior to autopsy. At the stations in the inner room, body parts were cataloged, and fingerprinting, X-rays, and dental examinations were performed. The atmosphere in this room was subdued. There was little conversation. Professionals as well as volunteers were exhausted, ashen, and silent. The volunteers remained with their escorted body during the examination and autopsy procedures. Nearly all volunteers experienced these stations as the most stressful. After the bodies were identified, volunteers escorted them through the mortuary stations where the remains were dressed in service uniforms and laid in caskets. The caskets were then sealed, crated, and shipped home to the family.

In addition to the exposure stress of burned and mutilated bodies, the participants frequently reported a personal identification with the dead soldiers and a tendency to think "it could have been me." The body postures of the dead often included an arm across the head or a facial expression that was easily interpreted as terror. A story circulated that black soot found in the trachea of an autopsied body meant that a soldier had survived the aircraft explosion and died in the ensuing fire. The horror, difficulty, and sheer exhaustion involved in the mortuary work resulted in emotional and behavioral changes for many of the participants. Anxiety reactions, zombie-like behaviors (e.g., blank stares, flattened affect, slowed movements, minimal speech), angry irritability, increased alcohol intake, and appetite and sleep disturbances were common. Both seasoned professionals and first-time volunteers experienced these reactions. Even those well trained or experienced were deeply affected by the magnitude of so many dead bodies in one room.

A team of medical and graves registration personnel from Ft. Bragg was deployed to Dover Air Force Base and to Gander to help identify the bodies. At Dover, this team included technicians who X-rayed the remains for dental and full-body data comparisons, and graves registration specialists responsible for photographing the bodies and collecting and cataloging the personal effects of the dead. At the Gander crash site, these individuals, often on hands and knees in the mud and melting snow, performed an exhaustive search of the extensive area strewn with body parts, wreckage, and debris from the exploded aircraft. National media coverage surrounding the crash added a sense of urgency to the recovery and identification process. The team often worked more than 16 hours a day in an effort to complete the work as soon as possible.

Twenty members of this team who worked 7 days under these conditions participated in a psychological debriefing program to evaluate and treat symptoms of PTSD. Debriefing is the process of collecting from a group the cognitive history of their experience. The goal of debriefing is to collect information to enable all involved to develop an accurate overview of the entire experience. Thus debriefing provides the opportunity to enlarge one's cognitive framework and also receive education about the normal responses to tragedies (Dunning 1988; Mitchell 1986). The soldiers who participated in this debriefing had two patterns of symptoms in response to the stress of body handling: 1) intrusive psychological reexperiencing of events associated with their exposure to body recovery and identification; and/or 2) diminished responsiveness to their current environment, with increased tendencies to seek isolation by avoiding family and friends (Garrigan 1987).

Garrigan (1987) summarized the intrusive pattern of symptoms:

> Often, common everyday experiences would evoke the intrusion. For example, a dental X-ray technician reported seeing skulls when he saw the teeth of smiling people. A young lieutenant could not enter a local fast food establishment because the smell of burning food elicited a vomiting response. Some intrusions did not require an external stimulus. Soldiers reported seeing bodies when they closed their eyes. Their dream content consisted of nightmarish horror shows where zombie-like bodies were coming to kill the dreamer. One soldier reported seeing himself in a dream where he searched through human body parts and found his own ID tag.
>
> The most striking characteristic of those experiencing intrusive phenomena was their personal identification with the suffering of the victims and their families. During the time they worked with the bodies at Gander and Dover, and as they discussed their experiences through the process of debriefing, they reported wondering about the kind of life the victim had led, the effects of the death on the victim's family and friends, and whether the victim had suffered much in dying. This group reported that they had not minded the long hours of work on-site because, ironically, they wanted to get the victims home for Christmas. (p. 8)

In the avoidance pattern, soldiers tended to deny that the experience had any personal impact, avoided discussion about what they had done, and avoided other soldiers who had been with them at Gander or Dover. Garrigan (1987) reported that the most striking characteristic about this group was their matter-of-fact, emotionally flat manner of discussing their experiences. He also noted that soldiers in this group tended to demonstrate increased disciplinary and/or substance abuse problems after their return from Dover, possibly a dysfunctional expression of anxiety and tension. Garrigan concluded that the intensity of the symptoms in this team had resulted from the pressure to complete the body recovery and identification as quickly as possible. Limited resources and overdedication had led to overwork and overexposure. Significantly, the psychological debriefing occurred several weeks after the exposure. Although little attention has been given to debriefing as a form of primary prevention (Williams et al. 1988), clinical experience suggests that earlier intervention might have been helpful in reducing symptom frequency and intensity.

The principles of preventive psychiatry indicate a number of interventions that may be useful for individuals and communities exposed to mass casualties. A prework briefing and orientation for body handlers should be mandatory to explain the body-handling task, to discuss normal responses to such tragedies and to the handling of bodies, and to provide the opportunity to decline participation without prejudice. Psychological debriefing of leaders, participants, and their support teams should be conducted as soon as possible after the work is completed. One of the goals of this debriefing is that, before returning to family and friends, participants should know that experiences such as nightmares, intrusive thoughts, and feelings of anger, fear, or empty numbness are normal and expected following exposure to a disaster. Participants should receive education about how to handle symptoms, how to respond to questions asked by families and friends, and how to contact an appropriate referral source if symptoms persist. Debriefing-rap groups should be available over the next 6 months for those who wish to talk. Spouses should also be encouraged to attend informational meetings to learn more about the participants' experiences so they can aid the natural recovery process.

Body handlers themselves should have limited exposure times, with frequent periods of respite, preferably at rest areas away from the immediate site. Records should be kept of those who participate in the body-handling experience—for how long and what they did. To monitor health, each participant's psychological well-being and available social supports should be assessed before, during, and at follow-up. Supervisors must be alert to body handlers who need a break, *despite* their wish to keep working. This may be indicated by anxiety reactions, inappropriate affect, withdrawal, blank stares, or "zombie-like" behaviors. Prebriefings for supervisors should emphasize their responsibility and the stress inherent in the supervisor's role under these conditions. Supervisors often tend to get overly involved in "doing" rather than monitoring in such settings and may neglect their own sleep requirements. The same mental health support recommended for participants should also be provided to supervisors. They are exposed to similar experiences, as well as to increased organizational demands and pressures. Individuals trained in the human responses to death and tragedy (e.g., mental health workers, hospital staff, chaplains, and family services workers) should be available and actively involved at a disaster site. Their visibility in the community and at the mortuary is critical. Being available at the office or clinic will not reach those involved in body handling who are unlikely to use typical mental health referral channels.

Appropriate recognition and commendations should be given by groups and communities to recognize those who help in such difficult tasks. Several months after the initial events, a reunion of volunteers may allow further debriefing and strengthen social supports within this group. Newspaper coverage can ensure that the community knows what its members are doing and can provide information on normal reactions to tragedy. At the end of each newspaper article, a contact person or agency can be mentioned so that participants may receive help if they have difficulties. Community health care personnel, particularly family practice physicians and medical person- nel in emergency rooms, should be alert to patients presenting with somatic complaints that may represent the effects of the stress of such work. Com- munity mental health teams should be adequately trained to offer counseling and support to all those involved in the body identification process. Educa- tion of the community should emphasize that recovery from the stress of a disaster and/or body handling is normal and expected, but may take months rather than days.

Grief Leadership

Loneliness at the top is never more evident among senior leaders than in times of organizational tragedy. This is frequently so because of senior leaders' age, accumulated experience, position, and ongoing leadership responsibilities. In their organizations they are simultaneously the principal mourners, orchestrators of solemn ceremonies, and symbols that life must go on. Several leaders in the Ft. Campbell community assumed key roles in the mourning process following the Gander air crash. For example, at the planned homecoming in the gymnasium where families were awaiting the soldiers, the brigade commander made emotion-laden announcements about the crash, assuring families that information would be passed on to the community as soon as it became available. He focused on the importance of not being alone in grief and empathized with those who had lost friends and family. His capacity to express his own grief helped both families and troops to do the same. Those assembled in the gymnasium that morning were able to respond to him, and subsequently to one another.

The presidential memorial service 4 days later was another significant example of grief leadership. Here, the division commander emphasized the importance of the President "sharing our sorrow" and joined the President in greeting each of the bereaved family members and expressing condolences. The President underscored that he represented the American people and that he had come to mourn with the community because the nation was grieving as well. He and the First Lady then proceeded to talk to and touch each of the family members and many of the task force soldiers gathered at the memorial service. The division memorial service, which occurred several days later, involved the entire Ft. Campbell community, including adjacent townspeople. At this service, the division commander remembered each "Fallen Eagle" by having his or her name, rank, and home state read, followed by a cannonshot. Finally, a number of months later, a service commemorated the burial of the last victim. Here, the division commander directed a 1-minute sounding of the post sirens, followed by a 2-minute silent tribute honoring the 248 soldiers who died in the air crash.

The expression of openly shared grief should be encouraged by leaders, emphasizing the normality and necessity for grieving. The use of social and family support systems can be stressed as avenues for sharing the pain of loss and as a means to avoid isolation in one's grief. The affirmation that bereavement is a painful process requiring time to heal can be asserted by leaders as a way to refocus thinking toward the future. Senior leaders must also reserve time for physical exercise, sleep, and other restorative activities, both during a disaster and in its aftermath, to maximize their own effective functioning over this stressful period. In addition, reaching outside the organization to good friends is important, even though senior leaders are reluctant to share their anguish. Useful information and reassurance may be provided by the temporary assignment of a consultant, mental health professional, or chaplain, adequately trained to offer consultation to senior leaders in mass casualty situations. Expert consultation may prove particularly useful for leaders dealing with their family members. They may have difficulty sharing what they have heard, seen, and felt, and their families in turn may be reluctant to participate in the leader's obvious pain. Consultation may also help leaders disengage from a tragedy by setting limits on their involvement.

FAMILY ASSISTANCE WORKERS

More than 250 Survivor Assistance Officers were appointed by the military to help bereaved family members after the Gander air crash. Many were young officers performing this duty for the first time. They filled an unusual and ambiguous role as boundary-crossers between the military and civilian society, and as emissaries of good will under tragic circumstances. Questionnaire, interview, and observational data were collected from these officers at two time points in the year following the air disaster by members of the research team (Bartone et al. 1989). Results showed three major task areas associated with their role: administrative assistance, emotional support, and official representative ("ambassador"). Current military organizational guidance covers only the first area, that of providing practical assistance to families in administrative matters (e.g., arranging death benefits and military funerals, disposing of personal effects, and providing transportation for next of kin).

The second task, that of providing emotional or psychological support to grieving relatives, is not a part of most Survivor Assistance Officer training. Many officers associated with the Gander crash had little experience along these lines. Usually they received no special training or guidance and had difficulty obtaining useful information over the course of their duties. Evidence from civilian disasters (Raphael 1986), as well as data collected by this research team, indicates that those who provide emotional support to grieving relatives of disaster victims are at risk for a variety of stress-related health problems. Roles that are ambiguously defined and confusing in crisis situations may increase that risk, since the organization becomes an additional source of stress in an already difficult situation.

The third important task area, that of serving as an official representative or emissary for the army, is also not presently a part of Survivor Assistance Officer training. The officers assumed the role of peacemaker between the army and those families whose sons and daughters had taken up a military occupation and who now had to accept the permanent loss of those loved ones. Death is not expected to occur in a peacetime, job-oriented army. The officers struggled to reconcile families to this unexpected loss and tried to help them derive some meaning from it. To the extent that they succeeded in this effort, anger, resentment, and bitterness toward the army was avoided or diminished. Gander Survivor Assistance Officers reported that little or no guidance was available on how to proceed with this task. They operated largely on their own. To be effective, they developed relationships of trust with the widows and families to whom they were assigned. However, this also had its cost, since many officers reported extreme difficulty disengaging from families when their support duties were completed.

Four major areas of stress were identified by Survivor Assistance Officers: 1) the family's grief, 2) the army, 3) the slow body-identification process, and 4) the proximity to sudden, violent, horrible death. First, these officers dealt closely with grieving and distraught family members. Second, Survivor Assistance Officers provided the interface between the family and the army. They confronted the army's bureaucracies in trying to obtain accurate and relevant information for the family and attended to various practical matters of concern (e.g., funeral arrangements, transportation). Third, in cases such as the Gander crash where bodies are badly disfigured, the body identification process is slow, painful, and laborious. During this difficult period, the Survivor Assistance Officer was powerless to provide the family with what they wanted most—the body of their loved one for burial. Fourth, Survivor Assistance Officers were in close proximity to death through the personal belongings, family members, and records of the dead. Since an officer was assigned to the family of only one victim, it was easy to personalize the experience and to come to know the victim very well, albeit posthumously. Since they shared similar jobs and circumstances, a psychological identification with the victim was easily made, resulting in fears and concerns about one's own mortality.

Although the role of Survivor Assistance Officer may be relatively unique to the military, the tasks and stressors inherent in this assignment are comparable to civilian service providers who work with bereaved families in disaster situations. These include medical and rescue teams, police and fire fighters, chaplains, the Red Cross, and other community service agencies established to assist survivors. Such service providers have come increasingly to the attention of disaster researchers as hidden, neglected victims of traumatic events (Duckworth 1986; Jones 1985; McFarlane 1984; Raphael 1986). Their intense involvement with those directly affected victims such as the dead, injured, or bereaved, identifies them as a part of the disaster community, at increased risk for stress reactions in the aftermath.

MENTAL HEALTH PROFESSIONALS

Mental health professionals were not immune to feelings of shock, anguish, and grief after news of the Gander tragedy reached Ft. Campbell. Additionally, they had the formidable responsibility for organizing the postdisaster interventions required to cover a multitude of individuals and groups affected by the air crash. Initial staff expectations centered on the probability of being overwhelmed by stressed and bereaved families. Planning focused on organizing and staffing the clinic in preparation. However, consistent with civilian experience (Quarantelli 1985), this expected reaction never materialized, and staff planning shifted to extensive community outreach, including consultation, support, and education about grief. Offers of help and support poured into Ft. Campbell from other military installations in the first days following the tragedy. The offers were appreciated but generally not accepted because it was feared that the inclusion of those outside the immediate community might contribute to the confusion and uncertainty. The reaction of closing ranks and forming a protective barrier around the affected community is also consistent with observations in the civilian disaster literature (Raphael 1986). Extreme ambivalence is typically found toward off-site participants. There is a need for their support and for their augmentation of stressed and exhausted service provider resources. This is, however, combined with a fear that "outsiders" will assume control or serve only to make a bad situation worse.

Despite the pressure and anxiety of mounting an extensive and immediate outreach program, the tragedy provided an opportunity for the development of close working relationships among the mental health staff. Typical territorial boundaries in a multidisciplinary staff and between troop and hospital elements dissolved in the face of the pressing community needs. With the realization that bereaved families would not flood the service, a unified staff planned outreach. Mental health teams were deployed throughout the community and maintained contact with daily briefing and planning sessions during the initial response to the air crash. This response focused on preventive interventions. The teams were sent to high-risk settings: the brigade gymnasium, where families were awaiting the return of the service members; the hospital's general medical clinic to help with triage; and the newly established Family Assistance Center, with the primary function to assist bereaved families.

Radke (1987) described a three-phase plan directed to prevention and early supportive interventions. Particular attention was given to the families of the victims, the soldiers who were the victims' friends and comrades, and the service providers (e.g., Survival Assistance Officers, Family Assistance Staff, chaplains). The principal interventions included consultation-liaison, education, group therapy, and the identification and treatment of high-risk individuals. The phases of grief provided a framework for organizing different outreach interventions in the aftermath of the tragedy. Previously established lines of communication afforded a significant inroad into the community. Crisis is not a time in which one can beat new pathways into the community; the mental health teams discovered that they could go only where they had been before.

CONCLUSIONS

An important outcome of the research at Gander is the development of a conceptual model of human responses to tragedy. Present models do not adequately describe the complexity, duration, and spread of the effects of a disaster across a "global community." As a result of information gathered in the aftermath of Gander, the degree of complexity of present disaster communities is clearer. An adequate model, at the very least, must consider four factors: time, level, location, and groups at risk.

Time.   Reactions and appropriate and inappropriate responses vary across time. For example, a community leader or unit commander in tears can symbolize strength at first, but later on may be viewed as a weak leader. Memorial services are useful to a point, after which people find them wearing and no longer helpful.

Level.   Military and civilian tragedies involve individuals, groups, and formal organizations. Individuals may do well while small groups fall apart, or small groups may save the day when organizations and individuals fail. Conversely, in some instances it may be only the formal organization that holds individuals and groups together at a time of intense pain.

Location.   Natural disasters are frequently restricted to one locale. Conversely, military tragedies involve more than one community, often the nation, as a result of the nature of military operations and organizational structures. The Gander crash directly affected three different community sites: the crash site at Gander, Newfoundland; the mortuary operation at Dover Air Force Base; and the soldiers' home base at Ft. Campbell, Kentucky. Although these three sites were predominant, families and friends of the victims were located in many different communities throughout the nation. Military communities in general are constantly alert to the risk of death due to war, combat, relocation, or training exercises. In part because of this, the military community as a whole was also dramatically affected by these deaths at the Christmas season. Thus the potential for unseen and unsuspected stress reactions in widely dispersed areas is multiplied in military settings.

Groups at Risk.   Those likely to experience extended stress over time include bereaved families and close friends of victims; senior leaders; family assistance workers and casualty affairs personnel; volunteer workers at the disaster and mortuary sites; and other service providers who come into direct contact with bereaved families, the dead, or the disaster sites.

Overall, greater knowledge about individual and group responses to disaster is needed to help the victims of such events, and to prepare for the undesired, unexpected, but inevitable next tragedy.

REFERENCES

Bartone P, Ursano R, Wright K, et al: The impact of a military air disaster on the health of assistance workers: a prospective study. J Nerv Ment Dis 177:317–328, 1989

Duckworth DH: Psychological problems arising from disaster work. Stress Medicine 2:315–323, 1986

Dunning C: Intervention strategies for emergency workers, in Mental Health Response to Mass Emergencies: Theory and Practice. Edited by Lystad M. New York, Brunner/Mazel, 1988, pp 284–307

Frazer DCJ, Taylor AJW: The stress of post-disaster body handling and victim identification work. Human Stress 8:5–12, 1982

Garrigan JL: Post traumatic stress disorder in military disaster workers, in The Human Response to the Gander Military Air Disaster: A Summary Report (Division of Neuropsychiatry Report No 88–12). Washington, DC, Walter Reed Army Institute of Research, 1987, pp 7–8

Harris SL: The Impact of the Gander Military Air Crash on the RCMP (Royal Canadian Mounted Police). Edmonton, Alberta, Canada, Health Services Officer, RCMP "K" Division (PO Box 1774), 1986

Hersheiser MR, Quarantelli EL: The handling of the dead in a disaster. Omega— The Journal of Death and Dying 7:195–209, 1976

Jones DR: Secondary disaster victims: the emotional effects of recovering and identifying human remains. Am J Psychiatry 142:303–307, 1985

McFarlane AC: Ash Wednesday and the C.F.S. firefighters. Emergency Response 1:34–35, 1984

Mitchell JT: Critical incident stress management. Emergency Response 5:24–25, 1986

Quarantelli BB: An assessment of conflicting views on mental health: the consequences of traumatic events, in Trauma and Its Wake. Edited by Figley C. New York, Brunner/Mazel, 1985, pp 173–215

Radke A: The mental health response, in The Human Response to the Gander Military Air Disaster: A Summary Report (Division of Neuropsychiatry Report No 88–12). Washington, DC, Walter Reed Army Institute of Research, 1987, pp 32–36

Raphael B: Rescue workers: stress and their management. Emergency Response 1:27–30, 1984

Raphael B: When Disaster Strikes. New York, Basic Books, 1986

Ursano R, Ingraham L, Wright K, et al: Psychiatric responses to death and body handling. Paper presented at the 141st annual meeting of the American Psychiatric Association, Montreal, May 1988

Williams C, Solomon SD, Bartone P: Primary prevention in aircraft disasters: integrating research and theory. Am Psychol 43:730–739, 1988

Wright K (ed): The Human Response to the Gander Military Air Disaster: A Summary Report (Division of Neuropsychiatry Report No 88–12). Washington, DC, Walter Reed Army Institute of Research, 1987

Chapter 11

Analgesia: A New Dependent Variable for the Biological Study of Posttraumatic Stress Disorder

Roger K. Pitman, M.D.
Scott P. Orr, Ph.D.
Bessel A. van der Kolk, M.D.
Mark S. Greenberg, Ph.D.
James L. Meyerhoff, M.D.
Edward H. Mougey, M.S.

D espite its appellation, understanding of the psychiatric condition post-traumatic stress disorder (PTSD) has as yet benefited little from insights into the biology of the stress response obtained with experimental work with animals. In this chapter, we will present evidence suggesting that a well-recognized dependent variable in animal stress research—pain sensibility—may prove useful in characterizing the stress response in combat-related PTSD.

As currently defined in DSM-III-R (American Psychiatric Association 1987), PTSD consists of a combination of tonic and phasic features. The "tonic" features are those that the patient manifests all or most of the time and that constitute part of his or her baseline mental functioning. The "phasic" features are manifested only from time to time, especially when they are evoked by some salient environmental event. The DSM-III-R criteria divide PTSD symptoms into three major categories: intrusion, avoidance (or numbing), and arousal. Although patients may complain of the frequency and intensity of their nightmares, flashbacks, and intrusive recollections, intrusion symptoms are phasic rather than tonic. The final symptom belonging to the intrusion category, "intense psychological distress at exposure to events that symbolize or resemble an aspect of the traumatic event" (p. 250), suggests classical Pavlovian conditioning as a mechanism for phasic PTSD symptoms (Pitman 1988).

In contrast to the intrusion symptoms, the avoidance symptoms of PTSD are tonic. Diminished interest, numbing, and estrangement characterize the PTSD patient's baseline functioning. Avoidance of reminders of the traumatic event derives from the painful phasic recollections that the reminders trigger, suggesting operant conditioning as a likely mechanism behind PTSD's avoidance symptoms (Pitman 1988).

The third category of PTSD symptoms, arousal, comprises a mixture of tonic and phasic symptoms. Examples of tonic arousal symptoms include insomnia and hypervigilance; examples of phasic arousal symptoms include exaggerated startle response and "physiological reactivity upon exposure to events that symbolize or resemble an aspect of the traumatic event" (American Psychiatric Association 1987, p. 250). This last symptom has served as the conceptual basis for psychophysiological studies of PTSD.

Biological studies of the tonic aspects of PTSD have included a variety of autonomic, endocrinologic, and neuroregulatory dependent variables measured in a baseline or resting condition (Giller 1990). Biological studies of the

This work was supported in part by a Merit Review Grant and a Research Career Development Award (Dr. Pitman) from the Veterans Administration.

phasic aspects of PTSD are more challenging because, in addition to whatever dependent variables are employed, unless one is prepared to wait for phasic changes to occur spontaneously, one or more independent stimulus variables are required to elicit them. Depending on the nature of the stimuli employed in such designs, Pavlovian terminology refers to the resulting phasic changes as conditioned or (less frequently) unconditioned responses.

Phasic studies may be considered biological if either the independent or dependent variables are biological. With the notable exception of research employing a biochemical stimulus (i.e., sodium lactate) in the elicitation of flashbacks and panic anxiety in PTSD (Rainey et al. 1987), it is the dependent variables that have been biological in phasic PTSD studies, and these have generally been limited to autonomic variables. The independent variables have consisted of audiovisual presentations of various types of trauma-related stimuli. A robust literature now exists documenting phasic autonomic hyperreactivity to combat stimuli in PTSD (Orr 1990).

Information is needed regarding the endocrinological, neuroregulatory, and other unstudied biological aspects of phasic change in PTSD. However, the spotty occurrence of significant findings in endocrinological studies of non-PTSD anxiety disorders (Curtiss and Glitz 1988; Stokes 1985) suggests that finding reliable endocrinological responses in PTSD studies may prove difficult. Designs that call for active rather than passive responding on the part of the subject may be more likely to yield positive results (Meyerhoff et al. 1988). Curtiss and Glitz (1988) noted a "paucity of the robust endocrine stress responses that one might intuitively expect where behavioral evidences of stress and distress are so marked" (p. 142). The explanation for this observation may be that the most critical components of the stress response in humans occur within the central nervous system (CNS), not necessarily accompanied by peripheral endocrinological changes. A complex CNS stress response system has been described (Stewart 1985) that, although it employs as neurotransmitters and neuromodulators a number of the same chemicals that act as peripheral hormonal mediators of the stress response—for example, adrenocorticotropic hormone (ACTH), beta-endorphin, vasopressin (Amir et al. 1980)—can function independently of the periphery. This makes a noninvasive means of detecting activity in the CNS stress response system a desideratum in the study of PTSD.

One component of the stress response in experimental animals is stress-induced analgesia (SIA) mediated by endogenous opioids (Akil et al. 1986; Lewis 1986). (Non-opoid SIA also exists but may be less relevant to PTSD.) Opioid-mediated SIA is to a large extent a CNS process independent of peripheral hormonal secretion. Opioid-mediated SIA in animals has been characterized as "hormonal" or "neural," depending on whether intact pituitary or adrenal function is necessary for its appearance (Watkins and Mayer 1986). SIA induced by Pavlovian conditioned fear stimuli (Fanselow 1986), or by an intraspecific aggressive encounter with a dominant animal (Miczek et al. 1986; Rodgers and Hendrie 1983), is neural (Watkins and Mayer 1986). The central mediation of conditioned SIA is demonstrated by the observation that it is reversed (or blocked) by peripheral administration of the opiate antagonist naloxone, which crosses the blood-brain barrier, and by intracerebroventricular but not peripheral administration of the opiate antagonist quatenary naltrexone, which does not cross the blood-brain barrier (Calcagnetti et al. 1987). SIA has been suggested as an experimental animal phenomenon with possible relevance to human traumatic stress (van der Kolk et al. 1985). Parallels between combat-related PTSD and the circumstances in which neural SIA is found in experimental animals suggest that neural SIA could accompany phasic changes in PTSD. PTSD symptoms have been characterized as classically conditioned fear responses (Kolb 1984; Pitman 1988), and military combat is indisputably an intraspecific aggressive encounter.

To investigate the utility of analgesia as a measurement of phasic response in PTSD, we exposed PTSD and control Vietnam veterans to a combat-related stimulus and measured changes in pain sensibility. This study has been reported in detail elsewhere (Pitman et al., submitted for publication) and will only be summarized here. Subjects were drug-free Vietnam veterans, eight with PTSD and eight with no mental disorder, matched for age and extent of combat exposure. Each subject viewed a 14-minute neutral videotape segment, followed by a 15-minute combat videotape segment from the movie *Platoon*, followed by a 30-minute neutral videotape segment, on two occasions separated by approximately 2 weeks. In one session, the subject received intravenous placebo; in the other session, intravenous naloxone, in random order under double-blind conditions. Autonomic measures were collected during each videotape, and emotion self-report, pain assessment, and blood samples for hormonal assays were collected immediately following each videotape. Pain assessments were completed by asking subjects to rate on an unmarked visual analog scale (VAS) subjective intensity and unpleasantness of a heat source applied to the forearm at four standard temperatures—45° C, 47° C, 49° C, and 51° C—in random order. Of the two pain dimensions, intensity is a more reliable indicator of opiate activity than unpleasantness (Gracely et al. 1979). Each VAS rating was converted to a number on a 0- to 100-point scale. This pain assessment methodology was well tolerated by all subjects.

In the placebo condition, the PTSD subjects showed a 30% decrease in reported pain intensity ratings of standardized heat stimuli after the combat videotape. No decrease in pain ratings occurred in the PTSD subjects in the naloxone condition. The non-PTSD subjects showed no decrease in pain ratings in either drug condition. These results are consistent with the occurrence of phasic opioid-mediated stress-induced analgesia in PTSD. They also support the status of pain intensity rating as a "biological" dependent variable. In this chapter, the question of the utility of analgesia as a dependent variable for assessing phasic change in PTSD, in comparison to other variables, will be examined. Because naloxone was found to block the analgesia, the analysis here will be confined to the placebo session data.

For a variable to serve as a useful dependent measure of phasic change in PTSD in the design employed here: 1) it should change in the predicted direction in PTSD subjects after exposure to the combat-related stimulus, and 2) the magnitude of the change in PTSD subjects should be greater than in control subjects. Table 11–1 lists the pain, autonomic, hormonal, and emotion self-report variables employed in the study. To address how well

Table 11–1. Point biserial correlations of responses to combat videotape

	PTSD [a]	PTSD versus control [b]
Pain ratings		
Intensity	−0.64*	−0.61**
Unpleasantness	−0.29	−0.18
Autonomic		
Heart rate	0.76**	0.21
Skin conductance	0.55	0.22
Hormonal		
Norepinephrine	0.79**	−0.15 [c]
Epinephrine	−0.50 [c]	−0.22 [c]
Met-enkephalin	0.19 [c]	0.26
Beta-endorphin	−0.19 [c]	−0.12 [c]
ACTH	0.00	−0.38 [c]
Cortisol	0.14	−0.06 [c]
Emotion dimensions		
Arousal	0.79**	−0.15 [c]
Valence (pleasantness)	−0.88***	−0.51*
Dominance	0.75**	−0.25
Emotion states		
Happiness	0.79**	−0.25
Sadness	0.86**	0.20
Fear	0.87**	0.35
Surprise	0.73*	0.14
Anger	0.91***	0.45*
Disgust	0.87**	0.27
Guilt	0.77**	0.46*

Note. PTSD = posttraumatic stress disorder. ACTH = adrenocorticotropic hormone.
[a] Within group: 7 df. [b] Between groups: 14 df, except for hormonal measures, 13 df (blood samples could not be drawn in one control subject). [c] The correlation was not in the predicted direction.
* $P < .05$. ** $P < .01$. *** $P < .001$. (All one-tailed.)

each dependent variable met the first criterion above, the responses to the combat videotape (i.e., the first neutral videotape level versus the combat videotape level) of the PTSD subjects were examined by means of within-group point biserial correlations for that dependent variable (Cohen 1965). To address how well each dependent variable met the second criterion, the responses to the combat videotape of the PTSD versus control subjects were subjected to between-group point biserial correlations for that dependent variable.

The point biserial correlations are given in Table 11–1. As a group, the emotion self-report variables were better measures of the PTSD subjects' phasic change (response to the combat videotape) than were the biological variables. Among the latter, pain intensity rating was better than pain unpleasantness rating, but not as good as heart rate or norepinephrine. However, where the dependent variables were required to serve as measures of the difference in response to the combat videotape between PTSD and control subjects, a very different picture emerged. Here pain intensity rating served as a better PTSD measure than all the other variables, biological and self-report. Six of the eight PTSD, but only one of the control subjects, showed an analgesic response to the combat videotape. The only hormonal dependent variable that served as a useful measure of phasic change in the PTSD subjects (i.e., norepinephrine) was not useful in the PTSD versus control comparison; the control subjects showed a larger mean norepinephrine response to the combat videotape than did the PTSD subjects.

The finding that the development of analgesia after the combat videotape successfully differentiated the responses of the PTSD and control groups, while peripheral hormonal changes did not, is consistent with the proposition that central and peripheral components of the stress response systems do not play an equal and parallel role in the phasic changes that characterize PTSD. Rather, the two appear to be dissociated, with only the central changes manifest. The results obtained in this small-sample study clearly require replication. However, the findings suggest that measurement of pain intensity may add a valuable dimension to the biological study of phasic change in PTSD that is worthy of further investigation.

REFERENCES

Akil H, Young E, Walker JM, et al: The many possible roles of opioids and related peptides in stress-induced analgesia. Ann NY Acad Sci 467:140–153, 1986

American Psychiatric Association: Diagnostic and Statistical Manual of Mental Disorders, 3rd Edition, Revised. Washington, DC, American Psychiatric Association, 1987

Amir S, Brown ZW, Amit Z: The role of endorphins in stress: evidence and speculations. Neurosci Biobehav Rev 4:77–86, 1980

Calcagnetti DJ, Helmstetter FJ, Fanselow MS: Quaternary naltrexone reveals the central mediation of conditional opioid analgesia. Pharmacol Biochem Behav 27:1529–1531, 1987

Cohen J: Some statistical issues in psychological research, in Handbook of Clinical Psychology. Edited by Wolman BB. New York, McGraw-Hill, 1965, pp 95–121

Curtiss GC, Glitz DA: Neuroendocrine findings in anxiety disorders. Neurol Clin 6:131–146, 1988

Fanselow MS: Conditioned fear-induced opiate analgesia: a competing motivational state theory of stress analgesia. Ann NY Acad Sci 467:40–54, 1986

Giller EL Jr (ed): Biological Assessment and Treatment of Posttraumatic Stress Disorder. Washington, DC, American Psychiatric Press, 1990

Gracely RH, Dubner R, McGrath PA: Narcotic analgesia: fentanyl reduces the intensity but not the unpleasantness of painful tooth pulp sensations. Science 203:1261–1263, 1979

Kolb L: The posttraumatic stress disorders of combat: a subgroup with a conditional emotional response. Milit Med 149:237–243, 1984

Lewis JW: Multiple neurochemical and hormonal mechanisms of stress-induced analgesia. Ann NY Acad Sci 467:194–204, 1986

Meyerhoff JL, Oleshansky MA, Mougey EH: Psychologic stress increases plasma levels of prolactin, cortisol, and POMC-derived peptides in man. Psychosom Med 50:295–303, 1988

Miczek KA, Thompson ML, Shuster L: Analgesia following defeat in an aggressive encounter: development of tolerance and changes in opioid receptors. Ann NY Acad Sci 467:14–29, 1986

Orr SP: Psychophysiologic studies of posttraumatic stress disorder, in Biological Assessment and Treatment of Posttraumatic Stress Disorder. Edited by Giller EL Jr. Washington, DC, American Psychiatric Press, 1990, pp 135–157

Pitman RK: Post-traumatic stress disorder, conditioning, and network theory. Psychiatric Annals 18:182–189, 1988

Pitman RK, van der Kolk BA, Orr SP, et al: Naloxone-reversible stress-induced analgesia in post-traumatic stress disorder (submitted for publication)

Rainey JM Jr, Aleem A, Ortiz A, et al: A laboratory procedure for the induction of flashbacks. Am J Psychiatry 144:1317–1319, 1987

Rodgers RJ, Hendrie CA: Naloxone partially antagonizes post-encounter analgesia and enhances defensive responding in male rats exposed to attack from lactating conspecifics. Physiol Behav 30:775–780, 1983

Stewart JM: ACTH neurons, stress and behavior: a synthesis, in Neuroendocrine Correlates of Stress. Edited by McKerns KW, Pantic V. New York, Plenum, 1985, pp 239–268

Stokes PE: The neuroendocrinology of anxiety, in Anxiety and the Anxiety Disorders. Edited by Tuma AH, Maser J. Hillsdale, NJ, Erlbaum, 1985, pp 53–76 van der Kolk BA, Greenberg MS, Boyd H, et al: Inescapable shock, neurotransmitters and addition to trauma: towards a psychobiology of post traumatic stress. Biol Psychiatry 20:314–325, 1985

Watkins LR, Mayer DJ: Multiple endogenous opiate and non-opiate analgesia systems: evidence of their existence and clinical implications. Ann NY Acad Sci 467:273–299, 1986

Chapter 12

Platelet Adenylate Cyclase Activity as a Possible Biologic Marker for Posttraumatic Stress Disorder

Bernard Lerer, M.D.
Avraham Bleich, M.D.
Zahava Solomon, Ph.D.
Arik Shalev, M.D.
Richard P. Ebstein, Ph.D.

A lthough DSM-III-R (American Psychiatric Association 1987) has established a clearly defined set of criteria for the diagnosis of posttraumatic stress disorder (PTSD), the empirical validity of the syndrome has yet to be conclusively demonstrated. Comorbidity, particularly alcohol and other substance abuse, is frequently observed in conjunction with PTSD among veteran populations in the United States, and antisocial behavior is often reported (Sierles et al. 1983; Yager et al 1984). Furthermore, a clinical overlap with anxiety and depressive states is commonly encountered and is, to some extent, encompassed within the DSM-III-R criteria for PTSD. The reported, although not uniformly replicated (Lerer et al. 1987a; Shestatzky et al. 1988), efficacy of monoamine oxidase inhibitors (Davidson et al. 1987; Hogben and Cornfield 1981) and tricyclic antidepressants (Bleich et al. 1986; Falcon et al. 1985) in alleviating the symptoms of PTSD is a further complicating factor. Positive reports in this regard do not clarify whether improvement is in features specific to PTSD or in the anxiety and depressive symptoms, which are the natural targets of such agents.

Biologic markers are an important potential avenue for characterizing PTSD and for establishing whether the syndrome can indeed be regarded as an independent diagnostic entity. The term *biologic markers* refers in this context to biological features that are a replicable concomitant of the syndrome. Such markers should be differentiated according to whether they are "state" characteristics, which are present in association with the clinical syndrome but do not necessarily indicate predisposition to it, or "trait" characteristics, which are also demonstrable in the remitted state and suggest an underlying biological vulnerability. Markers of either type are important in characterizing PTSD and in establishing its relationship to other psychiatric disorders. Trait markers are of particular importance in that they can provide direct clues as to the etiology and pathogenesis of the syndrome.

Biological marker studies in PTSD are still at a very preliminary stage. They are inevitably complicated by diagnostic limitations and subject to the concern that demonstration of specificity is problematic in the case of a syndrome whose clinical boundaries have yet to be clearly defined (Lerer et al., in press). Some interesting findings have nevertheless emerged. In a series of reports, Mason and colleagues (Kosten et al. 1987; Mason et al. 1986, 1989) found that the 24-hour urinary excretion of norepinephrine and epinephrine was higher in PTSD than in other diagnostic groups; cortisol levels were lower, and the norepinephrine/cortisol ratio was elevated. Also relevant is the finding of Kudler et al. (1987) that 50% of PTSD subjects with concomitant major depressive disorder were dexamethasone nonsuppressors as opposed to only 6% of nondepressed subjects with PTSD.

These findings suggest that PTSD and affective disorder patients can be biologically differentiated on some of the parameters examined.

In this chapter, we will focus on a biological parameter that has recently been of considerable interest in the context of affective disorder. In the nearly four decades since the original catecholamine hypothesis of affective disorder was proposed, research interest has shifted from the levels of biogenic amines and their metabolites in body fluids to the receptors for these amines and the second-messenger systems to which they are coupled. Because of the inaccessibility of brain tissue to direct study, peripheral blood cells have been used as a convenient model for such investigations. Studies examining the functional activity of beta-adrenergic receptors on lymphocyte and leucocyte samples of depressed patients have yielded remarkably consistent findings. To date, four groups of investigators have demonstrated reduced 3,5-cyclic adenosine monophosphate (AMP) accumulation in response to stimulation with isoproterenol (Ebstein et al. 1988; Extein et al. 1979; Mann et al. 1985; Pandey et al. 1979). Furthermore, Ebstein et al. (1988) have shown that isoproterenol-stimulated responses are lowest in patients with a subsequent poor response to antidepressant treatment.

The receptor-associated adenylate cyclase complex is now known to consist of three principal components: 1) the receptor to which the hormone or neurotransmitter binds, 2) a guanyl nucleotide binding unit (Sternweiss and Gilman 1982), and 3) a catalytic unit (Rodbell 1980). The availability of compounds that differentially stimulate these components has made the process of signal transduction distal to the receptors accessible to in vitro investigation. Stimulation with isoproterenol and prostaglandin E_1 (PGE_1) yields information as to beta-adrenergic receptor–mediated and PGE_1 receptor–mediated responsiveness, respectively. Aluminum chloride in the presence of sodium fluoride ($AlCl_3/NaF$) acts on the guanyl nucleotide binding unit (Sternweiss and Gilman 1982), and the diterpene compound, forskolin, interacts with the catalytic unit (Seaman et al. 1981). Abnormalities of response to agents acting distal to the receptor are of considerable interest. They could theoretically be a "downstream" manifestation related to alterations in receptor sensitivity induced by circulating amines or hormones. They could, however, reflect an intrinsic abnormality of one or more components of the adenylate cyclase complex, as has been demonstrated in certain disorders (Ebstein et al. 1986). In the case of depression, the work of Ebstein et al. (1988) showed reduced lymphocyte cyclic AMP production in response to forskolin stimulation in addition to that observed on stimulation with isoproterenol.

A preliminary study conducted in the Research Division of Ezrath Nashim Hospital raised the possibility that cyclic AMP signal transduction may be reduced in PTSD and that the defect may extend distal to the receptor (Lerer et al. 1987b). The mean ($\pm$ SD) age of the 12 subjects who gave informed consent to participate in the study was 35.9 ± 10.1 years. Five were military veterans in whom the precipitating traumatic event was combat related, three had been victims of terrorist activity, and four had been involved in motor accidents. None had suffered significant physical injury. All the subjects fulfilled DSM-III criteria for PTSD. Five patients fulfilled other DSM-III criteria, two for major depressive disorder, one for dysthymic disorder, and two for generalized anxiety disorder. None of the subjects had any history of alcohol or other substance abuse. Age- and sex-matched normal controls with no history of psychiatric illness were obtained from the hospital staff.

Lymphoctye and platelet preparations were obtained from 50-cc blood samples drawn into syringes containing preservative-free sodium heparin. Cyclic AMP accumulation in response to stimulation with isoproterenol (10 μM), forskolin (60 μM), and PGE_1 (1 μM) was determined in the lymphocyte preparations as described elsewhere (Lerer et al. 1987b). Platelet membranes were stored at $-100°C$ until assayed by the Salomon et al. (1974) procedure. Adenylate cyclase activity in response to forskolin (10 to 500 μM), aluminum chloride (50 μM) plus sodium fluoride (4 μM), and PGE_1 (10 μM) was determined as previously described (Lerer et al. 1987b).

In intact lymphocytes, significantly lower basal cyclic AMP levels and cyclic AMP responsiveness to isoproterenol and forskolin stimulation (after subtraction of basal values) were found in the patient group as compared to controls. No differences in PGE_1-stimulated cyclic AMP accumulation was observed between the two groups. Figure 12-1 shows the values for basal, forskolin, $AlCl_3$/NaF, and PGE_1-stimulated adenylate cyclase activity in platelet membranes; all four values were significantly lower for the patient group than the control group. Even when the five patients fulfilling criteria for concomitant DSM-III diagnoses other than PTSD were excluded from the data analysis, all the differences remained statistically significant.

These preliminary results suggest that drug-free patients with a DSM-III diagnosis of combat-related PTSD are characterized by abnormally low cyclic AMP signal transduction in intact lymphocytes and in platelet membrane preparations. Although the small sample size mandates caution in interpreting the results, the findings suggest a functional deficit similar to that found in depressed patients (Ebstein et al. 1988; Extein et al. 1979; Mann et al. 1985; Pandey et al. 1979). The significantly lower forskolin-stimulated activity suggests that this lower responsiveness extends distal to the receptor and involves the catalytic unit of the enzyme. Platelet membranes from the patients with PTSD showed, in addition, less response to $AlCl_3$/NaF stimulation, which acts on the nucleotide binding protein. Whereas no difference was observed in intact lymphocytes, PGE_1-stimulated activity in platelets was significantly lower in the PTSD group than in the normal controls. The reasons for this discrepancy are unclear. These results

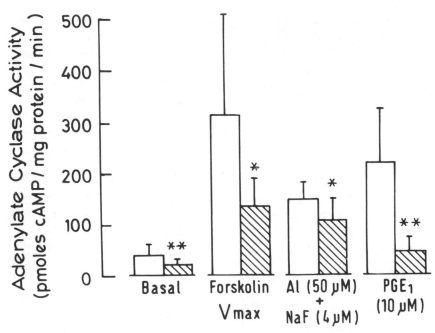

Figure 12-1. Basal and stimulated levels of adenylate cyclase activity in platelet
membranes from 10 subjects with PTSD (striped bars) and from 10
normal controls (open bars). *$P < .05$, Student's t test (two-tailed).
**$P < .01$, Student's t test (two-tailed).

raised the possibility that abnormally low cyclic AMP signal transduction
may be a biologic marker for PTSD. These findings have since been reevalu-
ated in a larger sample of subjects with PTSD as compared to an age- and
sex-matched control group. Subjects for this second study were male veterans of the 1982–1984 Lebanon War with combat-related PTSD. All were
reserve soldiers who had volunteered for a behavior modification program
aimed at improving their level of functioning in the military context. They
were examined for the present study while undergoing an intensive series of
psychological and physical evaluations prior to their participation in the
program. The assessments were conducted in a military clinic that performs
routine physical evaluations of military personnel. Age-matched servicemen
evaluated in the clinic on the same day as the PTSD subjects served as the
control group.

There were 19 subjects in the PTSD group (mean age, 34.2 ± 5.6
years) and 35 control subjects (mean age, 35.4 ± 4.2 years). The controls
were all psychiatrically healthy with no previous history of mental illness and
were all functioning adequately in their service duties. Neither group had
any evidence of physical illness or alcohol or other substance abuse, and

subjects were free of medication for at least 4 weeks before the examination. In the PTSD group, the diagnosis was confirmed according to DSM-III criteria. The PTSD subjects also completed the Symptom Checklist-90 (SCL-90) (Derogatis 1977) and the Impact of Event Scale (Zilberg et al. 1982). Blood for biochemical evaluations was obtained from both the PTSD group and control group as previously described (Lerer et al. 1987b). All the PTSD and control samples were collected over a period of 3 days. It was therefore not feasible to evaluate cyclic AMP accumulation in lymphocytes, since this procedure is performed on fresh cells. Platelets were, however, extracted, and their membranes prepared and frozen at $-100°C$ until assayed. Adenylate cyclase activity was determined as previously reported (Lerer et al. 1987b). Adenylate cyclase activity in the PTSD and control groups is shown in Table 12-1. Basal adenylate cyclase activity was lower in the PTSD group; this difference was marginally significant ($P = .07$). Stimulated values were therefore calculated after subtracting the basal values. Forskolin-stimulated adenylate cyclase activity in platelet membranes from the PTSD group was significantly lower than in the controls ($P = .02$), which was a result similar to the observations of our preliminary study. There was no difference in $AlCl_3/NaF$-stimulated adenylate cyclase activity or in PGE_1-stimulated activity between the PTSD group and the control group. The biochemical findings from the PTSD group were also examined in conjunction with data from the rating scales administered to these subjects. No relationship was observed between forskolin-stimulated adenylate cyclase activity, or the other biochemical parameters, and any of the subscales

Table 12-1. Mean ($\pm$ SD) basal and stimulated platelet adenylate cyclase levels in posttraumatic stress disorder (PTSD)

	Platelet adenylate cyclase level (pmol c-AMP/mg protein/minute)	
	PTSD ($n = 18$)	Controls ($n = 35$)[a]
Basal[b]	144.4 $\pm$ 84.0	196.2 $\pm$ 103.9
$AlCl_3$ (50 μM) + NaF (4 μM)[c]	635.7 $\pm$ 396.8	592.5 $\pm$ 247.6
Forskolin (V_{max})[d]	541.1 $\pm$ 140.3	720.1 $\pm$ 309.1
PGE_1 (10 μM)[c]	276.2 $\pm$ 118.2	299.6 $\pm$ 159.4

[a] $n = 34$ for PGE_1. [b] $t = 1.82$ (*S*tudent's two-tailed), $P = .07$. [c] Not significant, $P > .1$. [d] $t = 2.32$ (Student's two-tailed), $P = .02$.

of the SCL-90 (by Pearson r correlation coefficient). There was also no correlation between platelet adenylate cyclase activity and total scores in the Impact of Event Scale, the intrusion and avoidance subscales derived from this scale, and number of DSM-III items scored as present.

The present findings support our earlier suggestion that platelet adenylate cyclase activity may be a biologic marker for PTSD. In our preliminary study, basal platelet adenylate cyclase values were also significantly reduced as well as the response to stimulation with $AlCl_3$/NaF and PGE_1. Although basal values tended to be lower than control in the present study, stimulated values, other than those in response to forskolin, were not. The reason for this discrepancy is not immediately clear. PGE_1 activates platelet adenylate cyclase via the PGE_1 receptor and $AlCl_3$/NaF via the N protein. Forskolin acts distal to these two sites at the catalytic unit. One might therefore expect that low responsiveness at the catalytic unit should be associated with reduced responsiveness to agents acting proximal to this site (at the N protein or receptor level). It is, however, possible that this "upstream" effect might occur when forskolin-stimulated activity is more substantially reduced than in the present study. In our earlier work, forskolin-stimulated activity in the PTSD group was only 39% of control, whereas in the present study it was 75%.

The present findings raise the possibility that PTSD could be associated with an intrinsic dysfunction in cyclic AMP signal transduction at the level of the catalytic unit of the receptor-adenylate cyclase complex. An avenue for further investigating this possibility is to examine [^{3}H]forskolin binding in platelets from subjects with PTSD directly. As noted earlier, impaired cyclic AMP signal transduction in peripheral blood cells (lymphocytes and leucocytes) has also been reported in drug-free patients with depression (Ebstein et al. 1988; Extein et al. 1979; Mann et al. 1985; Pandey et al. 1979). Present evidence suggests that this is a beta-adrenergic receptor-mediated deficit; a primary defect distal to the receptor cannot, however, be excluded. Data of the type presented here on adenylate cyclase activity in platelets from depressed patients are not yet available. It is therefore not possible to speculate whether dysfunctional cyclic AMP signal transduction might be an intrinsic abnormality common to depression and PTSD and might predispose to the development of both syndromes. The latter possibility requires, of course, further characterization of the abnormality as a trait marker rather than as one simply associated with the clinical syndrome. The adenylate cyclase second-messenger system is a crucial factor in the transmission of neurotransmitter-stimulated signaling via a number of receptors in the brain. An abnormality of this system could have significant implications for the pathogenesis of PTSD and for the possible relationship of the syndrome to affective disorders.

REFERENCES

American Psychiatric Association: Diagnostic and Statistical Manual of Mental Disorders, 3rd Edition, Revised. Washington, DC, American Psychiatric Association, 1987

Bleich A, Siegel B, Garb R, et al: Post-traumatic stress disorder following combat exposure: clinical features and psychopharmacological treatment. Br J Psychiatry 149:356–369, 1986

Davidson J, Walker JI, Kilts C: A pilot study of phenelzine in post-traumatic stress disorder. Br J Psychiatry 150:252, 1987

Derogatis LR: The SCL-90 Manual: Scoring, Administration and Procedures for the SCL-90. Baltimore, MD, Johns Hopkins University School of Medicine, Clinical Psychometrics Unit, 1977

Ebstein RP, Oppenheim G, Ebstein BS, et al: The cyclic AMP second messenger system in man: the effects of heredity, hormones, drugs, aluminum, age and disease on signal amplification. Progress in Neuropsychopharmacology and Biological Psychiatry 10:323–353, 1986

Ebstein RP, Lerer B, Shapira B, et al: Cyclic AMP second-messenger signal amplification in depression. Br J Psychiatry 152:665–669, 1988

Extein I, Tallman J, Smith CC, et al: Changes in lymphocyte beta-adrenergic receptors in depression and mania. Psychiatry Res 1:191–197, 1979

Falcon S, Ryan C, Chamberlain K, et al: Tricyclics: possible treatment for posttraumatic stress disorder. J Clin Psychiatry 46:385–388, 1985

Hogben GL, Cornfield RB: Treatment of traumatic war neurosis with phenelzine. Arch Gen Psychiatry 39:1345, 1981

Kosten TR, Mason JW, Giller EL, et al: Sustained urinary norepinephrine and epinephrine elevation in post-traumatic stress disorder. Psychoneuroendocrinology 12:13–20, 1987

Kudler H, Davidson J, Meador K, et al: The DST and posttraumatic stress disorder. Am J Psychiatry 144:1068–1071, 1987

Lerer B, Ebstein RP, Shestatsky M, et al: Cyclic AMP signal transduction in posttraumatic stress disorder. Am J Psychiatry 144:1324–1327, 1987a

Lerer B, Bleich A, Kotler M, et al: Posttraumatic stress disorder in Israeli combat veterans: effect of phenelzine treatment. Arch Gen Psychiatry 44:976–981, 1987b

Lerer B, Braun P, Bleich A, et al: Pharmacotherapy trials in posttraumatic stress disorder: problems and prospects, in New Directions in Affective Disorders. Edited by Lerer B, Gershon S. New York, Springer-Verlag (in press)

Mann JJ, Brown RP, Halper JP, et al: Reduced sensitivity of lymphocyte beta-adrenergic receptors in patients with endogenous depression and psychomotor agitation. N Engl J Med 313:715–720, 1985

Mason JW, Giller EL, Kosten TR, et al: Urinary free-cortisol levels in posttraumatic stress disorder patients. J Nerv Ment Dis 174:1–5, 1986

Mason JW, Giller EL, Kosten TR, et al: Elevation of urinary norepinephrine/cortisol ratio in posttraumatic stress disorder. J Nerv Ment Dis 176:498–502, 1988

Pandey GN, Dysken MW, Garner DL, et al: Beta adrenergic receptor function in affective illness. Am J Psychiatry 136:675–678, 1979

Rodbell M: The role of hormone receptors and GPT-regulatory proteins in membrane transduction. Nature 78:3363–3367, 1980

Salomon Y, Londos C, Rodwell M: A highly sensitive adenylate cyclase assay. Anal Biochem 58:541–548, 1974

Seaman KB, Padgett W, Daly JW: Forskolin: unique diterpene activator of adenylate cyclase in membranes and in intact cells. Proc Natl Acad Sci USA 78:3363–3367, 1981

Shestatzky M, Greenberg D, Lerer B: A controlled trial of phenelzine in posttraumatic stress disorder. Psychiatry Res 24:149–155, 1988

Sierles FS, Jang-June C, McFarland RE, et al: Posttraumatic stress disorder and concurrent psychiatric illness: a preliminary report. Am J Psychiatry 140:1177–1179, 1983

Sternweiss PC, Gilman AG: Aluminum: a requirement for activation of the regulatory component of adenylate cyclase by fluoride. Proc Natl Acad Sci USA 79:4888–4889, 1982

Yager T, Laufer R, Gallops M: Some problems associated with war experience in men of the Vietnam generation. Arch Gen Psychiatry 41:327–333, 1984

Zilberg NJ, Weiss DS, Horowitz MJ: Impact of Event Scale: a cross-validation study and some empirical evidence supporting a conceptual model of stress response syndromes. J Consult Clin Psychol 50:407–410, 1982

Chapter 13

Psychoendocrinology of Posttraumatic Stress Disorder

Earl L. Giller, Jr., M.D., Ph.D.
Bruce D. Perry, M.D., Ph.D.
Steven Southwick, M.D.
Rachel Yehuda, Ph.D.
Victor Wahby, M.D., Ph.D.
Thomas R. Kosten, M.D.
John W. Mason, M.D.

P osttraumatic stress disorder (PTSD) has been a known syndrome characterized by fairly specific cognitive, anxiety, and autonomic nervous system (ANS) symptoms for many years (Bury 1918; Campbell 1918; DaCosta 1871; Frazer and Wilson 1918). Specific ANS hyperactivity was documented in soldiers from World War I in response to combat stimuli (Meakans and Wilson 1918). These individuals also appeared to be supersensitive to epinephrine, with greater increases in heart rate, blood pressure, and anxiety compared to controls following epinephrine administration (Frazer and Wilson 1918; Peabody et al. 1918). More current psychophysiologic studies have replicated and extended this work (Blanchard et al. 1982, 1986; Dobbs and Wilson 1960; Malloy et al. 1983; Pitman et al. 1987). Some of these studies (Blanchard et al. 1982; Pitman et al. 1987) reported higher baseline heart rate and systolic blood pressure in PTSD combat veterans compared to controls, suggesting ANS hyperactivity even at rest.

These findings in stress response disorders suggested that psychoendocrine studies of subjects with PTSD would be of interest. Alterations in catecholamine metabolism would be expected, reflecting a state of increased arousal and sympathetic nervous system functioning. Changes in cortisol metabolism are often found in acute and chronic stress responses. In addition, the psychoendocrine hypothesis is that a significant amount of the variance in hormonal levels, even within the "normal" range, can provide information about brain function as do the other effector systems: the autonomic and musculoskeletal systems. Endocrine measures, when compared to musculoskeletal system and ANS variables (which are the bases for the signs and symptoms currently used for diagnosis), can help to decide how much PTSD is similar to or different from other anxiety and mood disorders.

Although it would clearly be of interest to know whether localized alterations in brain neuronal activity are associated with symptoms of PTSD, we elected to concentrate initially on peripheral measurements, since these are measures of the actual effector systems (musculoskeletal, autonomic, and endocrine) and do not suffer from the problems of interpretation that occur with more indirect measures of neuronal activity, such as peripheral measures of neurotransmitter metabolites. A long history of psychoendocrine research has suggested that 24-hour urine excretions of catecholamines and cortisol, which provide an integrated sample of metabolism, are a more stable measurement than plasma samples, which can vary markedly from moment to moment. Thus we concentrated on 24-hour urinary excretion of norepinephrine, epinephrine, and cortisol—indices of sympathetic nervous system, adrenal medulla, and adrenal cortical activities, respectively.

In a pilot study, we found that a group of inpatients with PTSD showed significantly higher 24-hour urinary excretion of norepinephrine and epinephrine than comparison groups of other psychiatric patients (Kosten et al. 1987). The urinary norepinephrine and epinephrine remained relatively high over hospitalization, whereas the other group showing comparable levels at admission, bipolar manic subjects, showed a decrease in urinary norepinephrine and epinephrine excretion during hospitalization. Urinary catecholamine excretion in PTSD subjects remained relatively high even with some decrease in symptoms, although the reduction in symptoms in this group was not as great as the drop in symptoms in the comparison groups. Although we did not examine normal controls, these catecholamine levels are at the high end of normal. We also did not examine combat controls, veterans without PTSD but with combat exposure comparable to veterans with PTSD, which are an important comparison group. Thus PTSD is similar to depression in showing increased catecholamine excretion, although we found higher levels in PTSD compared to depressed patients, and our depressed patients did not show as high levels of catecholamine excretion as others have reported (Koslow et al. 1983).

Further, support of a hyperadrenergic state in PTSD comes from the study of alpha$_2$-adrenergic receptor binding sites on platelets from subjects with PTSD (Perry et al. 1987). We found that subjects with PTSD showed a significant reduction in total number of platelet alpha$_2$-receptor binding sites, primarily a decrease in high-affinity sites, and an increase in the ratio of low-affinity to high-affinity sites, compared to controls. These findings suggest that the platelet alpha$_2$-receptor sites show both down-regulation (decreased B$_{max}$) and desensitization (increased ratio of low-affinity to high-affinity sites) (Perry et al. 1990). Also, alpha$_2$-receptor sites on platelets from PTSD subjects, when incubated with epinephrine in the test tube (Perry 1988), showed a significantly more rapid and more extensive down-regulation than sites on platelets from controls (Figure 13-1). Although these results are consistent with chronic exposure to relatively high catecholamine levels, we are currently exploring the more interesting possibility that an alteration in receptor physiology may be the primary problem in PTSD. This finding of altered alpha$_2$-adrenergic receptor sites in PTSD is supported by the finding of decreased receptor-mediated second-messenger activation in blood cells from patients with PTSD (Lerer et al. 1987). Our pilot results thus suggest that alpha$_2$-adrenergic receptors are down-regulated and also show some desensitization in PTSD, while they only present desensitization in major depressive disorder (MDD). If such receptor changes also occur centrally, specifically in the locus coeruleus, it may make this area more sensitive to and less able to damp excitatory and possibly inhibitory inputs. That is, if alpha$_2$-receptors on the locus coeruleus are significantly down-regulated, locus firing would be disinhibited.

It is well-known that acute stress can result in increased output of

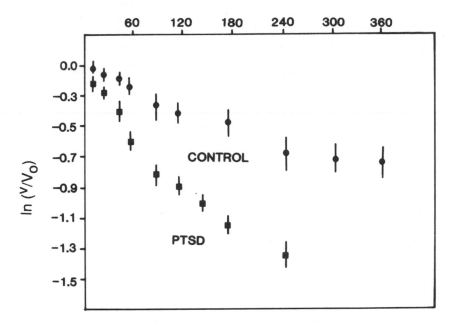

Figure 13-1. Platelet alpha$_2$-adrenergic receptor binding sites following in vitro exposure to epinephrine in five patients with posttraumatic stress disorder (PTSD) and in eight controls: increased rate of "down-regulation" in PTSD. Intact platelets were incubated for various times with 10^{-4} M (−)-epinephrine, and membranes were prepared as described elsewhere (Perry and U'Prichard 1984). The specific binding of 4.0 nM RAUW was then determined. Values are mean ± SEM.

cortisol, but less well-recognized that the cortisol stress response can be modulated by psychological variables such as denial (Mason et al. 1990). Also, chronic stress may be associated with low, rather than high, cortisol levels, although acute superimposed stress can increase cortisol levels. We found that the PTSD subjects described previously showed relatively low 24-hour urinary excretion of free cortisol (Table 13-1) compared to other patient groups and that this level of excretion remained relatively constant during the course of hospitalization. We have replicated this finding in a study of outpatient Vietnam veterans with PTSD compared to noncombat controls (Yehuda et al., in press). This is a marked difference from the high cortisol excretion often found in depression.

The catecholamine and cortisol variables can be combined in a bivariate analysis consisting of a norepinephrine/cortisol ratio, which more powerfully distinguishes subjects with PTSD from patients with other psychiatric disorders, including depression (Figure 13-2). While the discriminating ability of this ratio is a post-hoc finding, animal and clinical research has documented interactions between the hypothalamic-pituitary-adrenal (HPA) and the cat-

Table 13-1. Mean (± SE) urinary free cortisol excretion (μg/day) in patients with posttraumatic stress disorder (PTSD) versus other diagnostic groups

	PTSD (n=9)	PS (n=12)	BP (n=8)	MDD (n=8)	US (n=7)	Difference[a]
First[b]	34.9 ± 4.9	41.2 ± 9.5	77.4 ± 8.8	57.4 ± 5.6	71.7 ± 12.8	(PTSD = PS) < (BP = MDD = US)
Mean[c]	33.3 ± 3.2	37.5 ± 3.9	63.6 ± 7.6	49.6 ± 5.9	50.1 ± 8.9	(PTSD = PS) < (BP = MDD = US)
Last[d]	34.1 ± 4.7	41.5 ± 8.1	47.6 ± 6.3	40.0 ± 6.4	33.7 ± 8.5	Not significant
Change (first-last)[e]	−.8 ± 6.0	.0 ± 10.3	−34.1 ± 10.7	−17.4 ± 6.0	−38.0 ± 8.0	(PTSD = PS) < (BP = MDD = US)

Note: PS = paranoid schizophrenia, BP = bipolar disorder, MDD = major depressive disorder, US = undifferentiated schizophrenia.

[a] "=" indicates means are not significantly different; "<" indicates mean is significantly lower than the following value.

[b] $F = 4.36$, 4/43 df, $P < .0046$. [c] $F = 4.38$, 4/43 df, $P < .006$. [d] $F = .58$, 4/43 df, $P < .68$. [e] $F = 3.93$, 4/43 df, $P < .01$.

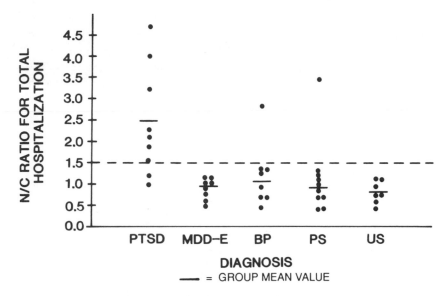

Figure 13-2. Mean urinary norepinephrine/cortisol (NC) ratio in individual patients by diagnosis. PTSD = posttraumatic stress disorder, MDD-E = major depressive disorder, endogenous, BP = bipolar disorder, PS = paranoid schizophrenia, US = undifferentiated schizophrenia. $F = 6.51$, 4/41 df, $P < .0005$.

echolamine systems (Yehuda et al. 1990). The interactions between these two systems are complex, however, and are different at the central nervous system, pituitary, peripheral, and receptor levels. In addition, stress may alter the interaction between these systems, and this interaction may also be different in acute compared to chronic stress. In general, the correlation between HPA and adrenergic activity has been reported as positive in depression as opposed to negative in PTSD.

Neuroendocrine challenge studies also support the dissimilarity between PTSD and depression. Kudler et al. (1987) reported that PTSD subjects with MDD showed a higher rate (5 of 10) of nonsuppression on the dexamethasone suppression test (DST) than did subjects with PTSD alone (1 of 18). Kauffman et al. (1987) found that 1 of 8 PTSD subjects showed DST nonsuppression and 4 of 8 had a blunted thyroid-stimulating hormone (TSH) response to thyrotropin-releasing hormone (TRH). These workers did not state whether or not subjects met criteria for MDD, although the mean Hamilton Depression Scale (Hamilton 1960) sum (number of items not specified) was 30. DST nonsuppression in PTSD is not surprising, given our finding of low cortisol excretion, although DST nonsuppression can occur even without high cortisol levels.

Our preliminary results (Kosten et al., in press) suggest that subjects with PTSD do not differ from normal controls in abnormalities on the DST and TRH (Figure 13-3). We studied 11 male veterans with PTSD (6 with concurrent MDD), 18 veterans with MDD (endogenous type) alone, and 28 controls. After receiving dexamethasone, the 4:00 P.M. serum cortisol was significantly higher in the MDD group (4.1 ± 1.8 μg/dl) than in the PTSD (1.8 ± 1.0 μg/dl) and control (1.9 ± 0.6 μg/dl) groups. When subjects were

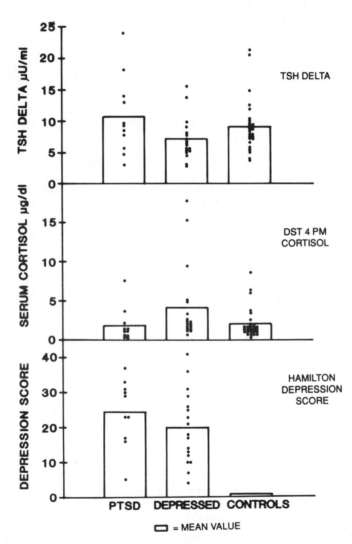

Figure 13-3. Thyroid-releasing hormone (TRH) and dexamethasone suppression test (DST) responses in inpatients with posttraumatic stress disorder (PTSD) in comparison with depressed inpatients and control subjects using first samples.

dichotomized into DST nonsuppressors and suppressors, the MDD group showed a 22% nonsuppression rate compared to a 10% rate in the PTSD and control groups. None of the six PTSD patients with concurrent MDD were DST nonsuppressors. On the TRH test, the peak TSH response to TRH was significantly lower in the MDD group (7.1 ± 0.8 $\mu IU/ml$) than in the PTSD (10.7 ± 1.8 $\mu IU/ml$) and control (9.4 ± 0.8 $\mu IU/ml$) groups. Baseline total thyroxine, free T_4, and TSH levels were equivalent across the three groups. When dichotomized into groups showing a blunted versus normal TSH response, a higher rate of blunting was seen in the MDD patients (67%) than in the PTSD (27%) or control (28%) subjects. Interestingly, four PTSD patients showed a relatively *high* TSH response, ranging from 13 to 24 $\mu IU/ml$, whereas only three controls (11%) and two MDD patients (11%) had TSH responses greater than 13 $\mu IU/ml$. Three of the six PTSD patients with concurrent MDD showed a blunted response to TRH; however, two of the four augmented TSH responses occurred among PTSD patients with concurrent MDD.

In conclusion, our psychoendocrine studies suggest that subjects with PTSD, even with concurrent MDD, show a different psychoendocrine profile from those with MDD alone when catecholamine excretion and receptor parameters, cortisol excretion, and neuroendocrine challenge test results are examined. These results are derived from a relatively small sample size and need to be tested in a larger sample. Factors that appear to be of importance in clinical research in PTSD include structured assessment of the diagnosis, with quantitative and qualitative assessment of intrusive, avoidance, and increased arousal symptoms; concurrent assessment of depressive and anxiety symptoms; separate analysis of subjects meeting criteria for other concurrent DSM-III-R (American Psychiatric Association 1987) Axis I disorders; possibly separate analyses of inpatients versus outpatients; and the use of both controls who have been exposed to similar traumatic events without developing PTSD and normal controls. Psychoendocrine studies, when coupled with measures of the other effector systems, such as psychophysiology studies (autonomic nervous system) and subjective and objective signs and symptoms (musculoskeletal system), can help to define the pathophysiology of PTSD, explore possible subtypes, and improve treatment strategies.

REFERENCES

American Psychiatric Association: Diagnostic and Statistical Manual of Mental Disorders, 3rd Edition, Revised. Washington, DC, American Psychiatric Association, 1987

Blanchard EB, Kolb LC, Pallmeyer TP, et al: A psychophysiologic study of post traumatic stress disorder in Vietnam veterans. Psychiatr Q 54:220–228, 1982

Blanchard EB, Kolb LC, Gerardi RJ, et al: Cardiac response to relevant stimuli as an adjunctive tool for diagnosing post traumatic stress disorder in Vietnam veterans. Behavioral Therapy 17:592–606, 1986

Bury JS: Pathology of war neurosis. Lancet 1:97–99, 1918

Campbell CM: The role of instinct, motion and personality in disorders of the heart. JAMA 71:1621–1626, 1918

DaCosta JM: Irritable heart: A clinical study of a form of functional cardiac disorder and its consequences. Am J Med Sci 71:17–52, 1871

Dobbs D, Wilson WP: Observations on persistence of war neurosis. Diseases of the Nervous System 21:686–691, 1960

Frazer F, Wilson RN: The sympathetic nervous system and the "irritable heart of soldiers." Br Med J 2:27–29, 1918

Hamilton M: A rating for depression. J Neurol Neurosurg Psychiatry 23:56–62, 1960

Kauffman CD, Reist C, Djenderedjian A, et al: Biological markers of affective disorders and posttraumatic stress disorder: a pilot study with desipramine. J Clin Psychiatry 48:366–367, 1987

Koslow SH, Maas JW, Bowden CL, et al: CSF and urinary biogenic amines and metabolites in depression and mania: a controlled, univariate analysis. Arch Gen Psychiatry 40:999–1010, 1983

Kosten TR, Mason JW, Giller EL, et al: Sustained urinary norepinephrine and epinephrine elevation in posttraumatic stress disorder. Psychoneuroendocrinology 12:13–20, 1987

Kosten TR, Wahby V, Giller E, et al: The dexamethasone test and TRH stimulation test in posttraumatic stress disorder. Biol Psychiatry (in press)

Kudler H, Davidson J, Meador K, et al: The DST and posttraumatic stress disorder. Am J Psychiatry 144:1068:1071, 1987

Lerer B, Ebstein RP, Shestatsky M, et al: Cyclic AMP signal transduction in PTSD. Am J Psychiatry 144:1324–1327, 1987

Malloy PF, Fairbank JA, Keane TM: Validation of a multimethod assessment of PTSD in Vietnam veterans. J Consult Clin Psychol 51:488–494, 1983

Mason JW, Giller EL Jr, Kosten TR, et al: Psychoendocrine approaches to the diagnosis and pathogenesis of posttraumatic stress disorder, in Biological Assessment and Treatment of Posttraumatic Stress Disorder. Edited by Giller EL Jr. Washington, DC, American Psychiatric Press, 1990, pp 65–86

Meakins JC, Wilson RN: The effect of certain sensory stimulations on respiratory and heart rate in cases of so-called "irritable heart." Heart 7:17–22, 1918

Peabody FW, Clough HD, Sturgis CC, et al: Effects of the injection of epinephrine in soliders with "irritable heart." JAMA 71:1912–1915, 1918

Perry BD: Placental and blood element neurotransmitter receptor regulation in humans: potential models for studying neurochemical mechanisms underlying behavioral teratology, in Biochemical Basis of Functional Neuroteratology:

Permanent Effects of Chemicals on the Developing Brain (Progress in Brain Research, Vol 73). Edited by Boer GJ, Feenstra MGP, Mirmiran M. Amsterdam, Elsevier, 1988, pp 189–207

Perry BD, Southwick SM, Yehuda R, et al: Adrenergic receptor regulation in posttraumatic stress disorder, in Biological Assessment and Treatment of Posttraumatic Stress Disorder. Edited by Giller EL Jr. Washington, DC, American Psychiatric Press, 1990, pp 87–114

Pitman RK, Orr SP, Forgue DF, et al: Psychophysiological assessment of PTSD imagery in Vietnam combat veterans. Arch Gen Psychiatry 44:970–975, 1987

Yehuda R, Southwick SM, Perry BD, et al: Interactions of the hypothalamic-pituitary-adrenal axis and the catecholaminergic system in posttraumatic stress disorder, in Biological Assessment and Treatment of Posttraumatic Stress Disorder. Edited by Giller EL Jr. Washington DC, American Psychiatric Press, 1990, pp 115–134

Yehuda R, Southwick S, Nussbaum G, et al: Low urinary cortisol excretion in patients with posttraumatic stress disorder. J Nerv Ment Dis (in press)

Treatment of Posttraumatic Stress Disorder

Chapter 14

Antidepressants in the Treatment of Posttraumatic Stress Disorder

Julia B. Frank, M.D.
Thomas R. Kosten, M.D.
Earl L. Giller, Jr., M.D., Ph.D.
Elisheva Dan, P.A.

The widespread use of drugs in the treatment of posttraumatic stress disorder (PTSD) dates back to World War II, when injecting barbiturates to facilitate recollection of repressed traumatic memories was a popular technique (Kolb 1985). During the next 25 years, professional interest in PTSD diminished, to be reawakened in the 1970s as the readjustment problems of Vietnam veterans brought the issue back into public awareness. The grass roots "rap group" movement (Lifton 1973) initially stressed social activism and psychological healing over pharmacotherapy. As more professionals became interested in traumatic stress, the similarity between PTSD and other disorders known to respond to drugs suggested the possibility that some posttraumatic symptoms might respond to medication. In particular, PTSD shares with depression symptoms of disturbed sleep, apathy, social withdrawal, sadness, guilt, and somatic complaints. However, when DSM-III (American Psychiatric Association 1980) appeared, PTSD was classified with the anxiety rather than the affective disorders. In part, this decision reflects the traditional classification of PTSD as a form of neurosis. It seems justified phenomenologically, since anxiety is also a frequent and disabling symptom. Moreover, many sufferers meet criteria for panic attacks during flashbacks (Mellman and Davis 1985), which are typically accompanied by hyperarousal (Kolb 1987; Pitman et al. 1987).

Clinical similarity to anxiety and depressive disorders has led both to open trials of numerous medications in PTSD and to research into possible biologic mechanisms subserving this disorder. Although uncontrolled studies support the use of lithium (Kitchner and Greenstein 1985; van der Kolk 1983), carbamazepine (Lipper et al. 1986; Wolf et al. 1988), benzodiazepines (Birkheimer 1985; Yost 1980), clonidine, and propranolol (Kolb et al. 1984) in PTSD, antidepressants have received the most systematic and thorough study to date. Table 14-1 summarizes the results of studies of antidepressants in PTSD (excluding our own) reported by early 1989.

On balance, these studies suggest that monoamine oxidase inhibitors (MAOIs) and tricyclic antidepressants (TCAs) may ameliorate symptoms of PTSD, especially in combat veterans. The dissenting reports merit further attention. The 15 patients reviewed by Birkheimer (1985) who did not respond to antidepressants were all inpatients, many of whom received combinations of drugs or inadequate doses. The Lerer et al. (1987) study, which found phenelzine to be of minimal benefit in the treatment of 25 Israeli combat veterans, lacked a placebo control and included many dropouts and subjects who received low doses of phenelzine. Although Shestatzky et al. (1988) did compare phenelzine to placebo, their finding of no significant benefit from active drug is inconclusive given the small size of their sample

171

Table 14-1. Trials of antidepressant drugs in posttraumatic stress disorder (PTSD)

Authors	N	Drug(s)	Results	Comments
Marshall (1975)	1	Imipramine	Decreased night terrors	
Hogben and Cornfield (1981)	5	Phenelzine	Decreased nightmares, flashbacks, startling, violent outbursts; enhanced psychotherapy	Combat veterans; inpatients refractory to tricyclics
Walker (1982)	3	Phenelzine	Decreased nightmares, flashbacks	Combat veterans
Levenson et al. (1982)	1	Phenelzine	Decreased nightmares, anxiety, anger, social withdrawal; enhanced psychotherapy	Combat veteran
White (1983)	18	Doxepin	Decreased nightmares	Combat veterans
Shen and Park (1983)	1	Phenelzine Tranylcypromine	Improvement despite sexual dysfunction	Combat veteran
	7	Phenelzine	Decreased intrusive recollection; increased reported memories (4/7)	
Burstein (1984)	10	Imipramine	Decreased intrusive recollections, nightmares, flashbacks; improved sleep	
Milanes et al. (1984)	6	Phenelzine	Improved sleep, anxiety, depressive, and PTSD symptoms	Combat veterans
Birkheimer et al. (1985)	15	Amitriptyline (10) Imipramine (7) Nortriptyline (2) Doxepin (7) Amoxapine (2) Maprotiline (2) Trazodone (1) Phenelzine (3)	Amitriptyline and imipramine improved sleep, decreased nightmares; no effect on flashbacks, depression; phenelzine improved sleep; diminished depression, anxiety (1/3)	Combat veterans, inpatients receiving combinations of drugs

Table 14-1. Trials of antidepressant drugs in posttraumatic stress disorder
(PTSD) *(continued)*

Authors	N	Drug(s)	Results	Comments
Falcon et al. (1985)	17	Amitriptyline Desipramine Doxepin	82% globally much improved	Combat veterans
Blake (1986)	3	Doxepin Imipramine	Decreased startle, dysphoria, nightmares; improved concentration	Civilians with acute PTSD
Bleich et al. (1986)	27	Amitriptyline (14) Doxepin (7) Maprotiline (2) Clomipramine (2) Phenelzine (2)	Good or moderate global improvement; improved concentration; decreased nightmares, stuttering (25/27) Poor response	Israeli combat veterans; minimal substance abuse (2/25)
Lerer et al. (1987)	25	Phenelzine	Modest improvement in sleep, intrusive recollection, nightmares; slight increase in flashbacks	Israeli combat veterans without history of substance abuse; no clinically significant remission; prospective study
Davidson et al. (1985)	11	Phenelzine	Marked improvement in flashbacks, intrusive recollection, estrangement; moderate improvement in sleep, nightmares, startle, guilt (7/11)	Combat veterans; prospective study
Shestatzky et al. (1988)	13	Phenelzine	No clinically significant response compared to placebo	Israeli combat veterans; 4-week trial; crossover design
Davidson et al. (1988)	46	Amitriptyline	Diminished depression	Combat veterans; placebo-controlled study
Reist et al. (1989)	18	Desipramine	Decrease in depressive symptoms; no changes in anxiety and other PTSD symptoms	Combat veterans; 4-week, double-blind, crossover, placebo-controlled study

and the 4-week length of their protocol. In a placebo-controlled study, David-son et al. (1990) showed that, in patients completing 8 weeks of treatment, amitriptyline was superior to placebo on the Hamilton Depression Scale (Hamilton 1960), the Hamilton Anxiety Scale (Hamilton 1959), the Clinical Global Impression Severity Scale and the Impact of Event Scale (IES) (Horowitz et al. 1979). There was, however, no evidence for amitriptyline effects on the Structured Interview for PTSD. In a 4-week, double-blind, placebo-controlled, crossover study, Reist et al. (1989) found that desipra-mine administration resulted only in reduction of depressive symptoms, without significant improvement of the overall PTSD symptomatology. The brief (4-week) administration of desipramine may account for their negative findings.

In the open-trial studies that did find medications to be beneficial, the small sample sizes and the dearth of rigorously measured outcome data leave many questions unanswered. Beyond the obvious problem of knowing how many of the apparent drug effects reflect spontaneous healing or placebo response, these studies do not address the problems of which aspects of PTSD may or may not respond to antidepressants, which class of antidepres-sant may be most effective, and whether coexisting anxiety or depressive disorders influence the drug effects. Only Blake's (1986) report offered any information about the possible use of antidepressants in acute rather than chronic PTSD. The largest studies all concern combat trauma specifically, limiting the extrapolation of the findings to other groups, particularly post-traumatic syndromes in women or children.

Design of the Current Study

The current study is a trial of either a TCA (imipramine) or an MAOI (phenelzine) for chronic PTSD in Vietnam veterans. Our design entails random assignment of subjects to one of the active drugs or placebo groups, with both subject and research clinician blind to the treatment condition. Our initial assessment includes quantification of traumatic events using the Combat Scale (Egendorf et al. 1981) and diagnosis of concurrent psychiatric illness by the Research Diagnostic Criteria (RDC) (Spitzer et al. 1978) using the Schedule for Affective Disorders and Schizophrenia (Endicott and Spitzer 1978). We diagnosed PTSD according to DSM-III-R (American Psychiatric Association 1987) criteria, using a portion of the Structured Clinical Interview for DSM-III-R (Spitzer and Williams 1985) for system-atic rating. The diagnosis is confirmed by an independent interview for which we have data showing excellent interrater reliability. In addition, baseline symptoms are rated on the Covi Anxiety Scale (Covi and Lipman 1984), the Raskin Scale for Depression (Raskin et al. 1969), and the IES. The IES is a well-established scale for measuring the symptoms of PTSD. It includes two eight-item subscales for intrusion and avoidance symptoms. We rated subjects weekly on the Covi Scale, Raskin Scale, and IES and made a global assessment at the end of the study using a five-point scale to rate symptom change as "none," "worse," or three levels of "improved."

We conducted this study through a Vietnam Veterans Outreach Center, and all subjects were male, outpatient Vietnam veterans. Subjects with current substance abuse (use of illicit drugs or heavy drinking within the past month) were excluded, as were subjects with a prior history of schizophrenia or bipolar disorder. Subjects with other concurrent psychiatric disorders were included. All gave informed consent before participating.

Of the 46 subjects screened, 10 refused to participate in the study or were excluded from the protocol for substance abuse, and 36 were randomly assigned to an 8-week trial of imipramine, phenelzine, or placebo. Of these 36, 2 dropped out within the first week, leaving 34 (11 placebo, 12 imipramine, and 11 phenelzine) for data analysis. Retention, which is a critical issue in antidepressant studies because of the length of time it takes for the drugs to have their full effect, was adequate in our study (mean ± SEM stay, 6.4 ± 0.3 weeks), with no significant differences across the three groups. All patients completed a minimum of 3 weeks of medication.

To summarize the relevant demographic and diagnostic data on our study population, the mean (± SEM) age was 38 ± 2 years, 15% were nonwhite, and all had combat scale scores above 3, which indicates substantial combat exposure (range, 3 to 14). Age, baseline symptoms, and severity of trauma were similar across the study groups. Although none had major depression, 15 (44%) had minor depression by RDC or dysthymia in DSM-III-R; 21 (62%) had a past history of substance abuse for at least 1 month before enrolling.

Medication was prescribed at the accepted dosage levels for treatment of depression (Glassman and Perel 1978; Robinson et al. 1978). For imipramine we aimed for a target dose of 200 to 300 mg/day and attained blood levels of about 150 ng/ml using individualized dosage adjustment. The target dose of phenelzine was 60 to 75 mg/day, enough to inhibit >90% of platelet monoamine oxidase activity (measured in week two). An independent physician reviewed the results and ordered appropriate changes in the number of 50-mg imipramine or 15-mg phenelzine pills to achieve the desired blood levels, which were measured again after the change. This physician also ordered changes in the number of pills taken by "yoked" placebo subjects. In this study, the mean (± SD) maximal dose of imipramine was 240 ± 40 mg/day and of phenelzine 71 ± 9 mg/day. The placebo group was given a mean maximal dose of 5.1 ± 0.3 pills/day. This was not significantly different from the mean number of pills taken by the imipramine group (4.8 pills) or the phenelzine group (4.7 pills), supporting the maintenance of the double-blind throughout the trial. Two subjects on imipramine and one each on phenelzine and placebo were maintained on chronic benzodiazepines—three on 15 mg/day of diazepam and one on 4 mg/day of alprazolam—but no other drug or medication use occurred during the study.

Results

Neither the Raskin depression score nor the Covi anxiety score decreased significantly on medication, relative to placebo (Table 14-2). However, the specific symptoms of PTSD measured by the IES declined significantly in the medicated groups, and rose in the placebo group, with the phenelzine group showing the greatest effect, a drop from 22 to 9 on the intrusion subscale ($F = 9.8$, 1/33 df, $P < .004$; contrast for phenelzine versus placebo plus imipramine). The avoidance subscale of the IES dropped, but not significantly, in both the phenelzine (19 to 11) and imipramine (19 to 14) groups. On the global assessment, the combined imipramine (75%) and phenelzine (64%) groups demonstrated significantly more improvement than placebo (27%) ($\chi^2 = 5.4$, $P < .05$). When the four subjects on benzodiazepines were excluded, findings were unchanged on the IES ($F = 6.5$, $P < .005$) and on the global assessment ($\chi^2 = 5.8$, $P < .05$). Improvement typically appeared within 3 to 4 weeks, with early effects on sleep and irritability.

Case Studies

The following case studies illustrate the quality of a good treatment response.

Case 1

ER is a 39-year-old, divorced, white veteran, currently employed. He completed high school and was trying to become a professional baseball player when he was drafted at age 19. ER served in Vietnam during 1967–1968 as an army medic, and he was wounded twice during his tour of duty. He participated in the Tet offensive, which involved many casualties, and described seeing truckloads of dead bodies doused with diesel fuel and burned.

On admission to the study, ER was experiencing intrusive thoughts about the war, vivid recollections stimulated by the smell of diesel fuel, and disturbed sleep with nightmares. Although steadily employed, he was extremely socially isolated, living alone and spending hours in his bedroom with the air conditioner on "enjoying the white noise and blanking out everything."

After randomization, ER received imipramine. In a week, he reported sound, restful sleep for the first time since leaving Vietnam. By the third week, he stated he felt generally more hopeful and less anxious. During week

Table 14-2. Posttraumatic stress disorder symptoms, depression, anxiety, and clinical global assessment changes with antidepressant treatment

Scale	Imipramine (n = 12)		Phenelzine (n = 11)		Placebo (n = 11)		F/χ^{2a}	P^b
	pre	post	pre	post	pre	post		
Impact of Event Scale (mean ± SEM)	40 ± 4.1	30 ± 4.6	41 ± 3.9	20 ± 4.1	35 ± 3.7	36 ± 4.3	7.0	<.003
Intrusion	21 ± 2.8	16 ± 4.3	22 ± 3.4	9 ± 2.8	19 ± 3.1	20 ± 2.7	6.2	<.006
Avoidance	19 ± 2.6	14 ± 1.9	19 ± 1.7	11 ± 1.8	16 ± 2.0	16 ± 2.5	2.7	<.08
Raskin Scale for Depression (mean ± SEM)	7.7 ± 0.8	6.4 ± 0.9	8.6 ± 0.8	6.6 ± 0.9	8.7 ± 1.1	8.3 ± 1.2	0.7	NS
Covi Anxiety Scale (mean ± SEM)	4.8 ± 0.4	4.2 ± 0.5	5.6 ± 0.7	4.3 ± 0.7	6.0 ± 1.1	6.6 ± 1.4	0.9	NS
Clinical global assessment (% improved)	—	75	—	64	—	27	5.7	<.06

[a] Ratio for repeated measures analysis of variance using "time by medication" interaction across the three medication groups (2/31 df).
[b] NS = not significant.

five, he became tearful describing the responsibilities of a medic—telling some wounded men to keep fighting and others to go to the rear. He began seeing a counselor at the Veterans Outreach Center to discuss these feelings further. ER's combat nightmares disappeared by the eighth week, and he also reported he had become the coordinator of his condominium association. Although the job involved many petty aggravations, he joked about it and seemed to enjoy interacting with his neighbors. ER elected to remain on imipramine after completing the study. At one year, he reports continued restful sleep with thoughts about the war "more in the background."

Case 2

MC is a 38-year-old, divorced, white, sporadically employed veteran who served in Vietnam during 1968–1969 as a helicopter crew chief in the army. His father had been an Air Force pilot during World War II, and MC enlisted after completing high school. During his tour of duty, he was frequently in combat and was shot down three times—the last time he was the only survivor of his crew. MC used heroin and opium in Vietnam, and in the last few months of his tour he was grounded, forbidden to leave his fire base or carry a weapon.

At screening, MC described pervasive sleep disturbance, nightmares, intrusive thoughts about the war, hyperarousal with exaggerated startle response and hypervigilance, and explosive aggressive reactions. He felt guilty about the period of disciplinary action when "I could have been doing more." He had had many jobs since the war and several intimate relationships that ended because of his ragefulness. He was living in relative isolation in the woods and stated that he always felt "driven up by people. I can't do any of the normal things people do every day without flying into a rage and wanting to hurt someone."

MC, who had a 17-year history of alcohol abuse, entered the study after achieving a full year of sobriety. He was randomized to phenelzine treatment, and he reported improvement in all phases of sleep after the first week. At the second visit, although he complained of mild dry mouth and light-headedness, he said he felt rested for the first time since returning from Vietnam. MC's sleep continued to improve, and by week four he said that while he still felt angry, he could control his behavior. Over the next several weeks, his mood continued to improve, and he reported less difficulty working with people on his job. He was less irritable and had to push himself less to get to work.

Throughout the study, MC participated in weekly group therapy, and after 8 weeks he chose to continue taking 75 mg of phenelzine daily. He tapered the medication about a year later, with return of his sleep disturbance and hyperactivity.

CONCLUSIONS

Although no single study can answer all the outstanding questions about the role of antidepressants in the treatment of PTSD, our findings indicate that both TCAs and MAOIs are superior to placebo in relieving intrusive symptoms such as flashbacks, unwanted recollections, and nightmares, as well as in improving global symptomatology. Although we studied a different TCA than did Davidson et al. (1988), we also found that avoidance symptoms such as emotional numbing, loss of feelings for others, or suppression of memory are relatively refractory. This differential efficacy for intrusive and avoidance symptoms, originally reported in case studies, merits further research.

Our work begins to address questions about the effect of comorbid psychopathology on treatment response. The issue is clinically important, given the high rates of other disorders, especially depression (40% to 70%) and substance abuse (40% to 83%), reported in patients with PTSD (Davidson et al. 1985; Helzer et al. 1987; Sierles et al. 1985; Wolf et al. 1987) and in our sample. To determine the effect of these conditions on response to treatment requires a large sample stratified by coexisting diagnoses. Unfortunately, our preliminary findings are based on too few subjects for such analysis and must be considered tentative. Although 44% of our subjects had dysthymia, none met criteria for major depression, suggesting that a severe depressive syndrome is not necessary for treatment response. Our failure to find significant differences in ratings of depressive symptoms between subjects and controls gives further weight to the specificity of the drug effects for PTSD symptoms other than depressed mood. Davidson et al. (1988) similarly concluded that, at least in younger combat veterans, the antidepressants significantly ameliorate posttraumatic symptoms but not depressive ones. The conclusion that a simple antidepressant response does not account for the efficacy of either TCAs or MAOIs in PTSD is particularly interesting in light of neurophysiologic and endocrinologic studies, suggesting that PTSD and major depression are biologically distinct (Mason et al. 1986). Further work on this disorder and the neurobiologic correlates of treatment may expand our knowledge of the action of these "antidepressant" medications.

We are cautious about generalizing our conclusions to more typical clinical populations with PTSD, many of whom have a more acute onset and less chronic course than do the subjects participating in our protocol. Our patients had experienced their trauma as long as 20 years ago, and many did not develop symptoms until several years after leaving the military. Furthermore, 26% (12 of 46) of those we screened refused to participate, either because of general refusal of medication, inability to forego substance abuse, or intolerance of side effects. Antidepressant treatment may not be acceptable or possible for everyone with PTSD. Even successful antidepressant therapy does not address the emotional numbing and social alienation associated with the disorder. Individual, group, and family therapies still constitute important treatment modalities for these and other aspects of PTSD, especially the destruction of patients' worldview and self-concept so well described by Horowitz (1974), Lifton (1973), and others.

In sum, although some studies do not support the view that antidepressants are efficacious in relieving the symptoms of chronic PTSD (Reist et al. 1989; Shestatzky et al. 1988), our research findings indicate that both TCAs and MAOIs are of significant benefit in the treatment of this disorder. Despite possible theoretical differences in the mechanism of action between various classes of TCAs, amitriptyline and imipramine (and presumably their derivatives) seem similarly effective. The recommended dosage range is similar to that used in the treatment of depression, and adjusting the dose according to blood level may be of value in patients who do not respond to typical doses of tricyclics. A fully adequate trial of medication would last for 8 weeks, and patients who do not respond to one class of drugs may respond to another. The choice of TCA or MAOI should be based on the patient's tolerance for the particular side effects and dietary restrictions of each type of drug. No reliable information is yet available about the appropriate duration of medical treatment when effective, so that patients who elect to discontinue taking antidepressants should be monitored for symptomatic relapse.

REFERENCES

American Psychiatric Association: Diagnostic and Statistical Manual of Mental Disorders, 3rd Edition. Washington, DC, American Psychiatric Association, 1980

American Psychiatric Association: Diagnostic and Statistical Manual of Mental Disorders, 3rd Edition, Revised. Washington, DC, American Psychiatric Association, 1987

Birkheimer LJ, DeVane CL, Muniz CE: Posttraumatic stress disorder: characteristics and pharmacological response in the veteran population. Compr Psychiatry 26:304–310, 1985

Blake DJ: Treatment of acute posttraumatic stress disorder with tricyclic antidepressants. South Med J 79:201–204, 1986

Bleich A, Siegel B, Garb R, et al: Post-traumatic stress disorder following combat exposure: clinical features and psychopharmacological treatment. Br J Psychiatry 149:365–369, 1986

Burstein A: Treatment of flashbacks by imipramine. Psychosomatics 25:683–687, 1984

Covi L, Lipman RS: Primary depression or primary anxiety: a possible psychosomatic approach to a diagnostic dilemma. Clin Neuropharmacol 7:S501, 1984

Davidson JRT, Swartz M, Storck M, et al: A diagnostic and family study of post-traumatic stress disorder. Am J Psychiatry 142:90–93, 1985

Davidson J, Walker JI, Kilts C: A pilot study of phenelzine in the treatment of post-traumatic stress disorder. Br J Psychiatry 150:252–255, 1988

Davidson J, Kudler H, Smith R, et al: Treatment of post traumatic stress disorder with amitriptyline: a double-blind study. Arch Gen Psychiatry 47:259–266, 1990

Egendorf A, Kadushin C, Laufer RS, et al: Legacies of Vietnam: Comparative Adjustment of Veterans and Their Peers, Vol 4. Washington, DC, U.S. Government Printing Office, 1981

Endicott J, Spitzer RS: A diagnostic interview: the Schedule for Affective Disorders and Schizophrenia. Arch Gen Psychiatry 35:837–844, 1978

Falcon S, Ryan C, Chamberlain K, et al: Tricyclics: possible treatment for posttraumatic stress disorder. J Clin Psychiatry 46:385–388, 1985

Glassman AH, Perel JM: Tricyclic blood levels and clinical outcome: a review of the art, in Psychopharmacology: A Generation of Progress. Edited by Lipton MA, DiMascio A, Killiam KF. New York, Raven, 1978

Hamilton M: The assessment of anxiety states by rating. Br J Med Psychol 32:50–55, 1959

Hamilton M: A rating scale for depression. J Neurol Neurosurg Psychiatry 23:56–62, 1960

Helzer JE, Robins LN, McEvoy L: Post-traumatic stress disorder in the general population: findings of the epidemiological catchment area survey. N Engl J Med 317:1630–1634, 1987

Hogben GL, Cornfield RB: Treatment of traumatic war neuroses with phenelzine. Arch Gen Psychiatry 38:440–445, 1981

Horowitz M: Stress response syndromes: character style and dynamic psychotherapy. Arch Gen Psychiatry 31:768–781, 1974

Horowitz M, Wilner N, Alvarez W: Impact of Event Scale: a measure of subjective distress. Psychosom Med 41:209–218, 1979

Kitchner I, Greenstein R: Low dose lithium carbonate in the treatment of post traumatic stress disorder. Milit Med 150:378–381, 1985

Kolb LC: The place of narcosynthesis in the treatment of chronic and delayed stress reactions of war, in The Trauma of War: Stress and Recovery in Viet Nam Veterans. Edited by Sonnenberg SM, Blank AS Jr, Talbott JA. Washington, DC, American Psychiatric Press, 1985, pp 211–226

Kolb LC: A neuropsychological hypothesis explaining posttraumatic stress disorders. Am J Psychiatry 144:989–995, 1987

Kolb LC, Burris BC, Griffiths S: Propranolol and clonidine in treatment of the chronic post-traumatic stress disorders of war, in Post-Traumatic Stress Disorder: Psychological and Biological Sequelae. Edited by van der Kolk BA. Washington, DC, American Psychiatric Press, 1984, pp 97–105

Lerer B, Bleich A, Kotler M, et al: Posttraumatic stress disorder in Israeli combat veterans: effects of phenelzine treatment. Arch Gen Psychiatry 44:976–981, 1987

Levenson H, Lanman R, Rankin M: Traumatic war neurosis and phenelzine. Arch Gen Psychiatry 39:1345, 1982

Lifton RJ: Home from the War: Vietnam Veterans, Neither Victims nor Executioners. New York, Simon & Schuster, 1973

Lipper S, Davidson JRT, Grady TA, et al: Preliminary study of carbamazepine in post-traumatic stress disorder. Psychosomatics 27:849–854, 1986

Marshall JR: The treatment of night-terrors associated with the post-traumatic syndrome. Am J Psychiatry 132:293–295, 1975

Mason JW, Giller EL, Kosten TR, et al: Urinary free-cortisol levels in posttraumatic stress disorder patients. J Nerv Ment Dis 174:145–149, 1986

Mellman TA, Davis GC: Combat-related flashbacks in posttraumatic stress disorder: phenomenology and similarity to panic attacks. J Clin Psychiatry 46:379–382, 1985

Milanes FJ, Mack CN, Dennison J, et al: Phenelzine treatment of post-Vietnam stress syndrome. VA Practitioner, June 1984, pp 40–49

Pitman RK, Orr SP, Forgue DF, et al: Psychophysiologic assessment of posttraumatic stress disorder imagery in Vietnam combat veterans. Arch Gen Psychiatry 44:970–975, 1987

Raskin A, Schulterbrandte J, Reating N, et al: Replication of factors of psychopathology in interview, ward behavior and self-report ratings of hospitalized depressives. J Nerv Ment Dis 148:87–98, 1969

Reist C, Kauffman CD, Haier RJ, et al: A controlled trial of desipramine in 18 men with posttraumatic stress disorder. Am J Psychiatry 146:513–520, 1989

Robinson DS, Nies A, Ravaris CL, et al: Clinical psychopharmacology of phenelzine: MAO activity and clinical response, in Psychopharmacology: A Generation of Progress. Edited by Lipton MA, DiMascio A, Killiam KF. New York, Raven, 1978, pp 961–973

Shen WW, Park S: The use of monamine oxidase inhibitors in the treatment of traumatic war neurosis. Milit Med 148:430–431, 1983

Shestatzky M, Greenberg D, Lerer B: A controlled trial of phenelzine in posttraumatic stress disorder. Psychiatry Res 24:149–155, 1988

Sierles FS, Chen J, McFarland RT: Posttraumatic stress disorder and concurrent psychiatric illness: a preliminary report. Am J Psychiatry 140:1177–1179, 1985

Spitzer RL, Williams JBW: Structured Clinical Interview for DSM-III-R. New York, New York State Psychiatric Institute, 1985

Spitzer R, Endicott J, Robins E: Research Diagnostic Criteria: rationale and reliability. Arch Gen Psychiatry 35:773–782, 1978 van der Kolk BA: Psychopharmacological issues in posttraumatic stress disorder. Hosp Community Psychiatry 34:683–684, 691, 1983

Walker JI: Chemotherapy of traumatic war stress. Milit Med 147:1029–1033, 1982

White NS: Post-traumatic stress disorder (letter). Hosp Community Psychiatry 34:1061–1062, 1983

Wolf ME, Alavi A, Mosnaim AD: Pharmacological interventions in post traumatic stress disorder. Research Communications in Psychology, Psychiatry and Behavior 12:169–176, 1987

Wolf ME, Alavi A, Mosnaim AD: PTSD in Vietnam veterans: clinical and EEG findings: possible therapeutic effects of carbamazepine. Biol Psychiatry 23:642–644, 1988

Yost J: The psychopharmacologic treatment of the delayed stress syndrome in Vietnam veterans, in Post-Traumatic Stress Disorders in the Vietnam Veteran: Observations and Recommendations for the Psychological Treatment of the Veteran and His Family. Edited by Williams T. Cincinnati, OH, Disabled American Veterans, 1980

Chapter 15

Carbamazepine in the Treatment of Posttraumatic Stress Disorder: Implications for the Kindling Hypothesis

Steven Lipper, M.D., Ph.D.

P harmacologic agents from a number of drug classes have been suggested to have clinical utility in the treatment of posttraumatic stress disorder (PTSD), particularly the tricyclic antidepressants and the monoamine oxidase inhibitors.

Among the tricyclic antidepressants, amitriptyline (Bleich et al. 1986; Falcon et al. 1985), imipramine (Blake 1986; Burstein 1984; Falcon et al. 1985), doxepin (Bleich et al. 1986; Falcon et al. 1985; White 1983), and desipramine (Falcon et al. 1985; Kauffman et al. 1987) have most frequently been reported to reduce symptomatology in patients with PTSD. However, these reports represent anecdotal observations, uncontrolled studies, and/or retrospective chart reviews that contain small numbers of patients. Additionally, rating scales, except for occasional use of the Impact of Event Scale (Horowitz et al. 1979, 1980), were generally not used, so that efficacy was usually assessed according to the investigators' global clinical impressions. A randomized, placebo-controlled, double-blind study of 12 patients found that imipramine treatment produced significant improvement on the intrusion subscale of the Impact of Event Scale (Frank et al. 1988). On the other hand, a double-blind study comparing amitriptyline to placebo in 46 veterans with chronic PTSD found no differences between treatments on a PTSD rating scale and an equivocal difference favoring amitriptyline on the Impact of Event Scale (Davidson et al. 1990). In a 4-week, double-blind study comparing the administration of desipramine with placebo in combat veterans, Reist et al. (1989) found that antidepressant treatment resulted only in reduction of depressive symptoms, without improvement of the overall PTSD symptomatology. Heterogeneity of the PTSD patient population (Reist et al. 1989) and length of treatment (Frank et al. 1988) may account for the variable findings in the literature on antidepressant efficacy in the treatment of PTSD.

Investigations subsequent to the initial report of Hogben and Cornfeld (1981), who observed favorable therapeutic responses to the monoamine oxidase inhibitor phenelzine in five patients with PTSD, have yielded results for phenelzine similar to those reported for the tricyclic antidepressants. Anecdotal reports (Levenson et al. 1982; Shen and Park 1983; Walker 1982) and small, uncontrolled studies (Davidson et al. 1987; Milanes et al. 1984) have indicated reductions in PTSD symptomatology following treatment with phenelzine. A placebo-controlled, randomized, double-blind study of 11 patients determined that phenelzine was significantly more effective than either imipramine or placebo in reducing PTSD symptoms, as measured on the intrusion subscale of the Impact of Event Scale (Frank et al. 1988). However, troublesome side effects, such as intensification of preexisting sleep disturbance, dizziness, and erectile failure, may limit the clinical utility of phenelzine or other monoamine oxidase inhibitors (Davidson et al. 1987) even if the efficacy of these agents were to be demonstrated in larger double-blind, placebo-controlled trials. Furthermore, the largest ($N = 25$) open, prospective study of phenelzine in PTSD found that while this agent may produce partial or transient symptomatic improvement, clinically significant remission was not achieved (Lerer et al. 1987).

In addition to the tricyclic antidepressants and phenelzine, lithium (Kitchner and Greenstein 1985) and the adrenergic-blocking agents clonidine and propranolol (Kolb et al. 1984) have been reported to ameliorate PTSD symptomatology in small, uncontrolled trials. Benzodiazepines have also been suggested to have clinical utility (Friedman 1988; van der Kolk 1987), and a retrospective review of the charts of 20 PTSD patients who had received alprazolam reported global improvement in 16 patients (Feldmann 1987). However, in addition to the absence of prospective, well-controlled studies of benzodiazepines with suitable rating scales, concerns about the use of benzodiazepines in the treatment of PTSD seem warranted because of the possibility of psychological and physical dependence, tolerance, benzodiazepine abuse, concomitant abuse of alcohol or other substances, episodes of disinhibition or paradoxical reactions, and withdrawal reactions (Juergens and Morse 1988).

In the absence of generally accepted and unequivocally effective pharmacotherapy, the prescription of medications to patients with PTSD has often been empirical and sometimes idiosyncratic. Additionally, treatment may be directed toward ameliorating possibly secondary or ancillary symptoms, such as anxiety, depression, avoidance, and rage, rather than toward what may be hypothesized to be the more "fundamental" or "core" experience of PTSD—namely the reexperiencing of the original trauma in memories, dreams, and flashbacks. These limitations in available pharmacologic treatments for PTSD, in conjunction with the work of Post and his colleagues (Post 1977; Post and Kopanda 1976) in the development of a kindling model for psychiatric disorders, led Lipper et al. (1986) to begin to study the efficacy of the tricyclic anticonvulsant carbamazepine in PTSD.

According to a kindling model (Post 1977; Post and Kopanda 1976), cumulative bioelectric changes, especially in the limbic area and secondary to repeated biochemical or psychological stresses, could result in abnormal limbic or neuronal sensitization and major psychiatric disturbances. Since the sine qua non of PTSD is "a recognizable stressor that would evoke significant symptoms of distress in almost everyone" (American Psychiatric Association 1980, p. 238), Lipper et al. (1986) speculated that a kindling model might be applicable to PTSD. As an extension of that idea, they further hypothesized that carbamazepine, which had been found to be effective in bipolar disorder (Okuma 1983; Post and Uhde 1985), might also be effective in the treatment of PTSD, particularly in ameliorating the "re-experiencing" symptoms, which tend to be repetitive and to recur under stress and which may be considered "kindled" or paroxysmal (Garbutt and Loosen 1983) phenomena.

Clinical trials of carbamazepine in PTSD also appeared worthwhile because of reports of improvement in a wide variety of psychiatric symptoms, many of which may occur as part of the clinical profile of individual patients with PTSD. In 40 published reports concerned with 2,500 epileptic patients, Ballenger and Post (1978) found that 50% improved psychiatrically while being treated with carbamazepine. In particular, they found improvement in the "affective" symptoms of mood instability, irritability, fits of anger, and states of anxiety and depression. Additionally, in phasic disorders of epilepsy, carbamazepine often seemed to result in dramatic improvement in a large percentage (33% to 90%) of patients, even without a reduction of seizures. Of particular interest, their literature review contained reports of favorable responses to carbamazepine in patients with behavioral problems and nonspecific electroencephalographic abnormalities in the absence of overt evidence of epilepsy (e.g., patients with gross psychopathology, especially with violent behavior). In such patients, carbamazepine had been said to decrease aggressiveness, emotional lability, agitation, restlessness, irritability, depression, hypo- and hyperactivity, and difficulties in social adaptation.

Although subsequent confirmatory reports from two independent groups of investigators have noted symptomatic improvement in carbamazepine-treated PTSD patients, particularly in regard to flashbacks (Brodsky et al. 1987) and poor impulse control and violent behavior or angry outbursts (Wolf et al. 1988), the preliminary work of Lipper et al. (1986) is, to date, the only study in which carbamazepine has been systematically evaluated in patients meeting DSM-III (American Psychiatric Association 1980) criteria for PTSD. The latter study[1] is reviewed and critically examined in the following sections of this chapter.

SUBJECTS

Ten inpatients completed a 5-week open trial of carbamazepine in the treatment of PTSD. All patients met DSM-III criteria for PTSD and were also evaluated for the presence of coexisting psychiatric disorders with DSM-III, the Schedule of Affective Disorders and Schizophrenia (Endicott and Spitzer 1978), Research Diagnostic Criteria (Spitzer et al. 1978), and the

---

[1]Material and tables, which have been revised, expanded, or updated, are reprinted from Lipper S, Davidson JRT, Grady TA, et al., *Psychosomatics* 27:849–854, 1986, with permission from the American Psychiatric Press, on behalf of the Academy of Psychosomatic Medicine.

Minnesota Multiphasic Personality Inventory (Hathaway and McKinley 1943). Nine patients, ages 32 to 39 years (mean $\pm$ SD = 36.2 $\pm$ 2.1), were Vietnam-era veterans; one, age 59, had served during the Korean War. Five were black and five were white. All patients but one had engaged in combat activities for at least 8 months, the longest duration being 18 months. The exception was a Vietnam-era veteran whose military stressor was not combat related. Military records of all 10 patients were obtained to verify length of overseas military service and, when possible, to corroborate combat duty.

Of the 10 patients, 4 had recent and 4 others had earlier histories (more than 1 to 5 years previously) of alcohol abuse with or without dependence; 2 had remote histories of drug abuse. Every patient had a personality disorder diagnosable by DSM-III, Research Diagnostic Criteria, and/or Minnesota Multiphasic Personality Inventory criteria: antisocial ($n = 2$), borderline ($n = 1$), narcissistic ($n = 1$), schizotypal ($n = 1$), or mixed ($n = 5$) with paranoid, antisocial, and/or borderline features. Apart from alcohol abuse and PTSD, an additional DSM-III Axis I diagnosis could be made for only one patient, that of generalized anxiety disorder in the Korean War veteran.

Among the medications with which the 10 patients had previously been treated, with variable therapeutic results, were: amitriptyline ($n = 2$), desipramine ($n = 1$), doxepin ($n = 1$), imipramine ($n = 1$), trazodone ($n = 1$), phenelzine ($n = 2$), alprazolam ($n = 3$), chlordiazepoxide ($n = 1$), hydroxyzine ($n = 1$), chlorpromazine ($n = 1$), fluphenazine ($n = 1$), loxapine ($n = 1$), perphenazine ($n = 1$), thioridazine ($n = 3$), thiothixene ($n = 1$), trifluoperazine ($n = 1$), and propranolol ($n = 1$).

In addition to the 10 patients whose results are reported here, 2 other subjects participated in the study. Carbamazepine was discontinued after 2 weeks in one patient who developed an erythematous, pruritic rash necessitating his withdrawal from the study. The second patient's military history could not be verified from official records and, in conjunction with observed behavior and unreliability, this inconsistency led to a diagnosis of factitious PTSD (Lynn and Belza 1984; Sparr and Pankratz 1983) and to the exclusion of his data from consideration.

METHODS

Each patient received a complete physical examination and underwent a series of baseline laboratory studies including a complete blood count with differential platelet and reticulocyte counts, serum iron, electrolytes, kidney and liver function tests, and a urinalysis. These tests were repeated after 1, 3, and 5 weeks of carbamazepine treatment. Prior to participation in the study, each patient also received an electrocardiogram and a sleep-deprived electroencephalogram with nasopharyngeal leads.

All patients provided written informed consent to participate in the study after the nature of the procedures had been fully explained. Prior to treatment with carbamazepine, patients were tapered off all psychotropic medication in accordance with standard clinical practice. Three patients who had been consuming alcohol excessively had successfully completed an alcohol withdrawal program before being considered for entry into the study. All patients had been drug-free for at least 1 week prior to initial assessment on rating scales. During the subsequent 5 weeks of carbamazepine treatment, patients received no other psychotropic medication, including hypnotic agents.

Before starting carbamazepine treatment and at weekly intervals thereafter, all patients were evaluated by a single rater on the Hamilton Rating Scale for Depression (Hamilton 1960), the Montgomery-Åsberg Depression Rating Scale (Montgomery and Åsberg 1979), the Hamilton Anxiety Scale (Hamilton 1959), the Brief Psychiatric Rating Scale (Overall and Gorham 1962), the Clinical Global Impression Scale (Guy 1976), and the PTSD Checklist. The PTSD Checklist is an unpublished scale consisting of the 12 symptoms listed in categories B, C, and D of the DSM-III diagnostic criteria for PTSD. Ratings for each of the 12 symptoms were on a 5-point scale (0, absent; 1, mild; 2, moderate; 3, severe; 4, very severe), with a total scoring range of 0 to 48. These severity ratings were based on the interviewer's clinical impression, derived from prior experience with veterans with PTSD.

On the same days on which interviews were conducted for rating purposes, each patient also completed seven self-report instruments to record subjective impressions: the Beck Depression Inventory (Beck et al. 1961), the IPAT Anxiety Scale (Cattell 1976), the Impact of Event Scale, the Zuckerman Sensation Seeking Scale (Zuckerman 1974), the Symptom Checklist-90 (SCL-90) (Derogatis et al. 1973), the Profile of Mood States (McNair et al. 1971), and a National Institute of Mental Health (NIMH) self-rating scale (van Kammen and Murphy 1975) devised for the assessment of antidepressant and activating drugs and their side effects.

Patients also completed a somatic symptom checklist and a PTSD Index. The PTSD Index is an unpublished rating scale containing 11 symptoms: dreams about combat, unwanted memories of combat, flashbacks, loss of temper, almost becoming violent, becoming violent, acting as if in combat, startle response, survivor guilt, avoidance of reminders, and becoming upset by reminders. The patients rated each symptom for both frequency and severity or intensity. For the purpose of this study, frequency was recorded as the number of days, from 0 to 7, during the preceding week, on which a particular symptom had occurred. Severity or intensity was recorded as the "average" magnitude of each symptom, during the preceding week, on a 6-point scale (0, absent; 1, very mild; 2, mild; 3, moderate; 4, severe; 5, very severe). The somatic symptom checklist is an unpublished tabulation of 39 items designed to reflect possible somatic and behavioral side effects of carbamazepine, on a 3-point scale (0, absent; 1, minimal; 2, marked).

After baseline laboratory tests and clinical ratings had been completed, oral carbamazepine was prescribed at a dose of 200 mg twice on the first day and three times daily for the next 6 days. Thereafter, the total daily dose of carbamazepine was adjusted after each weekly serum level to maintain serum carbamazepine levels between 5.0 and 10.0 μg/ml.

Comparisons of baseline data with corresponding values after 5 weeks of carbamazepine treatment were made with paired, two-tailed t-tests except for analyses of data from the PTSD Checklist, the PTSD Index, and the Clinical Global Impression scale, which could not be assumed to be normally distributed. To analyze data from the latter scales, two-tailed Wilcoxon matched-pairs signed-ranks tests (Siegel 1956) were employed. Statistical significance was accepted at the .05 level.

RESULTS

All laboratory studies, including the baseline sleep-deprived electroencephalograms with nasopharyngeal leads, were within normal limits throughout the course of the study. During the week prior to the study when all patients were drug-free, no change in their clinical condition was observed.

The mean daily doses of carbamazepine during each of the 5 weeks of treatment were: 577.1, 617.1, 637.1, 694.3, and 780.0 mg. The maximum daily dose prescribed was 1,000 mg. The mean serum concentrations of carbamazepine after each week of treatment were: 9.7, 8.2, 7.5, 7.3, and 8.4 μg/ml, with a range of 5.2 to 13.6 μg/ml.

The means of the total scores for all patients on the interviewer-rated PTSD Checklist (Table 15-1) and on the patient-rated PTSD Index for both frequency and intensity of symptoms (Table 15-2) were significantly lower after 5 weeks of carbamazepine treatment. The three individual items on the PTSD Checklist that were significantly improved, as compared with baseline, were recurrent and intrusive recollections, recurrent dreams, and sleep disturbance. On the PTSD Index, three symptoms were significantly reduced in both frequency and severity after carbamazepine treatment: dreams about combat, flashbacks, and becoming upset by reminders. Unlike recurrent and intrusive recollections on the PTSD Checklist, unwanted (intrusive) memories of combat as self-rated by patients on the PTSD Index were not significantly different after carbamazepine treatment. The mean score for the intrusive items, but not the avoidant items, on the Impact of Event Scale decreased significantly after carbamazepine treatment (Table 15-3).

The frequency but not the severity of "almost becoming violent" was

Table 15–1. Interviewer-rated scales: mean (± SD) scores before and after 5 weeks of treatment with carbamazepine ($N = 10$)

Rating scale	Pretreatment	Posttreatment
PTSD Checklist		
Total score (0–48)	26.1 ± 5.3	16.7 ± 7.5**
Individual items (0–4):		
Recurrent and intrusive recollections	2.8 ± 0.9	1.3 ± 1.2*
Recurrent dreams	3.1 ± 0.7	1.1 ± 1.3**
Acting as if the event were recurring	0.5 ± 1.0	0.3 ± 0.7
Loss of interest	1.9 ± 1.3	1.3 ± 1.1
Detachment	2.4 ± 0.7	1.6 ± 0.8
Constricted affect	1.0 ± 0.0	0.8 ± 0.4
Startle response	2.2 ± 0.4	1.8 ± 1.0
Sleep disturbance	2.9 ± 0.7	1.1 ± 0.7**
Survivor guilt	2.5 ± 0.9	1.8 ± 1.5
Poor memory	2.2 ± 1.0	1.6 ± 1.2
Avoidance	2.2 ± 0.9	1.9 ± 1.2
Symptoms intensification	2.4 ± 0.5	2.1 ± 1.0
Hamilton Rating Scale for Depression (0–74)	25.3 ± 7.2	16.5 ± 6.9**
Hamilton sleep items (initial, middle, and delayed insomnia; 0–6)	5.2 ± 1.1	1.6 ± 1.1***
Montgomery-Åsberg Depression Rating Scale (0–60)	25.8 ± 5.4	19.2 ± 10.4
Hamilton Anxiety Scale (0–56)	22.1 ± 4.8	13.1 ± 5.6**
Brief Psychiatric Rating Scale (18–126)	34.2 ± 7.5	26.7 ± 8.5**
Clinical Global Impression		
Severity (1–7)	4.7 ± 0.8	3.4 ± 1.1*
Improvement (1–6)	5.0 ± 0.0	2.6 ± 1.2**

Note. Numbers in parentheses indicate the range of possible mean scores.
* $P < .05$. ** $P < .01$. *** $P < .001$.
Source. Adapted from Lipper et al. 1986, with permission of the American Psychiatric Press, on behalf of the Academy of Psychosomatic Medicine. Copyright 1986.

significantly reduced according to mean PTSD Index scores (Table 15-2). While only two patients reported "becoming violent" during the week prior to treatment, and statistical significance was not achieved, this item was rated as zero at the end of the study. Also, the mean hostility subscale score on the SCL-90 (Table 15-3) was significantly decreased after carbamazepine treatment.

No statistically significant differences in mean depression ratings after carbamazepine treatment were found on the Montgomery-Åsberg Depression Rating Scale (Table 15-1), the Beck Depression Inventory (Table 15-3),

Table 15–2. Self-rating PTSD Index: mean (± SD) scores before and after 5 weeks of treatment with carbamazepine ($N = 10$)

	Number of days (0–7)		Severity or intensity (0–5)	
	Pretreatment	Posttreatment	Pretreatment	Posttreatment
Total score	3.8 ± 1.5	2.8 ± 1.3*	2.9 ± 0.7	2.0 ± 1.1*
Dreams about combat	3.9 ± 2.2	1.8 ± 2.3**	3.8 ± 0.9	1.9 ± 1.8*
Unwanted memories of combat	4.8 ± 2.2	4.6 ± 2.2	3.4 ± 1.1	2.7 ± 1.3
Flashbacks	5.2 ± 2.1	2.0 ± 1.5**	3.9 ± 1.0	2.1 ± 1.7**
Loss of temper	2.3 ± 2.5	1.5 ± 2.2	2.0 ± 1.4	1.3 ± 1.6
Almost violent	2.7 ± 2.1	1.4 ± 1.8*	2.6 ± 1.3	1.7 ± 1.8
Becoming violent	0.3 ± 0.7	0.0 ± 0.0	0.7 ± 1.5	0.0 ± 0.0
Acting as if in combat	2.0 ± 3.0	1.8 ± 2.1	1.9 ± 2.1	1.8 ± 1.6
Startle response	4.0 ± 3.0	4.0 ± 3.6	3.1 ± 0.6	3.0 ± 1.3
Survivor guilt	5.6 ± 2.3	4.8 ± 2.7	3.5 ± 0.9	2.7 ± 1.7
Avoidance of reminders	5.0 ± 2.8	4.8 ± 2.9	2.9 ± 1.5	2.4 ± 1.7
Upset by reminders	5.7 ± 2.2	3.3 ± 2.5*	3.9 ± 0.7	2.5 ± 1.8*

* $P < .05$. ** $P < .01$.
Source. Adapted from Lipper et al. 1986, with permission of the American Psychiatric Press, on behalf of the Academy of Psychosomatic Medicine. Copyright 1986.

the SCL-90 (Table 15-3), the Profile of Mood States (Table 15-4), and the NIMH self-rating scale (Table 15-4). While mean scores on the Hamilton Rating Scale for Depression were significantly reduced, most of this reduction could be attributed to a marked improvement on sleep items (see Table 15-1).

Anxiety was significantly reduced after carbamazepine treatment as rated on the Hamilton Anxiety Scale (Table 15-1), the "overt" subscale of the IPAT Anxiety Scale, and the SCL-90 (Table 15-3), but not as rated on the Profile of Mood States and the NIMH self-rating scale (Table 15-4).

Global improvement over baseline clinical status was statistically significant on the Brief Psychiatric Rating Scale (Table 15-1), the severity and improvement subscales of the Clinical Global Impression scale (Table 15-1), and the total SCL-90 score (Table 15-3).

The only other symptoms that were statistically significantly reduced

Table 15–3. Self-rating scales: mean (± SD) scores before and after 5 weeks of treatment with carbamazepine ($N = 10$)

Rating scale	Pretreatment	Posttreatment
Impact of Event Scale		
Intrusive items (0–21)	18.6 ± 2.2	14.5 ± 3.1***
Avoidant items (0–24)	18.3 ± 2.6	16.2 ± 5.1
Beck Depression Inventory (0–63)	26.3 ± 13.8	19.6 ± 14.0
IPAT Anxiety Scale		
Covert (0–40)	23.7 ± 5.1	22.4 ± 6.3
Overt (0–40)	30.6 ± 5.1	25.3 ± 9.2*
Symptom Checklist-90		
Total score (0–4)	2.0 ± 0.8	1.5 ± 1.0*
Somatization (0–4)	1.3 ± 0.9	0.9 ± 0.8*
Obsessive-compulsive (0–4)	2.5 ± 1.1	2.0 ± 1.3
Interpersonal sensitivity (0–4)	1.9 ± 0.9	1.5 ± 1.1
Depression (0–4)	2.4 ± 0.9	1.9 ± 1.3
Anxiety (0–4)	2.4 ± 1.0	1.6 ± 1.2*
Hostility (0–4)	1.9 ± 1.1	1.3 ± 1.2*
Phobic anxiety (0–4)	1.4 ± 0.8	1.0 ± 1.1
Paranoid ideation (0–4)	2.1 ± 1.1	1.7 ± 1.1
Psychoticism (0–4)	2.0 ± 0.9	1.3 ± 1.0*

Note. Numbers in parentheses indicate the range of possible mean scores.
* $P < .05$. *** $P < .001$.
Source. Adapted from Lipper et al. 1986, with permission of the American Psychiatric Press, on behalf of the Academy of Psychosomatic Medicine. Copyright 1986.

were somatization and psychoticism on the SCL-90 and confusion-bewilderment on the Profile of Mood States. No significant differences from baseline were found on the NIMH self-rating scale or on the Zuckerman Sensation Seeking Scale (Table 15-4).

The frequency and intensity of self-reported somatic symptoms over baseline levels at the end of 5 weeks of carbamazepine treatment are presented in Table 15-5. Headache and tremor, both of mild intensity, were the somatic symptoms most frequently ($n = 4$) reported to have increased over baseline levels.

Of the 10 patients studied, 7 were considered to have responded "moderately" to "very much" according to the Clinical Global Impression scale. Alternatively, if one defines carbamazepine responsiveness as at least a 30% reduction in the total scores on both the PTSD Index (either frequency or severity) and on the PTSD Checklist, 6 of 10 patients can be designated as "responders." Furthermore, if one specifically examines the "intrusive" symptoms (i.e., dreams, flashbacks, and recollections) on both the PTSD

Table 15–4. Additional self-rating scales: mean ($\pm$ SD) scores before and after 5 weeks of treatment with carbamazepine ($N = 10$)

Rating scale	Pretreatment	Posttreatment
Profile of Mood States		
Total score (0–200)	107.3 $\pm$ 45.9	83.2 $\pm$ 64.6
Tension-anxiety (0–36)	23.8 $\pm$ 7.8	20.1 $\pm$ 11.0
Depression-dejection (0–60)	35.4 $\pm$ 14.7	27.5 $\pm$ 19.0
Confusion-bewilderment (0–28)	17.2 $\pm$ 6.8	13.0 $\pm$ 9.0*
Vigor-activity (0–32)	9.1 $\pm$ 4.3	9.0 $\pm$ 5.8
Anger-hostility (0–48)	24.4 $\pm$ 11.5	18.9 $\pm$ 13.7
Fatigue-inertia (0–28)	15.6 $\pm$ 6.6	12.7 $\pm$ 8.6
NIMH self-rating scale		
Activation-euphoria (0–6)	1.6 $\pm$ 1.0	1.5 $\pm$ 1.3
Anxiety (0–6)	3.5 $\pm$ 1.7	2.8 $\pm$ 2.0
Depressive affect (0–6)	3.2 $\pm$ 1.9	2.7 $\pm$ 2.5
Dysphoria (0–6)	2.9 $\pm$ 1.6	2.8 $\pm$ 2.1
Altered self-reality (0–6)	2.5 $\pm$ 1.7	2.3 $\pm$ 2.1
Functional deficit (0–6)	3.1 $\pm$ 1.6	2.8 $\pm$ 2.3
Zuckerman Sensation Seeking Scale		
General (0–22)	9.1 $\pm$ 3.6	9.4 $\pm$ 4.2
Thrill/adventure seeking (0–14)	7.2 $\pm$ 4.9	8.4 $\pm$ 4.6
Experience seeking (0–18)	6.7 $\pm$ 2.8	6.1 $\pm$ 3.5
Disinhibition (0–14)	5.2 $\pm$ 2.0	4.5 $\pm$ 2.7
Boredom susceptibility (0–18)	7.4 $\pm$ 1.3	7.4 $\pm$ 2.6

Note. Numbers in parentheses indicate the range of possible mean scores.
* $P < .05$.
Source. Adapted from Lipper et al. 1986, with permission of the American Psychiatric Press, on behalf of the Academy of Psychosomatic Medicine. Copyright 1986.

Index and the PTSD Checklist, 7 of 10 patients had a 50% reduction on at least two of these three symptoms. With regard to rate of response to carbamazepine, some patients improved gradually during the 5 weeks of treatment, whereas others improved markedly after 1 week, with further but incrementally less response thereafter.

Discussion

Interpretation of the results of this study, as with any open study, is limited by the absence of a placebo-controlled, double-blind design. Responses to items on both self-rating and interviewer-rated scales may have potentially been confounded by a patient's desire for disability benefits or compensation. The latter difficulty is inherent, unfortunately, even in establishing a diagnosis of PTSD, since the majority of DSM-III criteria require accurate and

Table 15–5. Changes in self-reported symptoms during the fifth week of carbamazepine treatment in comparison with those reported prior to medication ($N = 10$)

Symptom	n	Average severity (0–2)
Headache	4	1.3
Tremor	4	1.0
Increased urinary frequency	4	1.3
Tiredness, poor memory, aching in legs, increased appetite, things taste different	3 [a]	1.0 [a]
Poor appetite	2	1.5
Constipation	2	1.5
Dizziness, weakness, clumsiness, stiffness, slurred speech, double vision, heart pounding, nausea	2 [a]	1.0 [a]
Unsteadiness in walking, blurred vision, stomachache, diarrhea, difficulty urinating, decreased libido, increased libido	1 [a]	1.0 [a]

[a] For each symptom.
Source.   Adapted from Lipper et al. 1986, with permission of the American Psychiatric Press, on behalf of the Academy of Psychosomatic Medicine. Copyright 1986.

unfalsified reporting of subjective symptoms by patients. In future studies, the use of objective assessment devices that include behavioral and physiologic measurements might enhance the reliability and validity of PTSD diagnoses (Malloy et al. 1983). In the present study, corroboration of the occurrence of a significant stressor required for a diagnosis of PTSD was attempted, insofar as was possible, from military records, and Minnesota Multiphasic Personality Inventory profiles were evaluated for characteristics reported to be confirmatory for the presence of PTSD (Fairbank et al. 1983, 1985, Keane et al. 1984). That all patients in the study met diagnostic criteria for a personality disorder and all but one had a history of alcohol abuse is not unexpected in view of reports of the frequent coexistence of PTSD with other psychopathology (Davidson et al. 1985; Sierles et al. 1983).

A notable difficulty in evaluating the efficacy of a psychopharmacologic treatment for PTSD is the absence of reliable, validated rating scales. The Impact of Event Scale is an exception, but does not address several symptoms frequently reported by combat veterans. Consequently, the interviewer-rated PTSD Checklist and the patient-rated PTSD Index were devised to assess symptomatic changes in response to pharmacologic treatment more comprehensively. The lack of reliability and validity assessments for these scales, which are important components of the present study, constitutes a possibly important limitation.

It should also be emphasized that even when the diagnosis is relatively unequivocal, PTSD is a complex disorder with symptoms that can be organized around three dimensions—reexperiencing, avoidance and numbing, and physiologic arousal—in addition to the frequent presence of other psychiatric disorders, including alcohol dependence, other substance abuse, and personality disorders. These are but a few of the factors that contribute to the heterogeneity existing among patients with PTSD and that make a universally effective treatment for PTSD unlikely to be found. Even from a solely biologic point of view, different neuroanatomic and neurophysiologic elements probably subserve different clinical features of PTSD. Consequently, it is perhaps not realistic to expect that a single psychotropic medication will alleviate all symptoms and features of PTSD. At best, psychotropic medication may alleviate some of the more prominent and distressing symptomatology and facilitate the possibility of further therapeutic benefit through psychological, behavioral, and social therapies.

It is conceivable that the kindling model advanced by Post (1977) and Post and Kopanda (1976) to explain the efficacy of carbamazepine in psychiatric disorders, particularly bipolar disorder (Ballenger and Post 1978, 1980; Post and Uhde 1985), may be applicable also to PTSD in view of the apparently selective effects of carbamazepine in ameliorating intrusive as contrasted with avoidant symptoms of PTSD in this study. All biologic research to date is consistent with the hypothesis that chronic PTSD is a hyperarousal state associated with excessive sympathetic nervous activity (Friedman 1988). Just as endogenous catecholamines might kindle limbic nuclei, thereby producing schizophrenic or biopolar psychoses (Post and Kopanda 1976), so too might the chronic hyperarousal observed in PTSD patients kindle limbic nuclei to produce a relatively stable neurobiologic alteration (Friedman 1988).

On both the PTSD Checklist and the PTSD Index, carbamazepine treatment was associated with a significant reduction in the frequency and/ or intensity of combat dreams, flashbacks, and intrusive recollections, coincident with a significant reduction in the mean score for intrusive but not avoidant items on the Impact of Event Scale. These particular intrusive symptoms can also be construed as "reexperiencing" phenomena, whether occurring during sleep (dreams) or wakefulness (intrusive recollections or flashbacks). According to a kindling hypothesis for PTSD, the initial psychologically traumatic event or events produce biochemical or bioelectric changes in the central nervous system, possibly within the limbic system, that result in abnormal neuronal sensitization and a resultant increased susceptibility (or lowered threshold) to psychic and physiological arousal during experiential states in which the original trauma or traumata are reevoked (e.g., in recollections, in dreams, or in environmentally similar circumstances). Carbamazepine's effects in the present study are consistent with such a formulation, whereby an anti-kindling or threshold-elevating effect of the medication may have been responsible for a selective amelioration of the intrusive or reexperiencing symptoms of PTSD.

Alternatively, carbamazepine seems to be effective in some paroxysmal disorders, such as trigeminal neuralgia, that do not appear to result from a kindling process, and carbamazepine's effects in the present study may represent an amelioration of paroxysmal phenomena in PTSD. Other current neurobiologic hypotheses (Burges Watson et al. 1988) consider that PTSD may represent a conditioned emotional response (Kolb 1984, 1987; Kolb and Mutalipassi 1982) or correspond to the behavioral sequelae of inescapable shock in animals (van der Kolk et al. 1985).

It is important to remember that baseline sleep-deprived electroencephalograms with nasopharyngeal leads were within normal limits for all patients in this study. This finding was corroborated in an independent study of 18 Vietnam veterans with PTSD, all of whose electroencephalograms, while asleep or awake, were found to be within normal limits (Wolf et al. 1988). In both studies, all patients had normal neurological examinations, and none presented symptoms of temporal lobe epilepsy. Consequently, it is not possible to attribute the clinical responses observed with carbamazepine in this study to alleviation of temporal lobe epilepsy (Devinsky and Bear 1984) or, in view of the patients' clinical profiles and histories, to treatment of temporal lobe syndrome (Blumer et al. 1988) in the absence of frank seizures. Flashbacks in patients with apparent PTSD and concomitant evidence of temporal lobe epilepsy, demonstrable by electroencephalogram and/or neuropsychological testing, have been reported to be responsive to carbamazepine (Brodsky et al. 1987).

The significant reduction in frequency and the (nonsignificant) decrease in intensity of self-reports of "almost becoming violent," along with both the absence of violent behavior during the study and a significant reduction on the hostility subscale of the SCL-90, are concordant with clinical observations of ward nursing staff who independently noted fewer and less serious instances of such behavior than usual. This impression of reduced hostility, aggressiveness, and violence-prone behavior was gained also in an independent study, in which eight Vietnam veterans with PTSD received carbamazepine in open fashion; according to staff observations and patients' self-reports, carbamazepine was especially useful in assisting the patients to exercise impulse control and in preventing violent behavior or angry outbursts (Wolf et al. 1988). Several small studies (Hakola and Laulumaa 1982; Luchins 1983; Mattes 1984; Neppe 1982) have reported a decreased incidence of aggressive or violent behavior among psychotic individuals receiving carbamazepine, a finding that is also consistent with the results of the present study from which psychotic patients were excluded. Additionally, carbamazepine has been found to produce a clear and dramatic reduction in the frequency and severity of episodes of behavioral dyscontrol in a small group of outpatient women with borderline personality disorder, characterized by prominent affective symptoms and serious behavioral dyscontrol (Cowdry and Gardner 1988).

Despite the similarity of the chemical structure of carbamazepine to that of imipramine, the antidepressant effect of carbamazepine was not evident on five of the six depression rating scales employed in the study. The significant reduction in Hamilton Rating Scale for Depression scores was largely attributable to this scale's characteristic of disproportionately weighting sleep difficulties in relation to other items. If confirmed, the improvement in sleep and reduction in the frequency and intensity of combat nightmares in association with carbamazepine may warrant further encephalographic study. Little is currently known about the possible effects of carbamazepine on the stages of sleep (Hasan et al. 1980; Jovanovic 1974), during any of which traumatic nightmares may occur (Fisher et al. 1970; van der Kolk et al. 1984).

Anxiety was significantly reduced during carbamazepine treatment on three of five scales, suggesting some anxiolytic activity of the medication. However, it is not clear whether this is a primary effect or secondary to reductions in reexperiencing symptomatology. Carbamazepine has been found to lack efficacy in the treatment of panic disorder (Uhde et al. 1988).

Carbamazepine treatment was not associated with significant changes on any of the five subscales of the Zuckerman Sensation Seeking Scale. This was an expected finding, since sensation seeking is considered to be largely a trait-dependent rather than a state-dependent characteristic of individuals. Furthermore, the mean baseline scores of the PTSD patients on the subscales do not seem to differ substantially from those of college undergraduates and high school students (Zuckerman 1975). In fact, the means for the patients are somewhat lower, suggesting that sensation seeking and possibly "impulsivity" were not characteristics of the PTSD patients who participated in this study. Further research is necessary to clarify whether this is broadly true of veterans suffering from PTSD.

In terms of global improvement, 7 of the 10 patients studied had improved after 5 weeks of treatment with carbamazepine. Furthermore, 9 of the 10 patients who participated in the study requested to continue taking carbamazepine after discharge. The lone exception was the Korean War veteran, who had a generalized anxiety disorder in addition to PTSD; he subsequently responded well to chlordiazepoxide. Unfortunately, many of the patients were lost to follow-up. Of the five for whom posthospital information is available, three resumed drinking and discontinued carbamazepine, and two stopped taking carbamazepine because of side effects (e.g., rash). Consequently, this study can shed no light on the long-term effectiveness of carbamazepine in the treatment of PTSD.

In conclusion, the present uncontrolled study suggests that carbamazepine might be of therapeutic benefit in the treatment of PTSD, with selective efficacy in ameliorating the symptoms concerned with re-experiencing the original trauma: nightmares, flashbacks, and intrusive recollections. If these findings are confirmed under placebo-controlled, double-blind conditions, important support might be afforded to the kindling hypothesis of PTSD.

REFERENCES

American Psychiatric Association: Diagnostic and Statistical Manual of Mental Disorders, 3rd Edition. Washington, DC, American Psychiatric Association, 1980

Ballenger JC, Post RM: Therapeutic effects of carbamazepine in affective illness: a preliminary report. Communications in Psychopharmacology 2:159–175, 1978

Ballenger, JC, Post RM: Carbamazepine in manic depressive illness: a new treatment. Am J Psychiatry 137:782–790, 1980

Beck A, Ward C, Mendelson M, et al: An inventory for measuring depression. Arch Gen Psychiatry 42:667–675, 1961

Blake DJ: Treatment of acute posttraumatic stress disorder with tricyclic antidepressants. South Med J 79:201–204, 1986

Bleich A, Seigel B, Garb R, et al: Post-traumatic stress disorder following combat exposure: clinical features and psychopharmacological treatment. Br J Psychiatry 149:365–369, 1986

Blumer D, Heilbronn M, Himmelhoch J: Indications for carbamazepine in mental illness: atypical psychiatric disorder or temporal lobe syndrome? Compr Psychiatry 29:108–122, 1988

Brodsky L, Doerman AL, Palmer LS, et al: Post traumatic stress disorder: a trimodal approach. Psychiatr J Univ Ottawa 12:41–46, 1987

Burges Watson IP, Hoffman L, Wilson GV: The neuropsychiatry of post-traumatic stress disorder. Br J Psychiatry 152:164–173, 1988

Burstein A: Treatment of post-traumatic stress disorder with imipramine. Psychosomatics 25:681–687, 1984

Cattell RB: The IPAT Anxiety Scale Questionnaire. Champaign, IL, Institute for Personality and Ability Testing, 1976

Cowdry RW, Gardner DL: Pharmacotherapy of borderline personality disorder: alprazolam, carbamazepine, trifluoperazine, and tranylcypromine. Arch Gen Psychiatry 45:111–119, 1988

Davidson J, Swartz M, Storck M, et al: A diagnostic and family study of post traumatic stress disorder. Am J Psychiatry 142:90–93, 1985

Davidson J, Walker JI, Kilts C: A pilot study of phenelzine in the treatment of posttraumatic stress disorder. Br J Psychiatry 150:252–255, 1987

Davidson J, Kudler H, Smith R, et al: Treatment of post traumatic stress disorder with amitriptyline and placebo. Arch Gen Psychiatry 47:259–266, 1990

Derogatis LR, Lipman RS, Covi L: SCL-90: an outpatient psychiatric rating scale: preliminary report. Psychopharmacol Bull 9:13–18, 1973

Devinsky O, Bear D: Varieties of aggressive behavior in temporal lobe epilepsy. Am J Psychiatry 141:651–656, 1984

Endicott J, Spitzer RL: A diagnostic interview: the Schedule for Affective Disorders and Schizophrenia. Arch Gen Psychiatry 35:837–844, 1978

Fairbank JA, Keane TM, Malloy PF: Some preliminary data on the psychological characteristics of Vietnam veterans with posttraumatic stress disorders. J Consult Clin Psychol 51:912–919, 1983

Fairbank JA, McCaffrey RJ, Keane TM: Psychometric detection of fabricated symptoms of post traumatic stress disorder. Am J Psychiatry 142:501–503, 1985

Falcon S, Ryan C, Chamberlain K, et al: Tricyclics: possible treatment for post traumatic stress disorder. J Clin Psychiatry 46:385–389, 1985

Feldmann TB: Alprazolam in the treatment of post traumatic stress disorder (letter). J Clin Psychiatry 48:216–217, 1987

Fisher C, Byrne J, Edwards A, et al: A psychophysiological study of nightmares. J Am Psychoanal Assoc 18:747–782, 1970

Frank JB, Kosten TR, Giller EL, et al: A randomized clinical trial of phenelzine and imipramine for post traumatic stress disorder. Am J Psychiatry 145:1289–1291, 1988

Friedman MJ: Toward rational pharmacotherapy for post traumatic stress disorder: an interim report. Am J Psychiatry 145:281–285, 1988

Garbutt JC, Loosen PT: Is carbamazepine helpful in paroxysmal behavior disorders? Am J Psychiatry 140:1363–1364, 1983

Guy W: ECDEU Assessment Manual for Psychopharmacology (DHEW Publ No 76-338). Washington, DC, U.S. Government Printing Office, 1976

Hakola HPA, Laulumaa VA: Carbamazepine in treatment of violent schizophrenics. Lancet 1:1358, 1982

Hamilton M: The assessment of anxiety states by rating. Br J Med Psychol 32:50–55, 1959

Hamilton M: A rating scale for depression. J Neurol Neurosurg Psychiatry 23:56–62, 1960

Hasan J, Bjorkqvist K, Bjorkqvist S-E, et al: Treatment of sleep disturbances during alcohol withdrawal with carbamazepine (Tegretol®). Abstract of paper presented at the 11th annual Nordic Meeting on Biological Alcohol Research, 1980

Hathaway SR, McKinley JC: Minnesota Multiphasic Personality Inventory. Minneapolis, MN, University of Minnesota, 1943

Hogben GL, Cornfeld RB: Treatment of traumatic war neurosis with phenelzine. Arch Gen Psychiatry 38:440–445, 1981

Horowitz M, Wilner N, Alvarez W: Impact of Event Scale: a measure of subjective distress. Psychosom Med 41:209–218, 1979

Horowitz MJ, Wilner N, Kaltreider N, et al: Signs and symptoms of post traumatic stress disorder. Arch Gen Psychiatry 37:85–92, 1980

Jovanovic UJ: Categories of psychotropic drug effects on sleep EEG and EOG. Act Nerv Super (Praha) 16:209–210, 1974

Juergens SM, Morse, RM: Alprazolam dependence in seven patients. Am J Psychiatry 145:625–627, 1988

Kauffman CD, Reist C, Djenderedjian A, et al: Biological markers of affective disorders and post traumatic stress disorder: a pilot study with desipramine. J Clin Psychiatry 48:366–367, 1987

Keane TM, Malloy P, Fairbank JA: Empirical development of an MMPI subscale for the assessment of combat-related post traumatic stress disorder. J Consult Clin Psychol 52:888–891, 1984

Kitchner I, Greenstein R: Low dose lithium carbonate in the treatment of post traumatic stress disorder: brief communication. Milit Med 150:378–381, 1985

Kolb LC: The post traumatic stress disorders of combat: a subgroup with a conditioned emotional response. Milit Med 149:237–253, 1984

Kolb LC: A neuropsychological hypothesis explaining post traumatic stress disorder. Am J Psychiatry 144:989–995, 1987

Kolb LC, Mutalipassi LR: The conditioned emotional response: a sub-class of the chronic and delayed post-traumatic stress disorder. Psychiatric Annals 12:979–987, 1982

Kolb LC, Burris BC, Griffiths S: Propranolol and clonidine in the treatment of the chronic post-traumatic stress disorders of war, in Post-traumatic Stress Disorder: Psychological and Biological Sequelae. Edited by van der Kolk BA. Washington, DC, American Psychiatric Press, 1984, pp 97–105

Lerer B, Bleich A, Kotler M, et al: Post traumatic stress disorder in Israeli combat veterans. Effect of phenelzine treatment. Arch Gen Psychiatry 44:976–981, 1987

Levenson H, Lanman R, Rankin M: Traumatic war neurosis and phenelzine (letter). Arch Gen Psychiatry 39:1345, 1982

Lipper S, Davidson JRT, Grady TA, et al: Preliminary study of carbamazepine in post-traumatic stress disorder. Psychosomatics 27:849–854, 1986

Luchins DJ: Carbamazepine for the violent psychiatric patient. Lancet 1:766, 1983

Lynn J, Belza M: Factitious post traumatic stress disorder: the veteran who never got to Vietnam. Hosp Community Psychiatry 35:697–701, 1984

Malloy PF, Fairbank JA, Keane TM: Validation of a multimethod assessment of post traumatic stress disorder in Vietnam veterans. J Consult Clin Psychol 51:488–494, 1983

Mattes JA: Carbamazepine for uncontrolled rage outbursts. Lancet 2:1164–1165, 1984

McNair DM, Lorr M, Droppleman LF: EdITS Manual for the Profile of Mood States. San Diego, CA, Educational and Industrial Testing Service, 1971

Milanes FJ, Mack CN, Dennison J, et al: Phenelzine treatment of post Vietnam stress syndrome. VA Practitioner 1:40–49, 1984

Montgomery SA, Åsberg M: A new depression scale designed to be sensitive to change. Br J Psychiatry 134:382–389, 1979

Neppe VM: Carbamazepine in the psychiatric patient. Lancet 2:334, 1982

Okuma T: Therapeutic and prophylactic effects of carbamazepine in bipolar disorders. Psychiatr Clin North Am 6:157–174, 1983

Overall JE, Gorham DR: The Brief Psychiatric Rating Scale. Psychol Rep 10:799–812, 1962

Post RM: Clinical implications of a cocaine-kindling model of psychosis. Clin Neuropharmacol 2:25–42, 1977

Post RM, Kopanda RT: Cocaine, kindling, and psychosis. Am J Psychiatry 133:627–634, 1976

Post RM, Uhde TW: Carbamazepine in bipolar illness. Psychopharmacol Bull 21:10–17, 1985

Reist C, Kauffman CD, Haier RJ, et al: A controlled trial of desipramine in 18 men with posttraumatic stress disorder. Am J Psychiatry 146:513–520, 1989

Shen WW, Park S: The use of monoamine oxidase inhibitors in the treatment of traumatic war neurosis: case report. Milit Med 148:430–431, 1983

Siegel S: Nonparametric Statistics for the Behavioral Sciences. New York, McGraw-Hill, 1956

Sierles FS, Chen J-J, McFarlane RE, et al: Post traumatic stress disorder and concurrent psychiatric illness: a preliminary report. Am J Psychiatry 140:1177–1179, 1983

Sparr L, Pankratz LD: Factitious post traumatic stress disorder. Am J Psychiatry 140:1016–1019, 1983

Spitzer RL, Endicott J, Robins E: Research Diagnostic Criteria: rationale and reliability. Arch Gen Psychiatry 35:773–782, 1978

Uhde TW, Stein MB, Post RM: Lack of efficacy of carbamazepine in the treatment of panic disorder. Am J Psychiatry 145:1104–1109, 1988

van der Kolk BA: The drug treatment of post-traumatic stress disorder. J Affective Disord 13:203–213, 1987 van der Kolk B, Blitz R, Burr W, et al: Nightmares and trauma: a comparison of nightmares after combat with lifelong nightmares in veterans. Am J Psychiatry 141:187–190, 1984

van der Kolk B, Greenberg M, Boyd H, et al: Inescapable shock, neurotransmitters, and addiction to trauma: toward a psychobiology of post traumatic stress. Biol Psychiatry 20:314–325, 1985

van Kammen DP, Murphy DL: Attenuation of the euphoriant and activating effects of d- and l-amphetamine by lithium carbonate treatment. Psychopharmacologica 44:215–224, 1975

Walker JI: Chemotherapy of traumatic war stress. Milit Med 147:1029–1033, 1982

White NS: Post traumatic stress disorder (letter). Hosp Community Psychiatry 34:1061–1062, 1983

Wolf ME, Alavi A, Mosnaim AD: Post traumatic stress disorder in Vietnam veterans: clinical and EEG findings: possible therapeutic effects of carbamazepine. Biol Psychiatry 23:642–644, 1988

Zuckerman M: The sensation-seeking motive, in Progress in Experimental Personality Research, Vol 7. Edited by Maher B. New York, Academic, 1974

Zuckerman M: Manual and Research Report for the Sensation Seeking Scale (SSS). Newark, DE, University of Delaware, 1975

Chapter 16

Interrelationships Between Biological Mechanisms and Pharmacotherapy of Posttraumatic Stress Disorder

Matthew J. Friedman, M.D., Ph.D.

It is no longer controversial whether there are biologic alterations associated with posttraumatic stress disorder (PTSD). During the past 5 years, a growing body of research findings has shown that patients with PTSD exhibit abnormalities in sympathetic nervous system arousal, in hypothalamic-pituitary-adrenocortical (HPA) axis function, in the endogenous opioid system, and in the physiology of sleep and dreaming (Friedman 1988, in press; van der Kolk 1987). Psychopharmacologic approaches to PTSD have progressed at a slower pace. Results from the few controlled drug trials that have been published to date are contradictory with respect to the efficacy and specificity of the drugs under consideration.

In this overview, I will evaluate the current status of basic and clinical research on PTSD and will show that biologic approaches to the diagnosis and treatment of PTSD clearly complement more traditional psychological approaches. In addition, I will focus on the most common concurrent psychiatric diagnoses associated with PTSD to determine whether such clinical comorbidities can be understood in terms of the pathophysiology of PTSD. Specifically, I will address biologic issues pertinent to the co-occurrence of PTSD and comorbid diagnoses such as alcoholism, drug abuse and dependency, personality disorders, major depression, and panic disorder. I will also review the current status of psychopharmacologic research on PTSD with regard to antidepressants, antipanic/anxiolytics, carbamazepine, lithium, and neuroleptics.

METHODOLOGICAL CONSIDERATIONS

Before evaluating the current status of work in the field, it is useful to reflect on three methodological issues specifically pertinent to PTSD: 1) PTSD can be produced in the clinical laboratory; 2) there are animal models of PTSD; and 3) PTSD comorbidities raise important questions about the relationship between PTSD and frequently associated disorders.

PTSD in the Clinical Laboratory

The hallmark of PTSD is a conditioned emotional response to meaningful stimuli that evoke thoughts, memories, and feelings uniquely associated with the trauma itself (Kolb 1987). Therefore, subjects with PTSD can be provoked to recreate a full-blown PTSD episode in a controlled laboratory setting by exposure to traumagenic stimuli. In the case of combat veterans with PTSD, a variety of traumagenic stimuli have reliably produced psychophysiologic arousal states that clearly differentiate PTSD patients from other groups of subjects. Traumagenic stimuli successfully employed in such experiments have included audiotapes of combat sounds (Blanchard et al. 1982), visual slides of Vietnam combat scenes (Malloy et al. 1983), videotape excerpts from the movie *Platoon* (Pitman et al. 1988), and autobiographical traumatic anecdotes read to the subject by the experimenter (Pitman et al. 1987). For this reason, it is methodologically possible to conduct A-B-A (off-on-off) experimental designs with PTSD patients in which various biologic (and psychological) parameters are monitored before, during, and after exposure to traumagenic stimuli. Such an approach should be the standard for laboratory biologic research on PTSD. Laboratory procedures for provoking and diagnosing PTSD are reviewed elsewhere (Friedman, in press).

Animal Models for PTSD

Van der Kolk et al. (1985) proposed that the animal model of learned helplessness to inescapable shock may be directly applicable to PTSD. Certainly the primacy of the Pavlovian paradigm, in which a conditioned stimulus becomes a sufficient condition for eliciting intense emotional arousal in experimental animals, suggests that this model may be much more applicable to PTSD than to affective disorders, as suggested by Siever and Davis (1985). Furthermore, the stimulus-driven behavior of PTSD can be explicated by classic psychological two-factor theory as originally proposed for traumatic avoidance learning in dogs by Solomon and Wynne (1954) and later extrapolated to traumatized war zone veterans by Keane et al. (1985). A recent comparison of inescapable versus escapable shock in rats suggests that the effect of the former condition is much more disruptive to learning through impairment of the hippocampal neural plasticity (Shores et al. 1989). Finally, van der Kolk (1987) and Friedman (1988) have independently hypothesized that chronic central sympathetic arousal in PTSD kindles limbic nuclei, thereby producing a stable neurobiologic abnormality. In other words, there is a wealth of psychological and neurobiologic theory and data that may be directly applicable to our understanding of PTSD. Furthermore, there are a number of well-developed animal research paradigms available for testing current clinical controversies about this disorder. Theoretical and animal models for PTSD are reviewed elsewhere (Kolb 1988; van der Kolk 1988).

PTSD Comorbidities

Other DSM-III-R (American Psychiatric Association 1987) psychiatric disorders are so frequently associated with PTSD that some have questioned whether PTSD itself is merely an artifact of observer bias (Behar 1987; Breslau and Davis 1987). Indeed, an epidemiologic survey of 2,348 Vietnam veterans (Kulka et al. 1988) demonstrated that 50% of veterans with a current diagnosis of PTSD had at least one other psychiatric disorder that met DSM-III (American Psychiatric Association 1980) criteria. Furthermore, within a self-selected Veterans Administration cohort of 107,107 patients seeking mental health treatment, at least one other diagnosis was reported in 80% of patients with PTSD (Friedman et al. 1987). Among the most frequent comorbid diagnoses are alcoholism, substance abuse or dependency, personality disorders, major depressive disorder (MDD), and panic disorder.

Such findings have obvious implications for research and treatment. First, since uncomplicated PTSD is such a rarity in clinical settings, any useful investigations must control for the likely co-occurrence of these other psychiatric disorders. Second, we must ask whether the co-occurrence of PTSD and, for example, MDD alters the biological expression of one or both disorders so that associated biological alterations indicate neither PTSD nor MDD but rather a hybrid of the two disorders. Finally, the clinical reality of comorbidities must be factored into psychopharmacological research on PTSD.

With this as a frame of reference, I will now review the relationship between PTSD and the most frequent comorbid diagnoses with respect to our emerging understanding of the pathophysiology of PTSD and possible implications for diagnosis and treatment.

PTSD AND CHEMICAL ABUSE AND DEPENDENCY

Published reports indicate that among clinical treatment-seeking cohorts, 60% to 80% of PTSD patients have concurrent diagnoses of alcohol or drug abuse or dependency (Branchey et al. 1984; Keane et al. 1988). An epidemiologic survey of Vietnam veterans reported that, among individuals currently suffering from PTSD, current and lifetime prevalence rates for alcoholism were 23% and 75%, respectively, and current and lifetime drug abuse or dependency rates were 6% and 23%, respectively (Kulka et al. 1988). Furthermore, Vietnam veterans with higher levels of war zone stress are more likely to exhibit chemical abuse or dependency than those who experienced considerably less combat exposure (Keane et al. 1988; Kulka et al. 1988). This latter finding suggests that neurobiological alterations associated with PTSD may make affected individuals more susceptible to alcohol and substance abuse or dependency.

Since patients with PTSD exhibit sympathetic hyperarousal both at baseline and especially following exposure to traumagenic stimuli (Friedman 1988; Kolb 1987; Pitman et al. 1988), it follows that any drug that can suppress adrenergic activity will produce temporary relief from PTSD intrusion and arousal symptoms. Therefore, self-medication with sedating drugs such as ethanol, marijuana, central depressants, or opiates should not be an unexpected behavioral consequence of PTSD. Furthermore, PTSD is associated with dysregulation of the endogenous opioid system, marked by lowered pain thresholds at rest and by stress-induced analgesia following exposure to traumagenic stimuli (Friedman, in press; Perry et al. 1987; Pitman et al. 1988). This suggests that PTSD patients may be biologically predisposed to reverse a chronic baseline endogenous opioid deficiency through self-medication with heroin, methadone, and other opiates.

In an elegant review of the biological basis for the comorbid occurrence of PTSD and chemical abuse or dependency, Kosten and Krystal (1988), invoking van der Kolk et al.'s (1985) inescapable shock model of PTSD, argued that the adrenergic arousal associated either with alcohol or opiate withdrawal will, itself, trigger a conditioned emotional response associated with PTSD symptoms during the vicious addiction-withdrawal cycle. They stated that the generic difficulties of treating any chemical dependency are amplified by the complex risk of exacerbating PTSD symptoms. It would appear, from this argument, that PTSD patients who are opiate addicts will be even more resistant to detoxification and rehabilitation than alcoholics, since the former addiction may reverse a chronic opioid deficiency associated with PTSD.

A final prediction from this hypothetical analysis is that PTSD patients will be less likely to self-medicate with cocaine, amphetamines, or other stimulants because such drugs will trigger sympathetic hyperarousal and thereby exacerbate PTSD intrusion and arousal symptoms. In my own clinical experience, PTSD patients tend to avoid central stimulants; this matter, however, has yet to be explored systematically.

To summarize, it is hypothesized that PTSD patients are especially susceptible to alcohol, marijuana, opiate, and central depressant abuse or dependency because of the biological abnormalities associated with their illness. This suggests that there may be a biologic basis for considering self-medication with such drugs a bona fide avoidant symptom of PTSD as originally proposed in DSM-III. With regard to treatment, it is clear that when PTSD and chemical abuse or dependency occur simultaneously, they must be treated simultaneously.

PTSD AND PERSONALITY DISORDERS

Among clinical treatment-seeking veteran cohorts, the co-occurrence of personality disorders with PTSD generally ranges between 40% and 60% (Boman 1986; Escobar et al. 1983; McFarland 1985; Sierles et al. 1983, 1986). Epidemiologic findings from the National Vietnam Veterans Readjustment Study showed a 20% lifetime prevalence rate of personality disorders among veterans who met DSM-III diagnostic criteria for PTSD (Kulka et al. 1988).

Lacking systematic, and especially longitudinal, studies on this matter, several issues come to mind that may be relevant to the biology of PTSD. First, presence of a personality disorder may predispose traumatized individuals to develop PTSD subsequently. Among the few studies on risk factors for PTSD, there is one report on traumatized Australian fire fighters showing higher neuroticism scores and greater prevalence of a personal history of psychiatric illness among individuals who later developed PTSD (McFarlane 1988). Other studies, however, show no such association (Friedman 1989).

Second, recent research on borderline personality disorder indicates that patients who carry this diagnosis have a high likelihood of having been physically and/or sexually traumatized during childhood (Herman et al. 1989; Zanarini et al. 1989). These data strongly suggest that patients with borderline personality disorder exposed to catastrophic stress during adulthood are actually being re-traumatized. If there are biologic alterations associated with borderline personality disorder and if they are similar to the abnormalities of PTSD, it follows that patients with borderline personality disorder may be especially vulnerable to developing PTSD following traumatic exposure.

Third, Cloninger (1987b) developed a systematic method for clinical description and classification of normal and abnormal personality variants in which he postulated an underlying genetic and neurobiological basis for the different personality disorders. Specifically, he proposed a tridimensional theory defined in terms of the basic stimulus-response characteristics of novelty seeking (dopaminergic), harm avoidance (serotonergic), and reward dependence (adrenergic). Some of his predictions regarding impulsivity, disinhibition, hostility, and type II alcoholism (Cloninger 1987a, 1987b) have been confirmed in patients with reduced central nervous system serotonergic function (Linnoila 1983, 1989). Such an approach obviously permits concurrent systematic investigation of PTSD and the various personality disorders to determine whether there is any overlap in observed biological abnormalities and whether such abnormalities in specific personality disorders might increase the risk for developing PTSD in traumatized individuals. In other words, such an approach provides a theoretical tool for understanding the high clinical comorbidity between PTSD and personality disorders.

PTSD AND MDD

Outpatient clinical cohorts show lifetime prevalence rates of MDD among PTSD patients ranging from 26% to 65% (Boman 1986; Escobar et al. 1983; Friedman et al. 1987; McFarland 1985). Epidemiologic data show that among Vietnam veterans with current PTSD, 20% meet DSM-III criteria for lifetime MDD (Kulka et al. 1988).

Table 16-1 shows that PTSD and MDD have many symptoms in com-

Table 16-1. Posttraumatic stress disorder and major depressive disorder: similarities

Dysphoria	Social withdrawal
Guilt	Insomnia
Grief	Decreased delta sleep
Anhedonia	Respond to tricyclic antidepressants
Irritability	Respond to monoamine oxidase inhibitors

mon. Indeed, one recent study's finding that 46% of hospitalized PTSD patients met DSM-III criteria for MDD (Reaves et al. 1989) is representative of other clinical reports. From the nosologic perspective of DSM-III-R, the major depression associated with PTSD is indistinguishable from the MDD observed in patients without PTSD. This is true both with regard to clinical symptomatology and with regard to responsivity to tricyclic antidepressants (TCAs) and to monoamine oxidase inhibitors (MAOIs). However, as will be shown below, this comparable psychopharmacologic responsivity may be more apparent than real.

As shown in Table 16-2, however, PTSD and MDD have a number of significant differences that can be detected using biological techniques. Psychophysiologic arousal provoked by exposure to traumagenic stimuli is the hallmark of PTSD and is unique to this disorder (Blanchard et al. 1982; Brende 1982; Dobbs and Wilson 1961; Gillespie 1942; Malloy et al. 1983; Pitman et al. 1987). Such traumagenic stimuli can produce a naloxone-reversible stress-induced analgesia in PTSD but not in MDD (Pitman et al. 1988, 1989). PTSD patients exhibit abnormally low beta-adrenergic binding in both intact lymphocytes and platelet membrane preparations as well as significant reductions in beta-adrenergic receptor-mediated cyclic adenosine monophosphate signal transduction (Lerer et al. 1987a), in contrast to depressed patients who characteristically exhibit up-regulation of beta-adrenergic receptors (Sulser et al. 1978). HPA function is reduced in PTSD and is excessive in depression as measured by the dexamethasone suppression test (DST), 24-hour urinary free cortisol levels, or serum cortisol levels (Halbreich et al. 1988; Kudler et al. 1987; Mason et al. 1986). Sleep research suggests that the sleep architecture in PTSD shows a different pattern of abnormalities than in MDD. Specifically, depressed patients exhibit reduced rapid eye movement (REM) latency, reduced delta sleep, and prolongation of the first REM period (Akiskal 1983; Dube et al. 1986; Kupfer and Thase 1983; Ross et al. 1990). On the other hand, most research to date suggests that PTSD patients exhibit excessive Stage 1 and Stage 2 sleep, reduced delta, reduced REM percentage, and increased REM latency (Friedman 1988; Kramer and Kinney 1985; Lavie et al. 1979; Schlossberg and Benjamin 1978). It should be noted, however, that some sleep researchers have observed sleep electroencephalogram findings in PTSD patients that look

Table 16-2. Posttraumatic stress disorder and major depressive disorder: differences

Posttraumatic stress disorder	Major depressive disorder
Stimulus-driven behavior	Not stimulus driven
Stress-induced analgesia	No stress-induced analgesia
Down-regulated beta-receptors	Up-regulated beta-receptors
HPA axis hypofunction	HPA axis hyperfunction
DST suppression	DST nonsuppression
Increased Stage 1 and Stage 2 sleep	Normal Stage 1 and Stage 2 sleep
Possible increased REM latency	Decreased REM latency
Probable decreased total REM period duration	Increased length first REM period
Responds to propranolol	Worsened by propranolol
Responds to carbamazepine	No response to carbamazepine
Responds to benzodiazepines	Worsened by benzodiazepines

Note: HPA = hypothalamic-pituitary-adrenal; DST = dexamethasone suppression test; REM = rapid eye movement.

much more like typical results in MDD (Greenberg et al. 1972; Kauffman et al. 1987; van Kammen et al. 1987). Finally, drug trials suggest that medications that ameliorate PTSD symptoms, such as propranolol, benzodiazepines, and carbamazepine, either exacerbate depressive symptoms or are without effect in MDD. (These pharmacologic results will be addressed in detail below.)

Given the differences between PTSD and MDD shown in Table 16-2, it would appear that the two disorders can be distinguished through a number of provocative diagnostic tests. For example, PTSD appears to be associated with HPA axis hypofunction, whereas MDD is characterized by HPA axis hyperfunction. Indeed, the work of Kudler et al. (1987) with the DST is consistent with this expectation, since PTSD patients exhibited DST suppression, whereas patients with both PTSD *and* MDD showed DST nonsuppression. This experiment also suggests that when PTSD and MDD occur concurrently, the biological abnormalities associated with MDD predominate over those associated with PTSD, hence DST nonsuppression. On the other hand, Halbreich et al. (1988) reached the opposite conclusion when they compared DST responses in patients with MDD alone versus a group of PTSD patients with MDD. As expected, the MDD patients were DST nonsuppressors, but, in contrast to Kudler et al.'s results, the PTSD patients with MDD were DST *suppressors*. Hence Halbreich et al. concluded that when PTSD and MDD occur concurrently, the biological abnormalities associated with PTSD predominate over those associated with MDD.

There are several tentative conclusions from these two studies. First, the DST may not be useful for distinguishing PTSD from MDD. Second, when

PTSD and MDD occur simultaneously, each may alter the biological expression of the other. Third, some MDD associated with PTSD may be qualitatively (biologically) distinct from true melancholia even though both meet DSM-III-R criteria for MDD. Perhaps it will be biologically meaningful to revive the distinction between primary and secondary depression in this regard. Primary depression (true melancholia) associated with PTSD is marked by HPA axis hyperfunction with DST nonsuppression and by characteristic depressive alterations in REM sleep. Secondary depression is actually a clinical manifestation of PTSD itself, rather than a separate disorder. It is characterized by normal-to-reduced HPA axis activity, with DST suppression, and by marked abnormalities in Stage 1 and Stage 2 sleep. Since the DSM-III-R cannot distinguish between primary and secondary depression, it may be necessary to utilize biological probes such as the DST and sleep electroencephalogram to categorize the associated depressive syndrome accurately. Finally, when MDD occurs in conjunction with PTSD, determining whether such depression is primary or secondary may explain discrepant psychopharmacological results with antidepressant medications.

ANTIDEPRESSANTS AND PTSD

Tricyclic Antidepressants

There is a general consensus that antidepressants help patients with PTSD. Open and controlled trials with TCAs and MAOIs have generally reported some sort of symptom relief. The question in evaluating this research is whether these drugs have a specific efficacy for PTSD symptoms rather than for depressive symptomatology. A number of open-drug studies have reported that TCAs effectively reduce DSM-III-R PTSD intrusive recollections and hyperarousal symptoms but have little effect on avoidant symptomatology (Blake 1986; Boehnlein et al. 1985; Burstein 1982; Embry and Callahan 1988; Falcon et al. 1985; Friedman 1981, 1988; Marshall 1975; Reaves et al. 1989; van der Kolk 1987). There is less unanimity, however, when one considers the three completed double-blind trials of TCAs in patients with PTSD.

Frank et al. (1988) performed a double-blind evaluation of imipramine, phenelzine, and placebo in 34 Vietnam combat veterans with PTSD. In their study, both the TCA and MAOI appeared to have a specific action against PTSD symptoms, since patients in both drug groups showed significant reduction in intrusion (but not avoidance) items, as measured by the Impact of Event Scale (Horowitz et al. 1979). Therapeutic efficacy of imipramine and phenelzine appeared to be specific for PTSD, since patients showed no significant improvement in depressive or anxious symptoms. It is important to note that no subjects in this study met DSM-III-R criteria for major depression.

Results from two other groups have contradicted these findings. Double-blind, placebo-controlled comparisons of amitriptyline (Davidson et al. 1988) and desipramine (Reist et al. 1989) have shown no improvement in PTSD symptoms. The only therapeutic effects of these TCAs were on depressive symptoms of subjects in both studies. There is an important sampling difference between these studies that may have affected the results. Whereas Frank et al. (1988) excluded all major depressive patients from their study, both Davidson et al. and Reist et al. included many patients with MDD. We will return to this point later.

Monoamine Oxidase Inhibitors

With regard to MAOIs, a number of open studies have also demonstrated that phenelzine is efficacious against intrusive (but not avoidant) symptoms as well as against depressive and generalized anxiety symptoms (Davidson et al. 1987; Hogben and Cornfield 1981; Lerer et al. 1987b; Milanes et al. 1984; Shen and Park 1983). In the comparison of imipramine, phenelzine, and placebo mentioned above, Frank et al. (1988) found that phenelzine was even more effective than imipramine against intrusive (but not avoidant) symptoms. On the other hand, in a double-blind, crossover comparison, Shestatzky et al. (1988) found no superiority of phenelzine over placebo.

Summary

Current research with TCAs and MAOIs is inconclusive with regard to efficacy of antidepressants against the specific symptoms of PTSD. Both drugs remain effective against depressive symptoms in patients with PTSD and MDD. Is this because TCAs and MAOIs are only marginally effective in PTSD? Or do these results suggest that the mechanism of action for antidepressants is primarily through an antipanic/anxiolytic effect that is obscured when MDD is present? These are obviously empirical questions that must await the accumulation of an adequate number of controlled studies before they can be answered with conviction. Sample sizes are small in the few double-blind trials conducted to date. On the other hand, these ambiguous research results with TCAs and MAOIs suggest other questions about the relationship between PTSD and depressive symptoms. Specifically, we must ask whether the difference between Frank et al.'s (1988) results in comparison with those of both Davidson et al. (1988) and Reist et al. (1989) has something to do with the fact that patients with MDD were excluded from the former study but included in relatively large numbers in the latter two studies.

PTSD AND PANIC DISORDER

Although the prevalence of panic disorder in a Veterans Administration outpatient treatment-seeking cohort of more than 100,000 veterans was only 1.2%, 21% of all veterans with panic disorder also met DSM-III criteria for PTSD (Friedman et al. 1987). This high comorbidity rate reflects the great symptomatic similarity between these two disorders and raises the question of overlapping pathophysiologic abnormalities.

Table 16-3 shows similarities between PTSD and panic disorder. Mellman and Davis (1985) have suggested that PTSD flashbacks actually meet DSM-III-R diagnostic criteria for panic attacks. Such an assertion, however, may actually obscure the important differences between the two disorders, listed in Table 16-4. PTSD episodes are psychological events driven by meaningful traumagenic stimuli that evoke stress-induced analgesia (Pitman et al. 1988) along with a sympathetic storm. Panic disorder, on the other hand, is marked by spontaneous physiological attacks devoid of psychological meaning in which stress-induced analgesia has not been demonstrated. Sodium lactate infusions can definitely precipitate panic attacks (Pitts and McClure 1967), but lactate has produced very ambiguous PTSD "flashbacks" in the only reported study on this matter (Rainey et al. 1987). Vietnam combat veterans who met DSM-III criteria for *both* PTSD and panic disorder responded to lactate infusion with "flashbacks" pertinent to a hospital setting or to the experimental laboratory rather than to the combat trauma that precipitated their PTSD. Sleep architecture (Hauri et al. 1989) is normal in panic disorder, whereas PTSD patients show a disturbance of the sleep architecture marked by increased Stage 1 and Stage 2 sleep, decreased delta sleep, increased REM latency, and probable reduction in total REM duration. HPA axis activity is apparently normal in panic disorder but diminished in PTSD. Finally, patients with panic disorder do not respond to carbamazepine (Uhde et al. 1988), whereas open trials with this drug in PTSD patients have been quite promising (Lipper et al. 1986; Wolf et al. 1988).

A number of questions remain. Can sodium lactate infusions precipitate bona fide PTSD episodes? If so, can they reliably distinguish panic disorder

Table 16-3. Posttraumatic stress disorder and panic disorder: similarities

Sympathetic hyperarousal	Often associated with major depressive
Sudden surges of anxiety	disorder
Flashbacks and panic attacks	Postulated locus coeruleus dysregulation
Increased sleep latency	Respond to tricyclic antidepressants
Decreased sleep efficiency	Respond to monoamine oxidase inhibitors
Increased movement during sleep	Respond to propranolol and clonidine

from PTSD? When panic disorder and PTSD occur simultaneously, will each alter the biological expression of the other? Is the panic disorder that occurs concurrently with PTSD qualitatively distinct from true panic disorder, even though both meet DSM-III-R criteria for the same disorder?

ANTIPANIC AND ANXIOLYTIC AGENTS AND PTSD

Medications efficacious in PTSD include sympatholytic drugs such as propranolol and clonidine in addition to TCAs and MAOIs. With one exception, all reports on clonidine, propranolol, benzodiazepines, and alprazolam have been descriptions of open-drug trials.

Propranolol

In the only controlled drug trial published to date, propranolol in doses up to 2.5 mg/kg/day was tested in 11 children with acute PTSD who had been physically and/or sexually abused. The study was an A-B-A design (off-on-off medication) in which patients exhibited significantly fewer symptoms during active treatment (Famularo et al. 1988). In an open propranolol trial with combat veterans with chronic PTSD who received 120 to 160 mg daily, Kolb et al. (1984) reported marked reductions in nightmares, intrusive recollections, hypervigilance, insomnia, startle responses, and angry outbursts. On the other hand, Kinzie (1989) reported that beta-blockers have been without effect on PTSD symptoms of traumatized Cambodian refugees. Given the high ratio of chemical abuse and dependency observed in PTSD patients (Branchey et al. 1984; Keane et al. 1988), the low abuse

Table 16-4. Posttraumatic stress disorder and panic disorder: differences

Posttraumatic stress disorder	Panic disorder
Attacks stimulus-driven	Attacks spontaneous
Attacks psychological	Attacks physiologic
Stress-induced analgesia	No stress-induced analgesia
Role of lactate unclear	Precipitated by lactate
HPA axis hypofunction	Normal HPA axis function
Increased Stage 1 and Stage 2 sleep	Normal Stage 1 and Stage 2 sleep
Decreased delta sleep	Normal delta
Possible increased REM latency	Normal REM latency
Probable decreased total REM duration	Normal REM duration
Responds to carbamazepine	No response to carbamazepine

Note: HPA = hypothalamic-pituitary-adrenal; REM = rapid eye movement.

potential of beta-blockers will make such drugs an attractive treatment option if their efficacy can be demonstrated conclusively.

Clonidine

There are two favorable reports on open trials with the alpha$_2$ agonist clonidine. From a theoretical standpoint, clonidine is an interesting agent to consider, since it will reduce the postulated central adrenergic arousal through inhibition of the locus coeruleus. Furthermore, clonidine would be expected to neutralize the opiate withdrawal-like symptoms of PTSD postulated by van der Kolk et al. (1985) in their inescapable shock model of PTSD. Kolb et al. (1984) reported that eight combat veterans experienced improved sleep, fewer nightmares, lessened explosiveness, reduced intrusion symptoms, and lessened hyperalertness following an open trial of clonidine 0.2 to 0.4 mg/day. Kinzie (1989) observed marked reductions in anxiety and autonomic arousal among Cambodian refugees with PTSD treated with clonidine. Results were even better when clonidine was combined with TCAs.

Benzodiazepines

In a report from one Veterans Administration hospital, 71% of PTSD patients received benzodiazepines either exclusively (36%) or in combination with other drugs (Ciccone et al. 1988). Certainly the proven anxiolytic potency of these drugs has led to their wide use despite clinical concerns about addiction as well as the complete absence of any controlled studies demonstrating their efficacy in PTSD. From a theoretical point of view, the kindling model of PTSD offers a neurobiological argument for prescribing benzodiazepines for appropriate patients. Since limbic kindling is associated with increased benzodiazepine receptor binding (McNamara et al. 1985; Morita et al. 1985; Tietz et al. 1985), it follows that benzodiazepines and other gamma-aminobutyric acid (GABA) agonists or synergists might be particularly useful in well-selected PTSD patients.

Alprazolam

Alprazolam shares the general properties of most benzodiazepines along with antipanic and possible antidepressant actions (Feighner et al. 1983; Sheehan 1982). Like other benzodiazepines, it has been widely prescribed for PTSD patients despite a complete lack of published double-blind trials demonstrating its efficacy. Alprazolam's short half-life raises, in addition to generic concerns about addiction, the possibility of clinical complications such as rebound anxiety and withdrawal symptoms (Higgitt et al. 1985; Noyes et al. 1985).

Summary

Current research with antipanic and anxiolytic agents is very sparse. There is only one controlled study with propranolol and a very low number of published open trials with beta-blockers, clonidine, benzodiazepines, or alprazolam.

OTHER DRUGS AND PTSD

Carbamazepine

Carbamazepine is particularly interesting from a theoretical point of view. It was introduced by Lipper et al. (1986) because it is an anticonvulsant that effectively counters the neurobiological changes produced by kindling. Van der Kolk (1987) and Friedman (1988) have independently hypothesized that the chronic central nervous system sympathetic arousal associated with PTSD produces an endogenous state in the brain that optimizes the conditions for limbic kindling. Therefore, the efficacy of carbamazepine in two open trials with PTSD patients is consistent with a kindling model of PTSD (Lipper et al. 1986; Wolf et al. 1988). Lipper et al. reported reduced intrusive symptoms such as traumatic nightmares, flashbacks, and intrusive recollections in 7 of 10 combat veterans with chronic PTSD. Wolf et al. reported alleviation of impulsivity, irritability, and violent behavior in 8 of 10 combat veterans with PTSD. Wolf et al. did not specifically report on PTSD symptoms, and their positive results could be due to carbamazepine's attentuation of anger and rage rather than on a specific improvement in PTSD. On the other hand, the fact that all of their patients had normal electroencephalograms and had no evidence of temporal lobe epilepsy suggests that their patients did not have complex partial seizures that had been misdiagnosed as PTSD (Stewart and Bartucci 1986). Obviously, there is a need for double-blind trials with carbamazepine in future research.

Lithium

According to van der Kolk (1987), the therapeutic response to lithium is indistinguishable from that to carbamazepine. Of 22 patients with PTSD treated with lithium, 14 reported reduced sympathetic arousal, better tolerance to stress, and diminished alcohol intake. Of note are clinical reports that lithium is an effective treatment for PTSD patients without a personal or family history of affective illness (Kitchner and Greenstein 1985; van der Kolk 1983). Again, controlled trials are needed to validate these open trials and clinical anecdotes.

Fluoxetine

Should lithium stand the test of double-blind trials, it would raise pertinent theoretical questions about the serotonergic system in PTSD. This possibility has not been investigated systematically. However, the impulsivity, disinhibition, hostility, and alcohol (and other chemical) abuse or dependency often associated with PTSD point to the serotonergic system as potentially important (Branchey et al. 1984; Carol et al. 1985; Cloninger 1987a; Hyer et al. 1986; Jelinek and Williams 1984; Keane et al. 1988; Penk et al. 1981; Yager 1976; Yager et al. 1984). Such questions would provide a useful theoretical context in which to evaluate vigorously serotonin reuptake inhibitors (e.g., fluoxetine) that are currently achieving anecdotal success in certain centers.

Neuroleptics

Psychiatrists have become much more reluctant to prescribe neuroleptics than they were 20 years ago. At that time, unrecognized PTSD appeared to be a bizarre and explosive psychotic disorder marked by agitation, paranoid thoughts, loss of control, potential for violence, and brief psychotic episodes now called flashbacks. Clinical observations that, in most cases, these symptoms could be controlled by antidepressants or antipanic and anxiolytic agents have relegated neuroleptics to second- or third-line drugs. Although neuroleptics have no place in the routine treatment, they do have a place in the treatment of refractory PTSD marked by paranoid behavior, aggressive psychotic symptoms, uncontrollable anger, self-destructive behavior, and frequent flashback episodes marked by frank auditory and visual hallucinations of traumatic episodes (Friedman, in press; Mueser and Butler 1987; Walker 1982). Neuroleptics should never be prescribed until other agents have been tried. As with other drugs mentioned above, there have been no controlled trials in PTSD with neuroleptic agents.

Summary

In this review, I have focused on biological aspects of the clinical treatment of PTSD. My starting point was current evidence that PTSD is associated with sympathetic nervous system hyperarousal, HPA axis hypofunction, endogenous opioid dysregulation, and abnormalities in the physiology of sleep. I accept the robust finding that PTSD is usually associated with other psychiatric disorders and question whether such clinical comorbidities can be understood in terms of the pathophysiology of PTSD.

Chemical abuse and dependency can readily be understood as a maladaptive coping strategy to neutralize the sympathetic hyperarousal and opioid dysregulation associated with PTSD. It follows that when PTSD and chemical abuse or dependency occur simultaneously, they must be treated simultaneously.

Certain types of personality disorders may eventually be shown to share some of the biological abnormalities seen in PTSD and thereby predispose affected individuals to develop PTSD following traumatic exposure.

Major depressive disorder is reviewed with respect to characteristics by which it both resembles and differs from PTSD. Data on HPA axis function and sleep physiology are cited to illustrate the unique patterns of biological abnormalities seen in MDD and PTSD, respectively. Despite such differences, use of biological tests to distinguish MDD from PTSD may have limited value, since it appears that when both disorders occur simultaneously, each may alter the biological expression of the other. Such findings raise the possibility that, in some cases, MDD associated with PTSD may be qualitatively (biologically) distinct from true melancholia even though both meet DSM-III-R criteria for MDD. Finally, current research on the specificity and efficacy of antidepressants (TCAs and MAOIs) in PTSD is reviewed. Although there are many published positive reports on the efficacy of TCAs and MAOIs in PTSD, results from controlled trials are inconclusive at this time.

Panic disorder is reviewed with respect to characteristics by which it both resembles and differs from PTSD. There is much less research on PTSD's relationship to panic disorder than the aforementioned studies on PTSD and MDD. The one study on sodium lactate infusion in PTSD is ambiguous. Clinical psychopharmacological studies on antipanic and anxiolytic agents are reviewed, with specific mention of propranolol, clonidine, benzodiazepines, and alprazolam. As with the literature on antidepressants, most positive reports are based on open trials or case reports.

Other drugs reviewed in the final section include carbamazepine, lithium, fluoxetine, and neuroleptics. Since none of these drugs have been tested in controlled trials, I focused the discussion on theoretical and practical issues rather than scientific data.

In conclusion, it appears that the high co-occurrence of other psychiatric disorders in conjunction with PTSD tells us something very important about PTSD itself. From a theoretical point of view, overlapping biological abnormalities between PTSD and some comorbid diagnoses suggest that PTSD patients may be particularly susceptible to develop certain other psychiatric disorders. Thus, the clinical reality of comorbidities must be factored into all of our treatment approaches to PTSD.

REFERENCES

Akiskal HS: Diagnosis and classification of affective disorders: new insights from clinical and laboratory approaches. Psychiatric Developments 2:123–160, 1983

American Psychiatric Association: Diagnostic and Statistical Manual of Mental Disorders, 3rd Edition. Washington, DC, American Psychiatric Association, 1980

American Psychiatric Association: Diagnostic and Statistical Manual of Mental Disorders, 3rd Edition, Revised. Washington, DC, American Psychiatric Association, 1987

Behar D: Flashbacks and posttraumatic stress symptoms in combat veterans. Compr Psychiatry 28:459–466, 1987

Blake DJ: Treatment of acute posttraumatic stress disorder with tricyclic antidepressants. South Med J 79:201–204, 1986

Blanchard EB, Kolb LC, Pallmeyer BA, et al: A psychophysiological study of post traumatic stress disorder in Vietnam veterans. Psychiatr Q 54:220–229, 1982

Boehnlein, JK, Kinzie JD, Ben R, et al: One-year follow-up study of posttraumatic stress disorder among survivors of Cambodian concentration camps. Am J Psychiatry 142:956–959, 1985

Boman B: Combat stress, post-traumatic stress disorder, and associated psychiatric disturbance. Psychosomatics 27:567–573, 1986

Branchey L, David W, Leiber CS: Alcoholism in Vietnam and Korea veterans: a long term follow-up. Alcoholism: Clinical and Experimental Research 8:572–575, 1984

Brende JO: Electrodermal responses in post-traumatic syndromes. J Nerv Ment Dis 170:352–361, 1982

Breslau N, Davis GC: Posttraumatic stress disorder: the stressor criterion. J Nerv Ment Dis 175:255–264, 1987

Burstein A: Treatment of post-traumatic stress disorder with imipramine. Psychosomatics 25:681–687, 1982

Carol EM, Rueger DB, Foy DW, et al: Vietnam combat veterans with post traumatic stress disorder: analysis of marital and cohabitating adjustment. J Abnorm Psychol 94:329–337, 1985

Ciccone PE, Mazarek A, Weisbrot M, et al: Letter. Am J Psychiatry 145:1484–1485, 1988

Cloninger CR: Neurogenetic adaptive mechanisms in alcoholism. Science 236:410–416, 1987a

Cloninger CR: A systematic method for clinical description and classification of personality variants. Arch Gen Psychiatry 44:573–588, 1987b

Davidson J, Walker JI, Kilts C: A pilot study of phenelzine in the treatment of post-traumatic stress disorder. Br J Psychiatry 150:252–255, 1987

Davidson J, Kudler H, Smith R, et al: Amitriptyline treatment of PTSD. Paper presented at 141st annual meeting of the American Psychiatric Association, Montreal, Quebec, May 7–12, 1988

Dobbs D, Wilson WP: Observations on persistence of war neurosis. Diseases of the Nervous System 21:40–46, 1961

Dube S, Jones DA, Bell J: Interface of panic and depression: clinical and sleep EEG correlates. Psychiatry Res 119:119–133, 1986

Embry CK, Callahan B: Effective pharmacotherapy for post-traumatic stress disorder. VA Practitioner 5:57–66, 1988

Escobar JI, Randolph ET, Puente G, et al: Post-traumatic stress disorder in Hispanic Vietnam veterans. J Nerv Ment Dis 171:585–596, 1983

Falcon S, Ryan C, Chamberlain K, et al: Tricyclics: possible treatment for post-traumatic stress disorder. J Clin Psychiatry 46:385–389, 1985

Famularo R, Kinscherff R, Fenton T: Propranolol treatment for childhood post-traumatic stress disorder, acute type: a pilot study. Am J Dis Child 142:1244–1247, 1988

Feighner JP, Aden GC, Fabre LF, et al: Comparison of alprazolam, imipramine and placebo in the treatment of depression. JAMA 249:3057–3064, 1983

Frank JB, Kosten TR, Giller EL, et al: A randomized clinical trial of phenelzine and imipramine for posttraumatic stress disorder. Am J Psychiatry 145:1289–1291, 1988

Friedman MJ: Post-Vietnam syndrome: recognition and management. Psychosomatics 22:931–943, 1981

Friedman MJ: Towards rational pharmacotherapy for posttraumatic stress disorder. Am J Psychiatry 145:281–285, 1988

Friedman MJ: Post-traumatic stress disorder. Current Opinion in Psychiatry 2:230–234, 1989

Friedman MJ: Biological approaches to the diagnosis and treatment of post-traumatic stress disorder. Journal of Traumatic Stress (in press)

Friedman MJ, Kolb LC, Arnold A, et al: Third Annual Report of the Chief Medical Director's Special Committee on Post-Traumatic Stress Disorder. Washington, DC, Veterans Administration, 1987, pp 46–94

Gillespie RD: Psychological Effects of War on Citizen and Soldier. New York, WW Norton, 1942

Greenberg R, Pearlman CA, Gampel D: War neuroses and the adaptive function of REM sleep. Br J Med Psychol 45:27–33, 1972

Halbreich U, Olympia J, Glogowski J, et al: The importance of past psychological trauma and pathophysiologic process as determinants of current biologic abnormalities. Arch Gen Psychiatry 45:293–294, 1988

Hauri PJ, Friedman MJ, Ravaris CL: Sleep in patients with spontaneous panic attacks. Sleep 12:323–337, 1989

Herman JL, Perry C, van der Kolk BA: Childhood trauma in borderline personality disorder. Am J Psychiatry 146:490–495, 1989

Higgitt AC, Lader MH, Fonagy P: Clinical management of benzodiazepine dependence. Br Med J 291:688–690, 1985

Hogben GL, Cornfield RB: Treatment of traumatic war neurosis with phenelzine. Arch Gen Psychiatry 38:440–445, 1981

Horowitz M, Wilner N, Alvarez W: Impact of Event Scale: a measure of subjective distress. Psychosom Med 41:209–218, 1979

Hyer L, Olary WC, Saucer RT, et al: Inpatient diagnosis of post traumatic stress disorder. J Consult Clin Psychol 54:698–702, 1986

Jelinek JM, Williams T: Post traumatic stress disorder and substance abuse in Vietnam combat veterans: treatment problems, strategies and recommendations. J Subst Abuse Treat 1:87–97, 1984

Kauffman CD, Reist C, Djenderedjian A, et al: Biological markers of affective disorders and posttraumatic stress disorder: a pilot study with desipramine. J Clin Psychiatry 48:366–367, 1987

Keane TM, Zimering RT, Caddell JM: A behavioral formulation of posttraumatic stress disorder in Vietnam veterans. The Behavior Therapist 8:9–12, 1985

Keane TM, Gerardi RJ, Lyons JA, et al: The interrelationship of substance abuse and posttraumatic stress disorder: epidemiological and clinical considerations. Recent Dev Alcohol 6:27–48, 1988

Kinzie JD: Therapeutic approaches to traumatized Cambodian refugees. Journal of Traumatic Stress 2:75–91, 1989

Kitchner I, Greenstein R: Low dose lithium carbonate in the treatment of post traumatic stress disorder: brief communication. Milit Med 150:378–381, 1985

Kolb LC: A neuropsychological hypothesis explaining posttraumatic stress disorders. Am J Psychiatry 144:989–995, 1987

Kolb LC: A critical survey of hypotheses regarding posttraumatic stress disorders in light of recent findings. Journal of Traumatic Stress 1:291–304, 1988

Kolb LC, Burris BC, Griffiths S: Propranolol and clonidine in the treatment of the chronic post-traumatic stress disorders of war, in Post-Traumatic Stress Disorder: Psychological and Biological Sequelae. Edited by van der Kolk BA. Washington, DC, American Psychiatric Press, 1984, pp 97–105

Kosten TR, Krystal J: Biological mechanisms in posttraumatic stress disorder: relevance for substance abuse. Recent Dev Alcohol 6:49–68, 1988

Kramer M, Kinney L: Is sleep a marker of vulnerability to delayed post traumatic stress disorder? Sleep Research 14:181, 1985

Kudler H, Davidson J, Meador K: The DST and posttraumatic stress disorder. Am J Psychiatry 144:1068–1071, 1987

Kulka RA, Schlenger WE, Fairbank JA, et al: Contractual Report of Findings from the National Vietnam Veterans Readjustment Study. Research Triangle Park, NC, Research Triangle Institute, 1988

Kupfer DJ, Thase ME: The use of the sleep laboratory in the diagnosis of affective disorders. Psychiatr Clin North Am 6:3–25, 1983

Lavie P, Hefez A, Halperin G, et al: Long-term effects of traumatic war-related events on sleep. Am J Psychiatry 136:175–178, 1979

Lerer B, Ebstein R, Shestatzky M, et al: Cyclic AMP signal transduction in posttraumatic stress disorder. Am J Psychiatry 144:1324–1327, 1987a

Lerer B, Bleich A, Kotler M: Posttraumatic stress disorder in Israeli combat veterans: effect of phenelzine treatment. Arch Gen Psychiatry 44:976–981, 1987b

Linnoila M, Virkkunen M, Scheinin M, et al: Low cerebrospinal fluid 5-hydroxyindoleacetic acid concentration differentiates impulsive from non-impulsive violent behavior. Life Sci 33:2609–2614, 1983

Linnoila M, Virkkunen M, deJong JB: Serotonin, impulse control and alcoholism. Paper presented at the 142nd annual meeting of the American Psychiatric Association, San Francisco, CA, May 6–11, 1989

Lipper S, Davidson JRT, Grady TA, et al: Preliminary study of carbamazepine in post-traumatic stress disorder. Psychosomatics 27:849–854, 1986

Malloy PF, Fairbank JA, Keane TM: Validation of a multimethod assessment of posttraumatic stress disorders in Vietnam veterans. J Consult Clin Psychol 51:488–494, 1983

Marshall JR: The treatment of night terrors associated with the posttraumatic syndrome. Am J Psychiatry 132:293–295, 1975

Mason JW, Giller EL, Kosten TR, et al: Urinary free-cortisol in posttraumatic stress disorder. J Nerv Ment Dis 174:145–149, 1986

McFarland RE: Post-traumatic stress disorder and concurrent psychiatric illness. Psychotherapy in Private Practice 3:55–58, 1985

McFarlane AC: The aetiology of post-traumatic stress disorders following a natural disaster. Br J Psychiatry 152:116–121, 1988

McNamara JO, Bonhaus DW, Shin C, et al: The kindling model of epilepsy: a critical review. CRC Critical Reviews of Clinical Neurobiology 1:341–391, 1985

Mellman TA, Davis GC: Combat-related flashbacks in posttraumatic stress disorder: phenomenology and similarity to panic attacks. J Clin Psychiatry 46:379–382, 1985

Milanes, FS, Mack CN, Dennison J: Phenelzine treatment of post-Vietnam stress syndrome. VA Practitioner, June 1984, pp 40–49

Morita K, Okamoto M, Seki K, et al: Suppression of amygdala-kindled seizures in cats by enhanced GABAergic transmission in the substantia innominata. Exp Neurol 89:225–236, 1985

Mueser KT, Butler RW: Auditory hallucinations in combat-related chronic post-traumatic stress disorder. Am J Psychiatry 144:299–302, 1987

Noyes R, Clancy J, Coryell WH, et al: A withdrawal syndrome after abrupt discontinuation of alprazolam. Am J Psychiatry 142:114–116, 1985

Penk WE, Rabinowitz R, Roberts WR, et al: Adjustment differences among male substance abusers varying in degree of combat experience in Vietnam. J Consult Clin Psychol 49:426–437, 1981

Perry SW, Cella DF, Falkenberg J, et al: Pain perception in burn patients with stress disorders. Journal of Pain and Symptom Management 2:29–33, 1987

Pitman RK, Orr SP, Forgue DF, et al: Psychophysiologic assessment of posttraumatic stress disorder imagery in Vietnam combat veterans. Arch Gen Psychiatry 44:970–975, 1987

Pitman RK, Orr SP, van der Kolk B, et al: Stress-induced analgesia in posttraumatic stress disorder. Paper presented at the 141st annual meeting of the American Psychiatric Association, Montreal, Quebec, May 7–12, 1988

Pitman RK, Orr SP, Forgue DF, et al: Physiology of PTSD in Vietnam combat veterans. Paper presented at the 142nd annual meeting of the American Psychiatric Association, San Francisco, May 6–11, 1989

Pitts FN Jr, McClure JN Jr: Lactate metabolism in anxiety neurosis. N Engl J Med 277:1329–1336, 1967

Rainey JM, Aleem A, Ortiz A, et al: A laboratory procedure for the induction of flashbacks. Am J Psychiatry 144:1317–1319, 1987

Reaves ME, Hansen TE, Whisenand JM: The psychopharmacology of PTSD. VA Practitioner, May 1989, pp 65–72

Reist C, Kauffman CD, Haier RJ, et al: A controlled trial of desipramine in 18 men with posttraumatic stress disorder. Am J Psychiatry 146:513–516, 1989

Ross RJ, Ball W, Sullivan KA, et al: Sleep disturbance in posttraumatic stress disorder (letter). Am J Psychiatry 147:374, 1990

Schlossberg A, Benjamin M: Sleep patterns in three acute combat fatigue cases. J Clin Psychiatry 39:546–549, 1978

Sheehan DV: Current perspectives in the treatment of panic and phobic disorders. Drug Therapy 7:179–193, 1982

Shen WW, Park S: The use of monoamine oxidase inhibitors in the treatment of traumatic war neurosis: case report. Milit Med 148:430–431, 1983

Shestatzky M, Greenberg D, Lerer B: A controlled trial of phenelzine in posttraumatic stress disorder. Psychiatry Res 24:149–155, 1988

Shores TJ, Seib TB, Levine S, et al: Inescapable versus escapable shock modulates long-term potentiation in the rat hippocampus. Science 244:224–226, 1989

Sierles FS, Chen JJ, McFarland RE, et al: Posttraumatic stress disorder and concurrent psychiatric illness: a preliminary report. Am J Psychiatry 140:1177–1179, 1983

Sierles FS, Chen JJ, Messing ML, et al: Concurrent psychiatric illness in non-Hispanic outpatients diagnosed as having posttraumatic stress disorder. J Nerv Ment Dis 174:171–173, 1986

Siever LJ, Davis KL: Overview: toward a dysregulation hypothesis of depression. Am J Psychiatry 142:1017–1031, 1985

Solomon RL, Wynne LC: Traumatic avoidance learning: the principles of anxiety conservation and partial irreversibility. Psychol Rev 61:353–385, 1954

Stewart JR, Bartucci RJ: Posttraumatic stress disorder and partial complex seizures. Am J Psychiatry 143:113–114, 1986

Sulser F, Vetulani J, Mobley PL: Mode of action of antidepressant drugs. Biochem Pharmacol 27:257–261, 1978

Tietz EI, Gomez F, Berman RF: Amygdala kindled seizure stage is related to altered benzodiazepine binding site density. Life Sci 36:183–190, 1985

Uhde TW, Stein MB, Post RM: Lack of efficacy of carbamazepine in the treatment of panic disorder. Am J Psychiatry 145:1104–1109, 1988

van der Kolk BA: Psychopharmacological issues in posttraumatic stress disorder. Hosp Community Psychiatry 34:683–691, 1983

van der Kolk BA: The drug treatment of post-traumatic stress disorder. J Affective Disord 13:203–213, 1987

van der Kolk BA: The trauma spectrum: the interaction of biological and social events in the genesis of the trauma response. Journal of Traumatic Stress 1:273–290, 1988

van der Kolk BA, Greenberg M, Boyd H, et al: Inescapable shock, neurotransmitters, and addiction to trauma: toward a psychobiology of post traumatic stress. Biol Psychiatry 20:314–325, 1985

van Kammen W, Christiansen C, van Kammen D, et al: Sleep and the POW experience: 40 years later. Sleep Research 16:291, 1987

Walker JI: Chemotherapy of traumatic war stress. Milit Med 147:1029–1033, 1982

Wolf ME, Alavi A, Mosnaim AD: Posttraumatic stress disorder in Vietnam veterans: clinical and EEG findings: possible therapeutic effects of carbamazepine. Biol Psychiatry 23:642–644, 1988

Yager J: Post combat violent behavior in psychiatrically maladjusting soldiers. Arch Gen Psychiatry 33:1332–1335, 1976

Yager T, Laufer R, Gallops M: Some problems associated with war experience in men of the Vietnam generation. Arch Gen Psychiatry 41:327–333, 1984

Zanarini MC, Gunderson JG, Marion MF, et al: Childhood experiences of borderline patients. Compr Psychiatry 30:18–25, 1989

Chapter 17

Psychotherapeutic Interventions in Chronic Posttraumatic Stress Disorder

Charles K. Embry, M.D.

P osttraumatic stress disorder (PTSD) continues to be one of the most devastating emotional health problems affecting today's United States veteran society. Although the number of World War II, Korean, and Vietnam veterans may be gradually declining, the far-reaching familial vibrations of this illness are manifesting themselves in an exponential manner as divorce, disrupted families, suicide, and homicide, with violence as an ever-common end product.

Even though there has not been a systematic investigation of the prevalence of PTSD in Vietnam veterans, it is estimated that 20% to 60% have readjustment problems (Friedman 1981). During the Vietnam War, approximately four million Americans were in Indochina; of these, 800,000 were assigned to the combat zone and are at high risk for development of PTSD (Lipkin et al. 1982). Patients with PTSD often do not respond to conventional psychopharmacological and psychotherapeutic approaches. In this chapter, I will describe psychotherapeutic reassessment and management strategies for chronic or delayed onset PTSD.

REASSESSMENT

The establishment of a PTSD diagnosis is complex, and the clinician should address issues such as comorbidity with personality disorders, substance abuse, and other psychiatric conditions, as well as shammed as opposed to genuine PTSD. Friedman (1981) gave us some of the best advice when he wrote: "The first rule in treating post-Vietnam syndrome is to take a careful and detailed history." This is important enough to warrant conduction of a complete and thorough anamnesis again and again.

The nature of the relationship between PTSD and personality disorders has been subject to considerable controversy, but the fact that they frequently coexist is accepted by practitioners in this field. In my experience, antisocial, borderline, and mixed personality disorder types are the most frequent. Green et al. (1985) found antisocial personality along with alcohol and drug dependence to be some of the most consistent diagnoses associated with PTSD. An in-depth discussion of the treatment of personality disorders is beyond the scope of this chapter. The reader is referred to Lion's (1981) book on diagnosis and management of personality disorders for a comprehensive discussion of this matter. However, there are general guidelines for working with these patients. Both Newman (1985) and Merback (1984) favor a reality-based therapy in assisting these individuals to gain insight into self-defeating ways, to develop limits surrounding externalization of anger and acting-out, to have more responsibility for their actions, and to make them more cognizant of their behavioral influence on those around them.

Several groups of investigators have reported a high rate of substance abuse disorders among PTSD patients, with rates varying from 40% to 83% (Davidson et al. 1985; Helzer et al. 1987; Wolf et al. 1988). The treatment of PTSD or substance abuse per se is complex, and the frequent coexistence of these two diagnoses, which further complicates patient management, has warranted the development in some Veterans Administration centers of joint PTSD and drug abuse programs. Denial of drug abuse, problems of negative interactions between prescribed psychotropic agents and illicit drugs, and noncompliance are often encountered in the PTSD population. Patients may abuse the prescription medications offered to alleviate their symptoms and may take larger dosages than recommended in attempts to free themselves from flashbacks, traumatic memories, and nightmares. Conversely, they may not take any medication, even though they have been instructed to do so, as a result of anger or paranoia toward governmental systems.

It has also been noted that other psychiatric diagnoses, such as depression and anxiety, frequently coexist with PTSD. Different investigators report rates of depression varying from 40% to 70% (Davidson et al. 1985; Helzer et al. 1987; Sierles et al. 1983). A Centers for Disease Control Vietnam experience study by Barrett et al. (1988) revealed depression, anxiety, and alcohol abuse or dependence to be more prevalent among Vietnam veterans than among non-Vietnam veterans.

Pary et al. (1987) addressed the issue of shammed and genuine PTSD and indicated that a careful premilitary, military, and postmilitary history is necessary to establish a diagnosis of PTSD. Hamilton (1985) supported these ideas by recommending that shammed PTSD in veterans is best substantiated by checking the veteran's claims folder, thus avoiding misdiagnosing a patient who may be presenting with malingering or factitious disorder. All veterans' health care providers should be familiar with the signs and symptoms of both malingering and factitious disorder, the former aimed at obtaining compensation and the latter focusing on hospital care.

Given the multivaried, nonspecific clinical manifestations of PTSD, as described in DSM-III-R (American Psychiatric Association 1987), and the above-mentioned issues, the differential diagnosis of PTSD is complex. Kaplan and Sadock (1988) included factitious disorder, malingering, adjustment reaction, depression, panic disorder, generalized anxiety disorder, mood disorder, chronic pain disorder, head injury, alcohol and drug dependence, and schizophrenia in their list of conditions to be considered in the differential diagnosis. A careful history, together with a thorough workup for organic pathology, may provide the basis for a proper PTSD diagnosis.

PSYCHOTHERAPEUTIC MANAGEMENT STRATEGIES

Perconte (1988) described a successful PTSD treatment protocol as consisting of six stages corresponding to the variety of problems experienced:

1. Preparation for treatment by individual support and education.
2. Verbalization of problem by group and individual education and supportive confrontation.
3. Abreaction/catharsis by supportive confrontation, guided examination of trauma, insight-oriented review and discussion, flooding, and desensitization.
4. Normalization of family relationships by communications training, social skills training, marital counseling, and family therapy.
5. Modification of stereotyped behavior by flooding and desensitization, relaxation training, stress management and problem-solving training, participant modeling and exposure therapy, and group and individual reinforcement techniques.
6. Social reintegration by social skills training, relaxation training, stress management training, vocational and educational counseling, and goal setting.

Veterans should not be led to expect to eliminate painful memories and nightmares but to learn how to defuse them. Quick therapeutic intervention often prevents escalation of the patient's PTSD symptoms. Kolb (1986) offers all PTSD patients immediate participation in an open stress group with other Vietnam veterans with similar problems. These veterans share their experiences with empathic fellow veterans, talk about problems in social adaptation, and are offered options for managing their aggression toward others. Severe cases of PTSD involving individuals who were unable to continue group therapy (i.e., those with severe depression and dissociative states) were selected out for individual treatment, since their intensely felt experiences surface only in the trusting relationship that individual psychotherapy can provide. The agitated PTSD patient is often a difficult management problem, especially when faced with severe organic disease and hospitalized on a medical or surgical ward. The quick-paced rounds and evaluation process are also anxiety-provoking in these individuals with low stress tolerance. These patients, as a result of increased frustration, may wish to leave against medical advice, may have misunderstandings with physicians or nursing staff, or may be reported as being manipulative or very agitated. The PTSD veteran often refuses medication or procedures and early on may prove difficult to manage.

PARAMETERS FOR EFFECTIVE PSYCHOTHERAPY

The following have emerged as parameters for effective psychotherapy with these chronic PTSD veterans: 1) investing extra energy in establishing rapport; 2) limit setting with supportive confrontation; 3) modeling of affect; 4) defocusing on stress; 5) processing of transference and countertransference issues; 6), understanding secondary gain; and 7) establishing a positive therapeutic attitude.

Rapport Building

Hendin (1983) was accurate when he related that even though veterans with PTSD are linked by common combat experiences, effective psychotherapy is based on more of an understanding of what the traumatic war experiences have meant to each veteran, the unique ways they defend themselves against the stress, and how this is reflected in their daily living. Veterans begin to trust gradually as they feel they are being understood. More than an average amount of energy and time invested early on in the development of rapport is needed to treat the PTSD patient who says he does not trust anyone.

These patients appreciate less time being spent on being told they can trust their physician and respond more to observing the physician's trustworthy behavior as the therapist makes appointments on time and actively listens with genuine interest and empathy. According to Jelinek and Williams (1987), openness and self-disclosure are necessary in forging therapeutic relationships with traumatized persons.

Limit Setting With Supportive Confrontation

As in any therapeutic situation, the patient should understand the ground rules of therapy clearly from the outset. Deviation from these rules can be confronted in a gentle, but expedient fashion.

> Mr. X, a heavy-set white male in his late 30s, was diagnosed with PTSD and chronic pain syndrome. He was referred for outpatient consultation after the neurology service had ruled out an organic basis for his pain. This patient entered the examiner's office and after introductions began beating on the desk and making demands for codeine to help relieve his pain and suffering. The patient finally stopped shouting and waited for a response. The response came slowly with a soft emphatic tone: "You seem to be in a great deal of pain and I want to help you but I can't understand your problem if you keep shouting and beating on the desk."

The patient must understand that threatening and hostile behavior is not permitted and only slows the therapist down in his or her attempt to provide care. It is reinforced that damaging office property is not allowed and that it is hoped that therapy can continue without this behavior, working together as a team to find out why all this came to surface. This helps the patient reflect on his misbehavior rather than ignoring it and letting it escalate. If rapport is sufficiently strong, many patients may apologize or begin to talk about their anger or reason for their conduct. PTSD patients trust therapists who appear to be in control of the therapy hour despite the patients' long-standing difficulties with authority figures. On occasion the patient may continue his threatening behavior, and the reasons for this need to be carefully thought through, since hospitalization may be necessary if the patient represents a danger to self or others. Even if the therapist is successful in setting limits initially, there will be many occasions to practice this therapeutic parameter and refine the technique, since PTSD patients usually test their therapist multiple times to see if they mean business.

Affective Modeling

Howard (1976) pointed out that the veteran will need help in regaining contact with a wide range of emotions before almost anything can be dealt with; this involves challenging and identifying defenses and actually giving the patient "permission" to feel and unlearn the "tough masculinity" of his upbringing and military experiences. As the patient is helped to recognize his affective state, care must be taken to prevent interventions or interpretations that are too early and could stimulate explosive outbursts.

This became clear during one session when a veteran of World War II, the Korean War, and the Vietnam War explained the difference in these wars. He explained that in World War II and in Korea it was more a war of men fighting men. He described Vietnam as "a slaughter, you killed men, women, children, and anything that moved, life itself. You have to lose all feeling and forget it to survive."

Many veterans with PTSD experience psychic numbing to various degrees. On the other hand, many of these patients abhor being told by friends or relatives that they don't feel anything for anyone.

One must remember abreaction for these patients can be extremely intense. The best suggestion here is to move slowly, not uncovering too much material at each session, but more importantly letting the patient ventilate feelings at his own rate. There should be more shoring up of defenses as therapy progresses rather than pushing or facilitating abreaction with early interpretations, which may lead to increased anxiety. This anxiety may be of overwhelming proportion, causing the patient to experience dissociative-like states during the therapy sessions.

Defocusing on Stress

The therapeutic maneuver of defocusing on stress deserves mention at this point. Many veterans dominate the therapy hour with continual revelations of PTSD-ridden issues. For a more balanced treatment process, defocusing on stress is needed from time to time. Occasional focusing away from stress-related and provocative areas and emphasis on the here and now (i.e., problems of the family and current everyday living) help the veteran become accustomed to a pattern conducive to minimizing stimuli that will heighten anxiety. This maximizes time spent dealing effectively with current life problems. Timing is important and must be individualized from one patient to the next. One patient may be able to defocus on stressful events for three to four sessions consecutively, whereas other patients may be able to do this only 20 minutes every 2 weeks.

> Mr. A had spent four sessions talking about certain war atrocities and appeared relieved after ventilating his feelings. During the fifth session the patient began as usual, except his anxiety began to increase as he talked. He remarked, "It's like I can't get away from it, it's with me all the time everywhere I go." Silence followed as the patient began to shake his legs and became more restless. The patient was then asked if he could tell the therapist what he had done with his family that week. As the veteran talked about his family, the muscle tension in his face gradually relaxed. Although he was describing family-related problems, he appeared more relaxed and was able to think about alternatives for coping more appropriately with his family problems. He remarked that he knows that he frustrates his wife and children but loves them very much and enjoys being with them and taking his son to football practice.

Appropriate fatherly activities are reinforced as well as helping the patient try to put into words how it made him feel to see his son get a first down on the first attempt. The value of helping the PTSD veteran appreciate his positive and negative behaviors in the home setting cannot be overemphasized.

Transference-Countertransference Issues

The key to unlocking transference and countertransference problems is found by appreciating that these patients have great difficulty with authority figures. Although therapists are usually well trained to recognize when feelings such as anger arise in them, they are somewhat less adept at being cognizant of hate, disgust, repugnance, condescension, and contempt. Egendorf (1978) emphasized that therapists need to try to see these adverse reactions in themselves and handle them so that productive therapy can continue.

The therapist walks a fine line, since he or she represents authority and is a setup for rejection from the beginning. Knowing this, however, one can use it to a therapeutic advantage by setting up a collaborative task between patient and therapist from the outset, relinquishing as much authority to the patient as can be handled, while still maintaining control.

Understanding Secondary Gain

Secondary gain in the Vietnam veteran population is often seen as monetary remuneration under the label of service-connected compensation or an increase in eligibility for care status. Veteran patients, due to their sense of entitlement and their feeling of not being recognized for what they perceive as their illness, tend to pursue the search for entitlement. Often this is fueled by their comrades' past experience of getting their compensation, and frequently one veteran will help another work his way through what veterans call "the maze of red tape," toward service connection. This quest for entitlement often takes on extreme proportions. Understanding secondary gain, and the dilemmas veterans face as a result of it, is essential in treating these patients.

> Patient Y entered the therapy hour stating that he is feeling better and would like to go back to work, but: "Doctor, who will hire someone who has been receiving compensation for 3 years. I've gotten better but I've been out of work for so long. I could never get a job making the kind of money I get for being ill; it's fun to be a Vietnam veteran, having flashbacks, it's really fun to be sick and get paid for it, isn't it; it's a hell of a job. I'm afraid to get well."

This particular patient had his service connection for some time and described going through the usual "red tape" to get it and of course felt extremely entitled. The veteran, as he was gradually improving over time, began to realize he was not as dysfunctional as he had once thought. This web of entitlement that encompasses secondary gain can cause the patient extreme problems. Since this patient has been 100% service connected for some years, it may be difficult for him to get back into the mainstream of the workplace if his compensation is reduced or discontinued. In addition, patients fear vocational rehabilitation programs, which may mean a future decrement in benefits as they become employable. Listening sensitively as the patient expresses his feelings regarding these issues is paramount. The patient feels very ambivalent toward the therapist and administration since he is dependent on them for emotional and financial support but often holds the system responsible for this dependence.

Positive Therapeutic Attitude

The area of therapeutic attitude is one of the most important in therapy with PTSD patients and carries over from therapist to patient. The therapist must not be frightened of the patients' violent and impulsive manner and must be sensitive to their unique position of dependence. The therapist's belief that he or she can really help these patients adjust to their postwar life and improve is one of the main ingredients of effective psychotherapy with the treatment-refractory patient. Once the patient sees that his therapist truly believes he can get better and is unfaltering in this positive therapeutic attitude over time, despite testing and impulsive patient behavior, then, with appropriate limit setting, progress can be made.

Perhaps the question here is what is progress? One of the best answers was given by a patient recently who said, "Doctor, for me, progress is living day to day. You know doctor, I believe I can get a job, making more money than I am getting now. Maybe I'm disabled, but even if I can only work part-time I want to give it a try. I won't give up!"

CONCLUSIONS

Are chronic PTSD patients addicted to trauma? If so, what can we do? Van der Kolk et al (1985) described a psychobiological hypothesis regarding this theme that may have important implications for future directions in PTSD treatment, whether primarily biological or psychosocial in orientation. The patient needs to learn a new nonaddictive life-style, substituting newly developed human relationship experiences and renewed spirituality parameters for alcohol and drug abuse and maladaptive interpersonal interactions.

Encouragement of one PTSD veteran to help another through group therapy at Veterans Administration centers and self-help groups redirects the patient's energy from self to others. Of great importance is the patient's relationship to his Higher Power or God as he understands Him, which may enable the veteran to develop a nonaddiction-seeking life-style that is not self-centered. Many PTSD patients are isolated emotionally and are at high risk for suicide. Marital and family therapies are often needed to reestablish and strengthen human relationships. To begin to heal the chronic PTSD patient, pharmacotherapy intervention may reduce symptoms and make individuals more amenable to psychological interventions (Friedman 1988). However, long-term improvement will rest on the ability of the patient to reintegrate into his family and community as soon as possible. Isolation must be replaced by a sense of belonging to all humanity. By addressing the multiple dimensions of pathology as outlined in the preceding sections, the therapist may not only be able to help the patient in coping with day-to-day living, but may also improve the quality of life for the veteran and his family.

REFERENCES

American Psychiatric Association: Diagnostic and Statistical Manual of Mental Disorders, 3rd Edition, Revised. Washington, DC, American Psychiatric Association, 1987

Barrett DH, Boyle CA, Decoufle P: Health status of Vietnam veterans, I: Psychosocial characteristics (the Centers for Disease Control Vietnam experience study). JAMA 259:2701, 1988

Davidson J, Swartz M, Storck M, et al: A diagnostic and family study of post-traumatic stress disorder. Am J Psychiatry 142:90–93, 1985

Egendorf A: Psychotherapy with Vietnam veterans: observations and suggestions, in Stress Disorders Among Vietnam Veterans: Theory, Research and Treatment. Edited by Figley CR. New York, Brunner/ Mazel, 1978, p 238

Friedman MJ: Post-Vietnam syndrome: recognition and management. Psychosomatics 22:931–943, 1981

Friedman MJ: Toward rational pharmacotherapy for PTSD. Am J Psychiatry 145:281–285, 1988

Green BL, Lindy JD, Grace MC: Post-traumatic stress disorder, toward DSM-IV. J Nerv Ment Dis 173:406–411, 1985

Hamilton JD: Pseudo-post-traumatic stress disorder. Milit Med 150:353–356, 1985

Helzer JE, Robins LN, McEvoy L: Post-traumatic stress disorder in the general population: findings of the epidemiological catchment area survey. N Engl J Med 317:1630–1634, 1987

Hendin H: Psychotherapy for Vietnam veterans with post traumatic stress disorders. Am J Psychother 37:86–99, 1983

Howard S: The Vietnam warrior: his experience, and implications for psychotherapy. Am J Psychother 30:121–135, 1976

Jelinek MJ, Williams T: Post-traumatic stress disorder and substance abuse: treatment problems, strategies and recommendations, in Post-traumatic Stress Disorders: A Handbook for Clinicians. Edited by Williams T. Cincinnati, OH, Disabled American Veterans, 1987

Kaplan HI, Sadock BJ: Anxiety disorders, in Synopsis of Psychiatry, 5th Edition. Baltimore, MD, Williams & Wilkins, 1988, pp 310–334

Kolb LC: Treatment of chronic post-traumatic stress disorder. Current Psychiatric Therapies 23:119–126, 1986

Lion JR (ed): Personality Disorders: Diagnosis and Management. Baltimore, MD, Williams & Wilkins, 1981

Lipkin JO, Blank, AS, Parson ER, et al: Vietnam veterans and post-traumatic stress disorder. Hosp Community Psychiatry 33:908, 1982

Merback K: A Vet center dilemma: post-traumatic stress disorder. Veterans Center Voice Newsletter, Aug 1984, pp 5–7

Newman J: Differential diagnosis in Vietnam veterans with PTSD: implications for treatment. Atlanta, GA, Founding Meeting Traumatic Studies, Sept 1985

Pary R, Tobias C, Lippmann S: Recognizing shammed and genuine post-traumatic stress disorder. VA Practitioner, July 1987, p 43

Perconte ST: Stages of treatment in PTSD. VA Practitioner, 1988, pp 47–57

Sierles FS, Chen JJ, McFarland RE, et al: Post-traumatic stress disorder and concurrent psychiatric illness: a preliminary report. Am J Psychiatry 140:1177–1179, 1983

van der Kolk BA, Greenberg M, Boyd H, et al: Inescapable shock neurotransmitters, and addiction to trauma: toward a psychobiology of post-traumatic stress. Biol Psychiatry 20:314–325, 1985

Wolf ME, Alavi A, Mosnaim AD: Pharmacological interventions in PTSD. Research Communications in Psychology, Psychiatry and Behavior 12:169–176, 1988

Chapter 18

Legal Aspects of Posttraumatic Stress Disorder: Uses and Abuses

Landy F. Sparr, M.D.

The term *posttraumatic stress disorder* (PTSD) has been embraced by the legal community. It has pulled together a previously diverse and heterogeneous nomenclature dating back more than 100 years. Early historical references to PTSD include a description of hysteria following injury by Abbercrombie in 1828 and by Broddie in 1837 (Millen 1966). The term *posttraumatic neurosis* was first coined by a neurologist named Oppenheim in about 1880 and became generally accepted in the medical community, but gradually became almost entirely a legal concept. So-called compensation neurosis appeared at the turn of the century with the proliferation of workers' compensation laws (Modlin 1986). Simultaneously, lawsuits for personal injury (torts) due to psychic injury were being pursued in the arena of civil law. At first, liability for psychic impairment was contingent on physical impact to the person (physical injury). Later, concepts of psychic impairment were liberalized to include nonimpact trauma. As a result, in the legal lexicon, multiple terms evolved for traumatic stress, such as disaster syndrome, American disease, accident neurosis, railway spine, reparation neurosis, and justice neurosis.

Early in the 20th century, psychoanalysts shed new light on emotional conflicts that were reactivated by accidents. Indeed, Freud himself proposed that all forms of neurosis represent a reaction or response to psychic trauma (Millen 1966). The two world wars introduced a variety of synonyms for traumatic stress, such as shell shock, war neurosis, combat exhaustion, flight fatigue, 3-day schizophrenia, prisoner-of-war syndrome, and soldier's heart. Many of these disorders also had legal ramifications. More recently, stress disorders have become a factor in the insanity defense (Sparr and Atkinson 1986) and in the Veterans Administration's (VA) consideration of service-connected disability (Atkinson et al. 1982).

There was an attempt in DSM-III (American Psychiatric Association 1980) to bring the varied stress syndromes under one generic medical heading: PTSD. Thus criteria were developed, and traumatic stress came back into the medical-psychiatric realm. The definition highlighted the theory that there was a single posttraumatic syndrome that is a final common pathway reached through a wide variety of relatively severe stressors. Several reports containing data about symptoms in survivors of extreme trauma had been published by the mid-1970s and were available to guide those who formulated the DSM-III PTSD diagnostic criteria. These included studies of survivors of fire (Adler 1943; Cobb and Lindemann 1943), explosion (Leopold and Dillon 1963), flood (Titchener and Kapp 1976), military combat (Archibald and Tuddenham 1965; Brill and Beebe 1955; Dobbs and Wilson 1960; Grinker and Spiegel 1945), concentration camps (Trautman 1964), and rape (Burgess and Holmstrom 1974), as well as more general studies, particularly Horowitz's (1976) work. As Horowitz summarized, the studies tend to depict a pattern of 1) overwhelming traumatic events, followed by 2) subsequent intrusive recollection of the trauma, together with arousal symptoms, such as startle and insomnia; and 3) restitutive efforts of denial and avoidance of the implications of the trauma and the intrusive symptoms.

Those who defined the criteria were mostly influenced by early studies of war neurosis. There was, in particular, a spate of articles in the late 1960s and early 1970s about the aftereffects of the Vietnam War (Fox 1972; Goldsmith and Cretekos 1969; Horowitz and Solomon 1975; Solomon et al. 1971; Van Putten and Emory 1973). Previously, with multiple terminology and multiple ideas of symptomatology, concepts of PTSD were exceedingly vague and emphasized the origin of the trauma (e.g., war, accident) rather than symptomatology. While the stimulus for the incorporation of PTSD in DSM-III was not forensic, the consolidation of the diagnosis quickly gained currency, especially among legal experts.

PTSD began to appear in a variety of forensic venues. The legal aspects of PTSD that will be discussed in this chapter include 1) the insanity defense, 2) disability, 3) duty to protect, 4) workers' compensation, and 5) personal injury (torts).

THE INSANITY DEFENSE

When not guilty by reason of insanity (NGRI) was conceived, tests of insanity were devised to enable the criminal justice system to avoid the death penalty for severely mentally disordered individuals charged with capital crimes. Prior to 1800 in England, "legal" insanity as a special verdict of acquittal did not exist. The Criminal Lunatics Act of 1800 provided for the automatic confinement "until his majesty's pleasure be known" of any defendant found NGRI. At first, standards were vague, and circular reasoning predominated (Halpern 1980). Insanity defense was considered if someone did something "insane." In other words, the nature of the criminal act itself became the primary evidence for a diagnosis of mental illness. Various diagnostic labels abounded, such as "moral insanity," "transitory mania," and "instantaneous mania." Mental illness was often seen to be secondary to some organic ailment, such as high pulse rate or congestion (Pankratz 1984). Still, there was controversy about the etiology of mental illness, as some favored physiologic explanations, while others representing the social theorists sought to understand the individual psyche (Smith 1983).

The modern antecedents of the insanity defense derive from the McNaughten case in England in 1843. Daniel McNaughten was brought to trial for the assassination of Edward Drummond, whom McNaughten had mistaken for Robert Peal, the British Prime Minister. The basis of the testimony was that McNaughten was suffering from persecutory delusions while committing the act. When McNaughten was called on to plead, there was confusion about the charges regarding the intent to kill Drummond, and as a result the judge entered an insanity plea. After the trial, the jury agreed and returned a verdict of NGRI, which immediately became the subject of considerable consternation and popular debate. The practical result of the decision came to be known as the "McNaughten Rule."

To establish a defense on the ground of insanity, it must be clearly proved that at the time of committing the act, the party accused was laboring under such a defect of reason, from disease of the mind, as not to know the nature and quality of the act he was doing; or if he did know it, that he did not know he was doing what was wrong.

The McNaughten decision rapidly became the primary approach to the insanity defense in England and in the United States. It focuses on the defendant's lack of intellectual cognitive capacity to appreciate the nature of the acts and their wrongfulness (Appreciation Test). This ruling or modifications of it are still in existence in 26 states today. However, as psychiatry has moved from the custodial era, NGRI has also changed. Perhaps the biggest impetus for change was the advent of the use of neuroleptic drugs, which became the harbinger of deinstitutionalization. A second factor was the rise of civil libertarianism, which in combination with shorter lengths of hospital stay changed NGRI from a life sentence to a judicial determination that was reviewed frequently with limitations on confinement.

The 1950s, known as the heyday of psychodynamic psychiatry, saw the advent of two new insanity defense interpretations that are based on a belief that psychiatrists and psychiatry offered rehabilitative promise to the criminally insane. The Modern Penal Code, first introduced in 1950, added a Volitional Test to the already existent Appreciation Test found in the McNaughten ruling. In legal parlance, the Volitional Test is a determination of an individual's ability or inability to control his actions and/or conform his conduct to the letter of the law. The Modern Penal Code, also known as the American Law Institute rule, was first applied in *United States v. Currens* (1961).

A person is not responsible for criminal conduct if at the time of such conduct as a result of mental disease or defect he lacks substantial capacity either to appreciate the criminality (wrongfulness) of his conduct or to conform his conduct to the requirements of the law.

The Modern Penal Code recommendation was followed by another standard in 1954 resulting from *Durham v. United States* (1954). Durham simply asked: Is the action (crime) a product of a mental disease or defect?

By establishing such a precedent, the court appeared to show a partiality toward a psychic determinism view of human behavior and broadened NGRI to include any psychiatric disorder. Surprisingly, the effect of these major changes in language was slight. It has been shown that the language used in instruction to the jury, which includes explanation of NGRI statutes, has less bearing on judicial outcome than such factors as sympathy toward the defendant, perceived reprehensibility of the crime, quality of the defense counsel, attitude of the trial judge, and ability of the expert witnesses (Pasewark 1981).

Public misconceptions regarding NGRI are staggering. The frequency and success of the pleas are grossly overestimated, and most people believe that the decision is solely a judgment of the psychiatrist (Pasewark et al. 1981). Paradoxically, it is a rare defense—one in a thousand defendants—and only 10% of those are successful (Stone 1982). Furthermore, most of the successful cases involve concurrence between prosecution and defense. These fallacies were further dramatized in a study by Steadman and Cocozza (1978) where people were asked to name someone found to be criminally insane. Of the persons named more than once by the general public, none had been adjudicated NGRI.

Cognizant of this rather imposing public relations problem and in the wake of the John Hinckley case, the American Psychiatric Association set up a work group that issued a report concluding that the insanity plea, although under siege, has clear practical utility. They agreed that alternative concepts, such as guilty but mentally ill, have received popular support, but when tried, the anticipated psychiatric treatment for the defendant has rarely been forthcoming (Criss and Racine 1980). In recognition of this issue, the work group suggested the following standard: A person charged with a criminal offense should be found NGRI if it is shown that as a result of mental disease or mental retardation, he was unable to appreciate the wrongfulness of his conduct at the time of the offense.

As used in this standard, the terms mental disease or mental retardation include only those severely abnormal mental conditions that grossly and demonstrably impair a person's perception or understanding of reality and that are not attributable primarily to the voluntary ingestion of alcohol or other psychoactive substances (Insanity Defense Work Group 1983).

The work group, therefore, suggested that mental disorders potentially leading to exculpation must be serious. Such disorders should be of the severity of conditions that psychiatrists diagnose as psychosis. Under this recommendation, conditions such as PTSD would ordinarily not be appropriate for an insanity plea.

PTSD as an Insanity Defense

Establishing a valid link between PTSD and criminal behavior is an imposing task. At least two levels of causation must be investigated: 1) causal connection between the traumatic stressor and psychiatric symptoms and 2) causal connection between psychiatric symptoms and the criminal act (Raifman 1983). Previously we have suggested that the insanity defense is appropriate only in the rare instance that a dissociative episode related to PTSD directly leads to unpremeditated criminal activity (Sparr and Atkinson 1986).

No one argues whether mental health experts are able to determine the symptoms of PTSD. At issue is whether their professional abilities extend to deciding whether the stressor occurred, if it was sufficiently traumatizing, and whether the designated stressor or some preceding or subsequent stressor or provocation is the cause of the complainant's symptoms. As Raifman (1983) stated: "A good poker player probably knows better than a mental health professional whether or not a person is lying. A psychiatrist is a doctor, not a lie detector." Yet in many such cases, psychiatrists have unwittingly represented themselves as master detectives, stating with certainty that reputed combat events as well as reputed symptoms happened as the veteran reported them. A great lesson of some (i.e., *Pard v. United States* [1984] and *State v. Jensen* [1985]) is the requirement for independent evidence to confirm the veteran's report of stressful events (Sparr and Atkinson 1986).

Wilson and Zigelbaum (1983) proposed specific psychological links between PTSD and criminal behavior: 1) the crime represents actual or symbolic repetition of war experiences; 2) the crime is an expression of conflicts about the war experiences; and 3) the crime is an attempt at the retrieval of experiences that have been intensely repressed with the unconscious goal of getting killed, venting rage, or getting caught in order to receive aid.

In addition, they propose that manifestations of PTSD include danger and sensation seeking or going into the so-called survivor mode in which the veteran reverts to the class of survival behaviors learned in combat. This line of reasoning has led to the argument that the veteran's personality has been so altered by the Vietnam War that he later engages in antisocial activities.

Packer (1983) questioned the validity of such a cause-and-effect relationship in the forensic setting because he believes it is irrelevant to the issue of legal accountability. If similar reasoning were to be generally accepted, no one would be responsible for his or her behavior. Risky and daring activity may be in the early history of most inner-city dwellers who commit crimes. Criminal behavior often is seen as a direct by-product of adverse childhood experiences. For instance, child abusers often have themselves been abused as children. The putative link between adult criminal activity and early formative experiences may contribute to understanding motivations for a particular behavior, but it does not absolve the individual of legal responsibility for that behavior. For an individual to be found NGRI, it is not enough just to demonstrate historical antecedents of the criminal activity. Instead, it must be shown that at the time of the commission of the crime the individual was experiencing a severely disturbed mental state.

Despite these problems, defense attorneys have increasingly introduced PTSD to support claims of self-defense, diminished capacity, or insanity. Additionally, PTSD has been used successfully in plea negotiations and in reduction of judicial sentences by virtue of reduction in criminal culpability, or, as in *State v. Jensen* (1985), there has been reconsideration on the basis of newly discovered evidence, since PTSD did not appear formally in DSM-III until 1980, many years after the end of the Vietnam War.

Finally, in a number of cases, defense attorneys have introduced the theory that at the time of the criminal offense the veteran was in an altered state of consciousness (dissociative state) brought on by reliving or reenacting his Vietnam experiences and, therefore, could not appreciate the nature of his acts or conform his conduct to the requirements of the law. Such psychological states typically feature impaired reality testing and unpremeditated behavior. When a dissociative state appears as a valid secondary manifestation of a DSM-III mental disorder (i.e., PTSD), the requirements for legal insanity may be met. In such circumstances, consideration of the dissociative state represents an intermediate step in deliberations over NGRI, not a starting point.

In some states there is an "unconsciousness" defense that comes under a separate statute and does not necessarily presume insanity (Apostle 1980). Unconsciousness defenses have been applied to persons who are "not conscious" of their actions at the time of the crime because of psychomotor seizures, febrile delirium, and so forth. The theoretical basis for this is the contention that acts performed nonvoluntarily do not satisfy minimal requirements for criminal activity. In practice, this sort of defense is very difficult to establish because the "unconscious" mental state is ephemeral and usually nonverifiable, and because of the clear potential for substantial secondary gain.

Criteria for diagnosis of unconscious flashbacks to war experiences in Vietnam veterans have been suggested by Blank (1985): 1) the flashback behavior is unpremeditated and sudden; 2) the flashback behavior is uncharacteristic of the individual; 3) there is a retrievable history of one or more intensely traumatic combat events that are reenacted in the flashback episode; 4) there may be amnesia for all or part of the episode; 5) the flashback behavior lacks current motivation; 6) the stimuli (trigger) for the flashback behavior may be current physical or environmental features that are reminiscent of original experiences in Vietnam; 7) the patient is mostly unaware of the specific ways he has repeated and reenacted war experiences; 8) the choice of victim may be fortuitous or accidental; and 9) the patient has or has had other symptoms of PTSD.

VETERANS ADMINISTRATION DISABILITY CLAIMS

Beginning in October 1980 the VA accepted the DSM-III diagnostic entity of PTSD delayed type as a potentially compensable disorder. This meant that for the first time since World War I, the Department of Veterans Benefits could consider disorders to be service connected when the symptoms first appeared more than 1 or 2 years after military discharge (Bitzer 1980). Many veterans—mostly Vietnam combatants but also a few from World War II and the Korean conflict—have responded by filing claims based on their belief that they suffer from PTSD related to traumatic war experiences. In Oregon alone, the number of claimants referred by the Department of Veterans Benefits for psychiatric diagnostic examination for this disorder rose to more than 40 per month (Atkinson et al. 1982).

To begin the process, a veteran must file a claim with the VA regional office. Often the veteran is represented by a service officer (e.g., Disabled American Veterans, Veterans of Foreign Wars) or a VA benefits counselor. Unlike personal injury and many workers' compensation claims, claimants are not represented by attorneys. Federal law limits attorneys' fees to 10 dollars in VA disability cases.

After the claim is filed, the local VA Rating Board asks the Department of Veterans Benefits to send the claimant's military service medical records, which include form DD 20, a chronologic history of military service and unit assignments. Particular attention is paid to military service medals, such as combat action ribbons and/or purple hearts. Most claimants are then sent a questionnaire asking for a description of traumatic events while in the military. If necessary, the rating board can request further verification and information from the United States Army and Joint Services Environmental Support Group in Washington, D.C. The group is able to research military unit logs, which may provide valuable information about the extent of the claimant's combat activity.

The claimant is also given an appointment for a psychiatric examination. Local VA psychiatric disability evaluation in Oregon had been limited to a half-hour session (range, 15–60 minutes) for review of records, patient interview, and dictation of a report that did not follow a written protocol. Social evaluation was possible but seldom used. Although this process was arguably adequate for reevaluation of veterans with major psychiatric disorders, it seemed inadequate for PTSD when the first cases were considered in early 1981.

Consequently, an evaluation protocol for PTSD cases was developed and put into effect during September 1981. The protocol included the following steps: 1) claimant contact by a social worker either by telephone or personalized letter; 2) interviews by the same social worker with the veteran and at least one family member; 3) social worker's report, according to a written protocol, based on the interviews, review of the Department of Veterans Benefits claim file, and a demographic questionnaire; 4) review of reports and records by the examining psychiatrist; 5) psychiatric interview at least 60 minutes long; and 6) psychiatric report according to a written protocol. The psychiatrists involved were private practitioners who conducted evaluations at the VA Medical Center on a fee-for-service basis and were selected because of their interest in evaluation of PTSD cases.

Disability determinations are made by two rating specialists and a physician who are members of the local VA Rating Board (eight members). First, there is a determination as to the presence or absence of PTSD. If PTSD is present, the rating board then assigns the claimant a percentage of disability. Disability is given along a percentile range (0% to 100% with gradations of 10%, 30%, 50%, and 70%). Zero percent disability confers eligibility for VA treatment of the disorder without monetary compensation. One hundred percent disability confers medical treatment plus full monetary compensation. Veterans have the right to a hearing before the rating board and the right of appeal to the Board of Veterans Appeals in Washington, D.C. From June 1, 1985, until October 23, 1987, there were 23,244 national PTSD disability claims; 54.7% were approved and 45.3% denied. During the same time period, the average percentage of disability was 33.47% (Department of Veterans Administration Affairs 1987).

After many years of experience in conducting disability examinations, the following problems have emerged (Atkinson et al. 1982).

Adverse Interactional Styles Between Claimants and Staff. The antipathy many Vietnam veterans feel toward the federal government may be exacerbated by the evaluation process, introducing artifact into the examination.

Lack of Corroboration of Data. This has improved with the development of the Environmental Support Group, but it has been quite difficult to acquire other third-party documentation of premilitary behavioral adjustment and exposure to noncombat-related stressors.

The "Silent" Claimant. Despite efforts of examiners to establish rapport, some veterans are not able to discuss either their war experiences or their symptoms in the psychiatric interview.

Exaggeration and Falsification of Data. Perhaps this is the first time that VA disability claimants have presented themselves to psychiatric examiners having read printed symptom checklists—from national service organizations—describing the diagnostic features of the disorder for which they seek compensation. Clinical judgment based on large case experience with PTSD is the best assessment method. Adjunctive strategies include more extensive contact with relatives and second evaluation by a colleague.

Partial PTSD (Stressors Without Full Symptoms). It is unlikely that anyone engaged in combat escaped without some psychological scars. The memories and reflections haunt the best adjusted veterans, but often these do not fulfill DSM-III-R (American Psychiatric Association 1987) criteria for PTSD. The Department of Veterans Benefits clearly requires strict adherence to DSM-III-R criteria. In cases where some but not all criteria are met, examiners are asked to report their findings but to refrain from making the PTSD diagnosis.

Idiosyncratic Disorders (PTSD Symptoms Without the Stressor). A vexing diagnostic dilemma arises when the claimant's symptoms and social behavior conform to criteria for PTSD but the military history fails to establish a stressor meeting the DSM-III-R requirement. Our protocol requires full description of military stressors and a rating on DSM-III-R Axis IV of their severity (usually Code 6 "catastrophic") whenever PTSD is diagnosed.

Intercurrent Civilian Stress. Years may have elapsed between military discharge and evaluation. In the interval, serious life stressors may occur. If the claimant's PTSD symptoms do not predate the civilian stress and the content of memories concerns civilian events, the examiner may make a PTSD diagnosis but unrelated to military service.

Either/or "Diagnostic Judgments." Psychiatric examiners and rating board members sometimes indulge in excessive diagnostic parsimony by reducing multifaceted cases to a single diagnosis. It has been reported that PTSD may mimic and be misdiagnosed as personality disorder (Van Putten and Emory 1973; Walker 1981), neurosis (Van Putten and Emory 1973), or psychosis (Domash and Sparr 1982). PTSD may also be complicated by or associated with another syndrome, for example, anxiety or depressive disorders or a substance abuse disorder (Wolf et al. 1988).

Impact on Examiners. Recounting gruesome events in Vietnam, expression of painful affects, and anger outbursts by claimants are stressful to examiners and may result in frequent examiner turnover. Measures to make this role bearable have included 1) examination of PTSD claimants only 1 day per week; 2) examination of other more routine claimants mixed among PTSD cases; and 3) regular opportunities for meeting with one another and with staff consultants.

DUTY TO PROTECT

The evolution of the duty to protect began with the California Supreme Court's *Tarasoff v. Regents of University of California* (1974) decision. The court's opinion enunciated a legal duty for psychotherapists to warn possible victims of their patient's potentially violent acts. The decision produced significant turmoil in the mental health community (Bloom and Rogers 1987). At the request of many professional organizations, the court agreed to reconsider its decision, reheard the case in 1976, and modified the original opinion. In so-called Tarasoff II (*Tarasoff v. Regents of University of California* 1976), the court held that the duty was to protect, rather than to warn, the intended victim. However, the court was vague about how the newly described duty could be discharged. The decision suggested that this duty might be performed by warning the victim or by calling the police, but it did not rule out conventional clinical interventions (e.g., medication changes, hospitalization, or civil commitment) that had long been made by psychotherapists dealing with potentially violent patients (Mills et al. 1987). Thus Tarasoff II affirmed a therapist's responsibility to take whatever steps are reasonably necessary to protect others and provided some flexibility as to the methods that could be used to accomplish such protection (Carlson et al. 1987).

Tarasoff was enacted despite the bulk of expert opinion and research data, which state that neither a psychiatrist nor anyone else can reliably predict the likelihood of a mentally ill patient's future violence (American Psychiatric Association 1974; Diamond 1975; Monahan 1981, 1984). The clinician willing to make such judgments is necessarily uncertain as to the accuracy of the prediction (Roth and Meisel 1977). Short-term predictions of violence are more exact than long-term predictions, and violence assessments based on observations in the patient's natural environment are more accurate than those performed in institutional settings (Monahan 1978). In general, however, whenever predictions of future violence are ventured by mental health professionals, they are wrong twice as often as they are right (Monahan 1981).

The ethical roots of the Tarasoff decision are found in the principles of medical confidentiality. The legal system has traditionally granted privileged communication status to certain special relationships, such as psychotherapist and patient. Although reporting a threat and warning the victim may sometimes give the therapist extra protection in a potential Tarasoff liability suit, if the danger proves to be nonexistent, reporting may leave the therapist open to a lawsuit for violation of confidentiality. Also, reporting and warning may further endanger a potential victim by so alienating the patient that he quits treatment at a time when it is most needed to help him control his actions (Weinstock 1988).

Unfortunately, fear of liability has led some psychiatrists to hospitalize patients who do not otherwise require inpatient care. Appelbaum (1988) believes that an unfortunate by-product of Tarasoff has been the creation of a de facto system of preventive detention that consumes resources intended to serve therapeutic ends and compels psychiatrists to share the social control responsibilities of the criminal justice system. Another problem has been therapist refusal to treat potentially dangerous or violent patients for fear of the legal repercussions if their patient acts out against a third party.

Mills et al. (1987) reviewed many post-Tarasoff court decisions and concluded that they largely turn on the issue of foreseeability. When the courts have imposed liability, the identity of the subsequently injured party was either known to the psychotherapist, or the victim could reasonably have been expected to be in close proximity to the target of violence. Furthermore, the threats were specific, and there were breaches of conventional practice, such as failure to obtain the patient's prior medical record or to examine the patient and the medical record carefully. When liability has not been imposed, the patient has, at the time of evaluation, been perceived as not being a threat to any individual or group, even when there was a history of violent behavior or alcoholism. In the majority of states, no cases involving the issue of third-party protection have been brought to the bar. A few states (e.g., Pennsylvania and Maryland) have considered the issue and decided against a Tarasoff policy. Nevertheless, the overall trend is toward a duty to protect. In states where the issue has not been litigated, the conservative assumption is that the court will find a Tarasoff duty when the issue arises (Mills et al. 1987).

In August 1985, the California legislature adopted the first state statute (California Assembly 1984) concerning the psychotherapist's duty to warn and protect third parties. The law states more clearly the circumstances in which the duty is applicable. The psychotherapist is liable only "where the patient has communicated to the psychotherapist a serious threat of physical violence against a reasonably identifiable victim or victims." The statute further directs that the duty to warn and protect shall be discharged by "reasonable efforts to communicate the threat to the victim or victims and to a law enforcement agency." After a decade of litigation, the current public policy dictates that the psychotherapist is required to use reasonable care to protect a third party from a potentially dangerous patient (Mills et al. 1987).

The issue of violence potential may be a strong consideration when working with PTSD victims. Various studies have found rage or anger to be a feature of PTSD, particularly in combat veterans. As a result, irritability or anger outbursts, formerly a DSM-III associated feature of PTSD, was added to DSM-III-R as a cardinal feature. Observers have commented on the role of externalized anger when working with PTSD patients (Egendorf 1975; Frick and Bogart 1982; Parson 1988; Perconte 1988; Rosenheim and Elizur

1977). During the first 2 or 3 months of group therapy, Vietnam veterans with PTSD characteristically ventilate their overwhelming anger toward society in general, and the VA in particular, for the injustices they claim to be experiencing (Frick and Bogart 1982). Fox (1974) found that 16% of a sample of 106 combat veterans manifested continuing violent behavior in civilian life. Therapists working with war survivors must have a high degree of tolerance for fantasized violence, although not for violence or criminal activity itself.

The above considerations have importance in treating PTSD. In short, violence, talk of violence, and preoccupation with violence are common and inevitable aspects of treatment. Since exposure to violence has such etiologic importance in many types of PTSD, its verbalization in treatment is important. Although it is not known whether PTSD patients are more violent than others, the therapist's decision to invoke a Tarasoff duty must be based on clinical circumstances. It is helpful if a therapist has a well-established relationship with the patient. Resorting to premature warnings or preventive detention may breach the patient's confidentiality and undermine trust.

Psychiatry's unwanted responsibility for the control of violence should not deter mental health professionals from treating victims of violence in an even-handed and rational way. Concern about liability should not prevent clinicians from allowing patients to deal with their violent propensities in an open manner. There is a tendency among clinicians to interpret duty to protect laws too restrictively; therefore, therapists should use reasonable care in assessing the patient's potential for violence, identifying possible victims, and informing a law enforcement agency. Duty to protect issues are best discussed with patients beforehand. In such circumstances, it has been shown that a Tarasoff warning or other protective actions may further the therapeutic alliance and contribute to the patient's progress in therapy (Beck 1982).

WORKERS' COMPENSATION

Each state has its own workers' compensation statutes. Most were passed in the early 1900s, around the time of World War I. In some basic respects, the various state statutes are similar and provide compensation to injured workers for certain consequences of their work injuries. Compensation includes medical expenses, lost wages during recuperation, and any permanent loss of earning capacity (Sersland 1984).

Before the first compensation law in 1911, employers were liable only for injuries resulting from negligence; hence, employees had to prove fault to receive an award for an injury arising in the workplace. To facilitate recovery and a quick return to work, injured workers were relieved from a legal burden of proof by workers' compensation laws, and, without fault, employers were responsible for all injury costs. Borrowing from the doctrine of proximate cause in tort law (see next section), workers' compensation law creates a two-part requirement for workplace causation: the injury must arise out of, and occur in, the course of employment (London et al. 1988).

The 1960 landmark Michigan case, *Carter v. General Motors* (1961), was the first case to compensate for a mental disorder precipitated solely by a mental stimulus. In common jargon, three basic terms are used to describe workers' compensation claims: *physical/mental, mental/physical,* and *mental/mental.* In a physical/mental claim, a physical injury leads to some sort of mental distress (e.g., depression or anxiety following a back injury). A mental/mental claim, of course, means that mental stress has resulted in a mental problem (Colbach 1982).

The injury must arise from the course of employment, but the employment contribution does not need to be the sole cause for the injury to be compensable. It is usually thought to be sufficient if the employment contribution is one cause among several. Moreover, the relative importance of the various causes is usually not weighted (Sersland 1984).

Another common concern about the mental/mental category of cases is preexisting vulnerability to mental illness. Since a significant percentage of adults in the United States have suffered from at least one psychiatric disorder (Robins et al. 1984), the potential exists for much greater liability under workers' compensation laws for mental disabilities than has ever existed for physical disabilities. Both in personal injury cases and workers' compensation, a claimant's predisposition to, or preexisting, mental illness is legally irrelevant. The worker is taken as is. As Justice Oliver Wendell Holmes remarked: "The law is not for the protection of the physically sound alone" (Modlin 1983).

Throughout the United States, worker's claims for stress-related disorders have proliferated during the past 15 years (Appleson 1983). In part, this is because of growing epidemiologic evidence of the relationship between workplace stressors and pathophysiology (Leavitt 1980). While stress claims represented only 4.7% of the occupational disease cases in 1980, they more than doubled in the following 3 years and have continued to rise ever since (Blodgett 1986). The economy is moving away from claims for physical injury—the kind that often occur working with machines—to stress claims arising out of office work. In the state of Oregon, from 1980 to 1986, the number of disabling mental stress claims rose from 159 to 683, an increase of more than 300%; in the same time period, total claims decreased (Department of Insurance and Finance 1987). Mental stress claimants are typically younger than other claimants, and a significantly higher proportion are female. Stress claims are increasing as the work force continues to shift from manufacturing to service sector jobs.

It has been suggested that highly publicized workers' compensation claims spur similar claims. This may be particularly important in mental stress claims because stress is acknowledged to be a universal condition. Since dissatisfaction with working conditions commonly underlies mental stress, some of the recent claim increases may be related to increases in unemployment, plant closings, and relocations.

A portion of the increase in mental stress claims may simply reflect the increasing legal recognition of compensation for mental injuries in contexts other than workers' claims. There is an increasing legal tendency to allow tort recovery for both intentional and negligent infliction of emotional distress. Tort recoveries, which were previously limited to narrow and extreme situations, have expanded considerably (National Council on Compensation Insurance 1985).

In some states, if there is no physical stimulus, compensability is denied. There are 10 states that quite clearly apply this requirement; 27 states do not impose a physical injury requirement; and the remainder have not clearly addressed the issue. In 16 states, the standard for compensability in the mental/mental category requires that the mental injury result from a situation of greater dimensions than day-to-day on-the-job stress. There is a requirement in some states that the mental stimulus be a sudden or dramatic event. In a few states, to be compensable, the mental disability must be peculiar to the unique facets of the employment and not due to such factors as on-the-job interpersonal relationships. In Maine, if the claimant is predisposed to mental illness and might succumb to ordinary work stress, it must be proved that his or her employment predominated in producing the mental disorder. In Oregon, when employment conditions are compared with non-employment factors, the major contributing causes of the claimant's disorder must be job related. The stressful conditions, however, must be real and not imaginary (Sersland 1984). Recently, a handful of states have been granting compensation for workers' stress caused by job termination, demotion, or disciplinary action (Blodgett 1986). This has caused considerable controversy; in California, an amendment was written to the state employer's liability insurance specifically excluding claims due to termination of employment, demotion, reassignment, or disciplinary action (California Employer's Liability Insurance Amendment 1988).

Basically there are four categories of reasoning adopted by courts regarding mental/mental compensability standards (National Council on Compensation Insurance 1985): 1) no compensation; 2) compensation if the stress is a sudden, frightening, or shocking event; 3) compensation if the stress exceeds the stress of everyday life or employment; and 4) compensation even if the stress is not in excess of the stress of everyday life or employment.

The reluctance on the part of many states to compensate for mental stress dates back many decades. There were many journal articles about "compensation neurosis" from the 1930s to the 1960s (Kamman 1951; Miller 1959; Pokorny and Moore 1953; Ross 1966; Weighill 1983). Accident victims were formerly categorized as those with legitimate injuries and claims, and those with disability out of proportion to the tissue damage they sustained. The latter were suspect and regularly labeled by conjugated neuroses: injury, industrial, occupational, indemnity, compensation, litigation, or accident neurosis. Many physicians, attempting to understand and treat workers with compensation claims, became cynical. They were puzzled by, if not suspicious of, the considerable disability some persons manifested after seemingly minor or even trivial stresses (Modlin 1986).

Kennedy (1946) stated that "a compensation neurosis is a state of mind, born out of fear, kept alive by avariciousness, stimulated by lawyers, and cured by a verdict." This theme, supported by Miller's (1961) influential accident neurosis article, has ensured that generations of patients have been regarded with suspicion if they dared to present with psychological symptoms following an accident. This view remained unchallenged for more than a decade and is still presented, and accepted by courts, despite the fact that recent studies dispute Miller's findings and the concept of compensation neurosis has lost legitimacy. Various authors have clearly shown that monetary compensation does not remove stress symptoms (Burstein 1986; Kelly and Smith 1981; Modlin 1986; Sprehe 1984). In this decade, an impetus for legitimization of mental stress claims has been the PTSD designation, which has been a helpful counterpoint to claims often burdened with pejorative diagnostic designations. Despite this current affirmative direction, I shall suggest in the concluding section that the DSM-III-R diagnosis of PTSD usually does not apply to workers' compensation cases.

PERSONAL INJURY (TORTS)

In a personal injury lawsuit or tort action, the plaintiff claims that a trauma has caused damages that have resulted from the negligent or intentional action of the defendant and asks for a money award in reparation for the damage. The law on torts is concerned with the allocation of losses arising out of human activities (Slovenko 1985). Most personal injuries are pursued under the theory of negligence, that is, unintentional breach of tort.

To press a lawsuit successfully, the plaintiff must assume the burden of proof and show that the defendant had a legal duty of care that was fulfilled negligently, and that, as a result, the plaintiff experienced substantial damage. A psychiatrist's legal involvement in such cases is usually occasioned by a victim's decision to bring suit against another individual or individuals for damages due to psychic injury. The plaintiff's attorney must be satisfied on the first two points of liability before the mental health professional is called on to determine the extent of psychic damage to the claimant. This third point is crucial: if there is no damage, there is no case. The testimony of medical experts, whether expressed in written report, deposition, or trial appearance, makes or breaks the plaintiff's lawsuit (Modlin 1983).

In the past, liability for psychic impairment was contingent on physical impact or physical injury. Other than that, there was no tort liability for a "broken mind." In a famous English case, *Lynch v. Knight* (1861), the judge said: "The law does not pretend to redress mental pain when the unlawful act complaint consists of that pain alone." The first case that involved the intentional infliction of "extreme mental suffering" was litigated in 1897 (*Wilkinson v. Downton*). In this seminal case, the defendant was held liable for intentional infliction of mental suffering in "outrageous circumstances" that exceeded the bounds of decency. This has come to be called the tort of "outrage" (Lambert 1978). The law then moved from the intentional infliction of extreme mental distress to the area of negligent infliction. At first it was not possible to recover for mental distress from fright or shock without physical impact—the so-called impact rule (*Spade v. Lynn 1897*). The theory seemed to be that the impact afforded the desired guarantee that the mental disturbance was genuine.

In the past 20 years, the courts have been tracing a somewhat irregular line between compensable and noncompensable psychic impairment (Slovenko 1985). With psychic injury becoming more widely recognized, the courts have become increasingly willing to compensate for emotional distress in the absence of physical injury or impact. Three types of rulings have resulted (Lambert 1978): 1) zone of danger cases, in which the plaintiff is within the radius of risk from negligent physical contact and suffers emotional disturbance without impact; 2) bystander recovery (e.g., *Dillon v. Legg* 1968), in which the plaintiff is outside the zone of physical impact, but suffers emotional distress from witnessing the peril or harm of a third person, such as a spouse, child, or near relative; and 3) beyond bystander (e.g., *Prince v. Pittston* 1974), in which the plaintiff does not actually see the physical injury of a third person (e.g., child) but suffers severe shock when hearing of it or seeing the results.

In consideration of the above situations, the trend of the law has been to give increasing and extensive protection to feelings and emotions of injured parties and to enlarge redress in reparation for psychic injury.

These cases, as well as workers' compensation cases, often involve complex scientific issues of causation. Lawyers usually divide the idea of causation into two parts: 1) cause in fact, or factual cause, and 2) proximate cause, or legal cause. It is the former that is closely related to the concept of medical causation that would encompass, for example, the scientific question of whether cigarette smoking causes lung cancer. Cause in fact can be formulated by the "but for" rule, which states that one event is a cause of another when the first event would not have occurred but for the second event. Another rule for cause in fact is the "substantial factor" test, which states that a defendant's action is the cause of the damage if it was a material element in bringing it about (Goldstein 1987).

Proximate cause, on the other hand, often revolves around the question of whether or not the defendant has a legal duty of care. If the defendant has a legal duty to protect the plaintiff and could reasonably have foreseen a risk of harm to the plaintiff, the defendant would then be held liable for any damages. Once the plaintiff suffers any foreseeable injury, even if relatively minor, as a result of the defendant's negligent conduct, the defendant is then liable for any additional consequences. This consideration extends liability to encompass injury that causes a disability, activates a latent condition, or worsens a preexisting condition (Modlin 1983). An example is the hypothetical case of a plaintiff who, unbeknownst to the defendant, has a skull of eggshell thinness. If the defendant inflicts even a minor impact on this skull, the defendant will then be liable for any injury. The rule is sometimes expressed by saying the defendant "takes his plaintiff as he finds him" (Goldstein 1987).

Physicians sometimes have difficulty understanding legal approaches to causation that include not only the initiation of physical or psychological injury, but also the production of additional damage or dysfunction in individuals with preexistent problems. A causal role may be legally significant if it can be shown to have played some part, not necessarily the major one, in initiating, contributing to, accelerating, or aggravating the plaintiff's injury. Most jurists also have difficulty empathizing with this view. An astute defense attorney, therefore, endeavors to draw opinions from expert witnesses about the plaintiff's preexistent susceptibility to stress in an effort to influence the jury despite the letter of the law (Modlin 1986).

In personal injury litigation, psychiatrists typically offer opinions about whether or not a traumatic event—physical injury, psychological stress, and/ or exposure to a noxious substance—is the proximate cause of the plaintiff's ensuing psychic injury. The court follows the reasoning that the test for allowing a plaintiff to recover in a tort suit is not scientific certainty but legal sufficiency. Thus a cause in fact relationship need not be conclusively proven before a psychiatrist can testify that, in his or her opinion, a causal relationship exists. The following case (*Wotalewiez v. Gallagher* 1986) is illustrative.

The plaintiff, a 33-year-old female parking patrol officer, was involved in an altercation with an irate male citizen after issuance of a parking ticket. The defendant grabbed the plaintiff's right arm and verbally abused her for writing the ticket. The plaintiff, suing for $150,000 with punitive damages of $100,000, asserted that the defendant intentionally and willfully attempted to do violence to her. Furthermore, "as a direct and proximate result of the defendant's assault and battery, plaintiff was caused to suffer permanent injuries including acute PTSD with some associated regression, partial personality decompensation, depressive reaction, pain, suffering, stress and anxiety." The defendant's anger and physical force reminded the plaintiff of previous physical and sexual abuse that she had sustained as a child. The developmental history indicated that the plaintiff's mother had died when she was a young girl and that she also had lost a child several years earlier from medical complications of a premature birth. Medical history was remarkable for a right shoulder injury in an auto accident 3 years prior, with subsequent surgery for thoracic outlet syndrome. The clinical evaluations by several mental health professionals described a variety of symptoms and signs, such as tearfulness, wringing of hands, stuttering, and a pervasive feeling of helplessness. Although there was no systematic inquiry for objective symptoms, all clinicians for the plaintiff diagnosed PTSD. At trial, the defendant was found negligent, but there was no battery and no intentional tort established. The final financial settlement was approximately 10% of what the plaintiff had originally requested.

The Diagnosis of PTSD in Torts and Workers' Compensation

A thorough understanding of the diagnosis of PTSD is important, not only for clinical purposes but also because of the forensic implication (Brett et al. 1988). The diagnosis has evolved since DSM-I (American Psychiatric Association 1952) from an acute reaction in an individual with good premorbid adjustment (gross stress reaction) to a specific syndrome occurring as an acute or chronic response with or without preexisting or concurrent pathology. The DSM-III-R PTSD definition includes emphasis on the rare occurrence of the stressor and its nearly universal ability to evoke symptoms. However, it adds a list of generic characteristics of traumatic stressors. Some stressors "frequently produce the disorder" (e.g., combat, torture), and others produce it only "occasionally" (e.g., natural disasters, car accidents). The most common traumas involve either a "serious threat to one's life or physical integrity; serious threat or harm to one's children, spouse, or other close relatives and friends; sudden destruction of one's home or community; or seeing another person who has recently been, or is being, seriously injured or killed as the result of an accident or physical violence" (American Psychiatric Association 1987, p. 250). DSM-III-R states that the disorder is apparently more severe and longer lasting when the stressor is of "human design."

Many of the early diagnostic formulations regarding PTSD were influenced by work with combat veterans and emphasized the process of reexperiencing severe trauma. Symptomatology was observed as long as 20 years after combat participation (Archibald and Tuddenham 1965). As Marin (1981) pointed out, genuine victims of PTSD are often struggling with profound moral issues, including realization of the consequences of human aggression and of evil in themselves and others. These moral issues also have applicability to victims of rape (Burgess and Holmstrom 1974). The chronicity of the symptoms appears to be primarily related to the profundity of the moral pain.

The tenor of DSM-III-R discussion on the severity of a stressor required to produce PTSD suggests that events must be serious or severe to warrant the diagnosis. It is noted that the precipitating event is "outside the range of usual human experience" (p. 250). It is further stated that the stressor producing this syndrome would be "markedly distressing to almost anyone, and is usually experienced with intense fear, terror, and helplessness" (p. 247). Forensic fact finders should compare the DSM-III-R descriptions to the actual events purported to cause PTSD in psychic injury claimants. For example, when a claim is made following a minor or moderate car accident, one might look at the DSM-III-R statement, suggesting that even car accidents with serious physical injury only "occasionally" produce PTSD.

As in the case example, it appears that many claims of PTSD that follow stressors that are not particularly usual or severe would be more properly classified as adjustment disorder or some other psychiatric disorder. By definition, an adjustment disorder disturbance begins within 3 months of the onset of a stressor and lasts longer than 6 months. If the stressor persists, however, as in chronic physical illness, it may take much longer to achieve a new level of adaptation. In some forensic venues, however, an adjustment disorder may not be compensable, which may be the crux of the problem. A claimant has to suffer "stress." Platt and Husband (1986) believe that there exists a "mutually exclusive gap" between the PTSD and adjustment disorder diagnoses. This gap includes individuals who reexperience a traumatic event even though the trauma is a relatively common occurrence (e.g., a motor vehicle accident). In such cases, adjustment disorder does not appear to be the appropriate diagnosis because of the presence of intrusive recollections or recurrent nightmares of the accident, yet the stressor is not severe enough to justify a diagnosis of PTSD. Slovenko (1984) aptly stated that the meaning of the trauma to the individual and the resolution of trauma are so varied that it cannot be said that the effects of a stressor are the same for all. The best conclusion seems to be a statistical probability that people exposed to trauma develop stress symptoms to a greater extent than those not exposed to trauma. To add to the diagnostic difficulty, DSM-III-R states that in adjustment disorder, "the stressor is usually less severe and within the range of common experience; and the characteristic symptoms of Post-traumatic Stress Disorder, such as reexperiencing the trauma, are absent" (p. 249).

Hoffman (1986) reviewed nearly 100 litigation cases following car accidents; fewer than 10 patients seemed to meet the criteria for PTSD. McFarlane (1986) reported on the consequences of a disastrous fire in Australia in which 2,697 adults and children were registered as victims, 28 individuals were killed, and 385 houses were destroyed or extensively damaged. He noted that although special, widely publicized clinical services were set up for possible victims, not a single victim initiated psychiatric contact on his or her own. A survey of 36 patients showed that many suffered from chronic pain syndromes, depression, and specific phobias as well as symptoms of PTSD. Platt and Husband (1986) examined approximately 150 personal injury cases arising from automobile accidents and discovered only two instances where the "hitter" in the accident sought psychiatric treatment for accident-attributable symptomatology. Hoffman stated that the most common applicable DSM-III diagnosis after motor vehicle accidents is psychological factors affecting physical condition. Other Axis I diagnoses that occur after trauma may include the somatoform disorders (conversion disorder and psychogenic pain disorder), phobic disorder, generalized anxiety disorder, major depression, dysthymic disorder, and occasionally factitious disorder. Rutter (1986) believes that psychiatric symptoms precipitated by severe physical illness such as may be seen in natural disasters can also be viewed as normal stress responses rather than a psychiatric disorder.

In the courtroom setting, the term PTSD has DSM-III-R "legitimacy," and the concept of stress following trauma is easily understandable to the lay person (e.g., juror, compensation board member). The PTSD diagnosis may elicit more sympathy for, and identification with, the patient because of perceived external causation as opposed to internal causation (e.g., personal weakness) in the case of depression, anxiety, or adjustment disorder. Also, the previously discussed gap between the PTSD and adjustment disorder diagnoses might tempt some clinicians to overdiagnose by erring on the side of giving a patient the PTSD diagnosis whenever intrusive reexperiencing is present. This temptation may be particularly strong in the case of automobile accident victims. In contrast to individuals with more resilient personality structures, it has been shown that predisposed individuals may react to a minor to moderate traumatic event, such as an automobile accident, with a cluster of symptomatology that is a mixture of PTSD and depressive symptoms (Platt and Husband 1986).

There is absolutely no doubt that victims of various accidents and trauma manifest stress. Insurance carriers frequently shortchange patients who undergo psychiatric care following an accident (Resnick 1988). Suspicions of malingering may help to explain why damages awarded for posttraumatic psychological symptoms are substantially less than those for physical injury, despite the fact that limitations on the patient's life may actually be greater (Trimble 1981).

Continued incapacity, despite apparent medical recovery after an injury, may be due to factors other than malingering. Resnick (1988) contended that physical injury and pain often produce a regression, characterized by breakdown of more mature coping mechanisms. Injured patients may become totally dependent even though they were formerly quite autonomous. Injury that causes incapacity is a stress on one's psychological integrity, a challenge to one's mature self-concept, and a fundamental threat to one's sense of personal worth. The resultant depression and dependency may be seen as a psychological reaction to physical illness (Resnick 1988). Intrusive reexperiencing may occur if the individual psychologically fixates on the accident.

Perhaps forensic psychiatrists and other clinicians should follow the advice of Tanay (1986) in rendering forensic diagnostic opinions. Tanay stated that it is important to differentiate between diagnostic accuracy and diagnostic precision. In the context of a forensic evaluation for stress compensation, it is necessary only to address the issue of whether or not the claimant experiences stress. When the examiner is able to state that psychic injury has occurred, an adequate level of precision has been gained. One could go beyond that and make a specific diagnosis, which in my opinion ordinarily would not be PTSD. A specific diagnosis may be important for therapeutic purposes, but in a legal setting this is a distinction without difference.

Psychic injury, particularly in the forensic context, casts a broad net. The definition of mental stress for legal purposes does not require a level of precision of a Swiss watch. PTSD should be diagnosed if the facts fit, but only if they fit. To do otherwise dilutes and trivializes the diagnosis. When mental stress due to an auto accident is called PTSD, one wonders whether or not we are questioning if human beings can adapt to anything. It is most important for the diagnostician to communicate to insurance carriers, attorneys, or other fact finders that the claimant is experiencing stress. The precise diagnosis is less important than a thorough description of the symptoms. PTSD should not be the only admission ticket to the ballpark.

REFERENCES

Adler A: Neuropsychiatric complications in victims of Boston's Coconut Grove disaster. JAMA 123:1098–1101, 1943

American Psychiatric Association: Diagnostic and Statistical Manual of Mental Disorders. Washington, DC, American Psychiatric Association, 1952

American Psychiatric Association: Clinical aspects of the violent individual (Task Force report 8). Washington, DC, American Psychiatric Association, 1974

American Psychiatric Association: Diagnostic and Statistical Manual of Mental Disorders, 3rd Edition. Washington, DC, American Psychiatric Association, 1980

American Psychiatric Association: Diagnostic and Statistical Manual of Mental Disorders, 3rd Edition, Revised. Washington, DC, American Psychiatric Association, 1987

Apostle DT: The unconsciousness defense as applied to post-traumatic stress disorder in a Vietnam veteran. Bull Am Acad Psychiatry Law 8:426–430, 1980

Appelbaum PS: The new preventive detention: psychiatry's problematic responsibility for the control of violence. Am J Psychiatry 145:779–785, 1988

Appleson G: Stress on stress: compensation cases growing. American Bar Association Journal 69:142–143, 1983

Archibald HC, Tuddenham RD: Persistent stress reaction after combat: a 20 year follow-up. Arch Gen Psychiatry 12:475–481, 1965

Atkinson RM, Henderson RG, Sparr LF, et al: Assessment of Vietnam veterans for post-traumatic stress disorder in Veterans Administration disability claims. Am J Psychiatry 139:1118–1121, 1982

Beck JC: When the patient threatens violence: an empirical study of clinical practice after Tarasoff. Bull Am Acad Psychiatry Law 10:189–201, 1982

Bitzer R: Caught in the middle: mentally disabled veterans and the Veterans Administration, in Strangers at Home: Vietnam Veterans Since the War. Edited by Figley CR, Leventman S. New York, Praeger Publications, 1980

Blank AS Jr: The unconscious flashback to the war in Viet Nam veterans: clinical mystery, legal defense, and community problem, in The Trauma of War: Stress and Recovery in Viet Nam Veterans. Edited by Sonnenberg SM, Blank AS Jr, Talbott JA. Washington, DC, American Psychiatric Press, 1985, pp 293–308

Blodgett N: Legal relief from tension—work-induced stress spurs workers' compensation claims. American Bar Association Journal 17:17–18, 1986

Bloom JD, Rogers JL: The duty to protect others from your patients—Tarasoff spreads to the Northwest. West J Med 148:68–74, 1987

Brett EA, Spitzer RL, Williams JB: DSM-III-R criteria for post-traumatic stress disorder. Am J Psychiatry 145:1232–1236, 1988

Brill NQ, Beebe GW: A follow-up study of war neuroses (Veterans Administration Medical Monogram). Washington, DC, U.S. Government Printing Office, 1955

Burgess AW, Holmstrom LL: Rape trauma syndrome. Am J Psychiatry 131:981–986, 1974

Burstein A: Can monetary compensation influence the course of a disorder (letter)? Am J Psychiatry 143:112, 1986

California Assembly Bill 1133, McAllister, 1984

California Employer's Liability Insurance Amendment 413181, State Compensation Insurance Fund, Jan 13, 1988

Carlson RJ, Friedman LC, Riggert SC: The duty to warn/protect: issues in clinical practice. Bull Am Acad Psychiatry Law 15:179–186, 1987

Carter v General Motors, 106 NW2d (361 Mi 1961)

Cobb S, Lindemann E: Neuropsychiatric observations during the Coconut Grove fire. Ann Surg 117:814–824, 1943

Colbach EM: The mental-mental muddle and work comp in Oregon. Bull Am Acad Psychiatry Law 10:165–169, 1982

Criss ML, Racine DR: Impact of change in legal standard for those adjudicated not guilty by reason of insanity 1975–1979. Bull Am Acad Psychiatry Law 8: 261–271, 1980

Department of Insurance and Finance: Mental Stress Claims in Oregon 1980–1986. Salem, OR, Department of Insurance and Finance, Research and Statistics Section, 1987

Department of Veterans Administration Affairs: Factsheet. Portland, OR, Veterans Administration Regional Office, December 14, 1987

Diamond BL: The psychiatric prediction of dangerousness. University of Pennsylvania Law Review 123:439–452, 1975

Dillon v Legg, 441 P2d 919 (Cal 1968)

Dobbs D, Wilson WP: Observations on persistence of war neurosis. Diseases of the Nervous System 21:686–691, 1960

Domash MD, Sparr LF: Post-traumatic stress disorder masquerading as paranoid schizophrenia: a case report. Milit Med 147:772–774, 1982

Durham v United States, 214 F2d 862 (DC Cir 1954)

Egendorf A: Vietnam veterans rap groups and themes of postwar life. Journal of Social Issues 31:111–124, 1975

Fox RP: Post-combat adaptational problems. Compr Psychiatry 13:435–443, 1972

Fox RP: Narcissistic rage and the problem of combat aggression. Arch Gen Psychiatry 31:807–811, 1974

Frick R, Bogart L: Transference and countertransference in group therapy with Vietnam veterans. Bull Menninger Clin 46:429–444, 1982

Goldsmith W, Cretekos C: Unhappy odysseys: psychiatric hospitalizations among Vietnam returnees. Arch Gen Psychiatry 20:78–83, 1969

Goldstein RL: The twilight zone between scientific certainty and legal sufficiency: should a jury determine the causation of schizophrenia? Bull Am Acad Psychiatry Law 15:95–104, 1987

Grinker RR, Spiegel JP: Men Under Stress. Philadelphia, PA, Blakiston, 1945

Halpern AL: The fiction of legal insanity and the misuse of psychiatry. J Leg Med (Chicago) 2:18–74, 1980

Hoffman BF: How to write a psychiatric report for litigation following a personal injury. Am J Psychiatry 143:164–169, 1986

Horowitz MJ: Stress Response Syndromes. New York, Jason Aronson, 1976

Horowitz MJ, Solomon GF: A prediction of delayed stress response syndromes in Vietnam veterans. Journal of Social Issues 31:67–80, 1975

Insanity Defense Work Group: American Psychiatric Association statement on the insanity defense. Am J Psychiatry 140:681–688, 1983

Kamman GR: Traumatic neurosis, compensation neurosis or attitudinal pathosis? Archives of Neurology and Psychiatry 65:593–603, 1951

Kelly R, Smith BN: Post-traumatic syndromes: another myth discredited. J R Soc Med 74:275–277, 1981

Kennedy I: Mind of the injured worker: its effect on disability neurosis. Compensation Medicine 1:19–24, 1946

Lambert TF: Tort liability for psychic injuries: overview and update. Journal of the Association of Trial Lawyers of America 37:1–31, 1978

Leavitt SS: Determining compensable workplace stressors. Occup Health Saf 49: 38–46, 1980

Leopold RL, Dillon H: Psychoanatomy of a disaster: a long-term study of post-traumatic neurosis in survivors of a marine explosion. Am J Psychiatry 119: 913–921, 1963

London DB, Zonana HV, Loeb R: Workers' compensation and psychiatric disability, in Psychiatric Injury in the Workplace. Edited by Larson R. Philadelphia, PA, Hanley and Belforth, 1988

Lynch v Knight, 11 Eng. Rep. 854, 863 (HL 1861)

Marin P: Living in moral pain. Psychology Today 6:68–74, 1981

McFarlane AC: Post-traumatic morbidity of a disaster: a study of cases presenting for psychiatric treatment. J Nerv Ment Dis 174:4–14, 1986

Millen FJ: Post-traumatic neurosis in industry. Industrial Medicine and Surgery 35:929–935, 1966

Miller MH: The compensation neurosis. J Forensic Sci 4:159–166, 1959

Miller MH: Accident neurosis. Br Med J 1:919–925, 1961

Mills MJ, Sullivan G, Eth S: Protecting third parties: a decade after Tarasoff. Am J Psychiatry 144:68–74, 1987

Modlin HC: Traumatic neurosis and other injuries. Psychiatr Clin North Am 6: 661–682, 1983

Modlin HC: Compensation neurosis. Bull Am Acad Psychiatry Law 14:263–271, 1986

Monahan J: Prediction research and the emergency commitment of dangerous mentally ill persons: a reconsideration. Am J Psychiatry 135:198–201, 1978

Monahan J: The Clinical Prediction of Violent Behavior. Washington, DC, U.S. Government Printing Office, 1981

Monahan J: The prediction of violent behavior: toward a second generation of theory and policy. Am J Psychiatry 141:10–15, 1984

National Council on Compensation Insurance: Emotional Stress in the Workplace: New Legal Rights in the 80's. New York, National Council on Compensation Insurance, 1985

Packer IK: Post-traumatic stress disorder and the insanity defense: a critical analysis. Journal of Psychiatry and the Law 11:125–136, 1983

Pankratz LD: Murder and insanity: 19th century perspectives from the "American Journal of Insanity." International Journal of Offender Therapy and Comparative Criminology 28:37–43, 1984

Pard v United States, 589 F Supp 518 (D Ore 1984)

Parson ER: The unconscious history of Vietnam in the group: an innovative multiphasic model for working through authority transferences in guilt-driven veterans. Int J Group Psychother 38:275–301, 1988

Pasewark RA: Insanity plea: a review of the research literature. Journal of Psychiatry and Law 9:357–401, 1981

Pasewark RA, Seidenzahl D, Pantle MA: Opinions about the insanity plea. Journal of Forensic Psychology 8:63–72, 1981

Perconte ST: Stages of treatment in PTSD. VA Practitioner 5:47–57, 1988

Platt JJ, Husband SD: Post-traumatic stress disorder in forensic practice. American Journal of Forensic Psychology 4:29–56, 1986

Pokorny AD, Moore FJ: Neurosis and compensation. Archives of Industrial Hygiene and Occupational Medicine 8:547–563, 1953

Prince v Pittston, 63 FRD 28 (SD WVa 1974)

Raifman LJ: Problems of diagnosis and legal causation in courtroom use of post-traumatic stress disorder. Behavioral Science Law 1:115–130, 1983

Resnick TJ: Malingering of post-traumatic stress disorders, in Clinical Assessment of Malingering and Deception. Edited by Rogers R. New York, Guilford, 1988

Robins LN, Helzer JE, Weissman MM, et al: Lifetime prevalence of specific psychiatric disorders in three sites. Arch Gen Psychiatry 41:949–958, 1984

Rosenheim E, Elizur A: Group therapy for traumatic neuroses. Current Psychiatric Therapies 17:143–148, 1977

Ross WD: Neuroses following trauma and the relation to compensation, in American Handbook of Psychiatry, Vol 3. Edited by Arieti S. Basic Books, New York, 1966

Roth LH, Meisel A: Dangerousness, confidentiality, and the duty to warn. Am J Psychiatry 134:508–511, 1977

Rutter M: Depressive feelings, cognitions, and disorders: a research postscript, in Depression in Young People: Developmental and Clinical Perspectives. Edited by Rutter M, Izard CE, Read PB. New York, Guilford, 1986

Sersland SJ: Mental disability caused by mental stress: standards of proof in workers' compensation cases. Drake Law Review 33:751–816, 1984

Slovenko R: Syndrome evidence in establishing a stressor. Journal of Psychiatry and Law 12:443–467, 1984

Slovenko R: Law and psychiatry, in Comprehensive Textbook of Psychiatry, 4th Edition. Edited by Kaplan HI, Sadock BJ. Baltimore, MD, Williams & Wilkins, 1985

Smith R: Criminal insanity: from a historical point of view. Bull Am Acad Psychiatry Law 11:27–34, 1983

Solomon GF, Zarcone VP, Yoerg R, et al: Three psychiatric casualties from Vietnam. Arch Gen Psychiatry 25:522–534, 1971

Spade v Lynn, 47 NE 88 (Mass 1897)

Sparr LF, Atkinson RM: Post-traumatic stress disorder as an insanity defense: medicolegal quicksand. Am J Psychiatry 143:608–613, 1986

Sprehe DJ: Workers' compensation: a psychiatric follow-up study. Int J Law Psychiatry 7:165–178, 1984

State v Jensen, CR 75687 (Superior Court of Arizona, Maricopa County, 1985)

Steadman HJ, Cocozza JJ: Selective reporting and the public's misconceptions of the criminally insane. Public Opinion Quarterly 41:523–533, 1978

Stone AA: The insanity defense on trial. Hosp Community Psychiatry 33:636–640, 1982

Tanay E: Forensic diagnosis: accuracy or precision. American Academy of Psychiatry and the Law Newsletter 11:15, 1986

Tarasoff v Regents of University of California, 118 Cal Rptr 129 (1974)

Tarasoff v Regents of University of California, 131 Cal Rptr 14 (1976)

Titchener JL, Kapp FT: Family and character change at Buffalo Creek. Am J Psychiatry 133:295–299, 1976

Trautman EC: Fear and panic in Nazi concentration camps: a biosocial evaluation of the chronic anxiety syndrome. Int J Soc Psychiatry 10:134–141, 1964

Trimble MR: Post-traumatic Neurosis from Railway Spine to the Whiplash. New York, John Wiley, 1981

United States v Currens, 290 F2d 751, 744 (3d Cir 1961)

Van Putten T, Emory WH: Traumatic neuroses in Vietnam returnees—a forgotten diagnosis? Arch Gen Psychiatry 29:695–698, 1973

Walker JI: Vietnam combat veterans with legal difficulties: a psychiatric problem? Am J Psychiatry 138:1384–1385, 1981

Weighill VE: "Compensation neurosis": a review of the literature. J Psychosom Res 29:97–104, 1983

Weinstock R: Confidentiality and the duty to protect: the therapist's dilemma. Hosp Community Psychiatry 39:607–609, 1988

Wilkinson v Downton, 2 QB 57 (1897)

Wilson JP, Zigelbaum SD: The Vietnam veteran on trial: the relation of post-traumatic stress disorder to criminal behavior. Behavioral Science Law 1:69–83, 1983

Wolf ME, Alavi A, Mosnaim AD: Posttraumatic stress disorder in Vietnam veterans: clinical and EEG findings: possible therapeutic effects of carbamazepine. Biol Psychiatry 23:642–644, 1988

Wotalewiez v Gallagher, CR 831–207779 (Circuit Court of Oregon, Multnomah County, 1986)

Index